BEDSIDE CARDIOLOGY

BEDSIDE CARDIOLOGY

Fifth Edition

Jules Constant, M.D., F.A.C.C.
Associate Clinical Professor
Department of Medicine
State University of New York at Buffalo
School of Medicine
Buffalo, New York

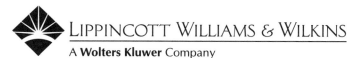 LIPPINCOTT WILLIAMS & WILKINS
A **Wolters Kluwer** Company

Philadelphia • Baltimore • New York • London
Buenos Aires • Hong Kong • Sydney • Tokyo

Acquisitions Editor: Ruth W. Weinberg
Developmental Editor: Jennifer Kowalak
Production Editor: Jonathan Geffner
Manufacturing Manager: Kevin Watt
Cover Designer: Marker Lerner
Compositor: Maryland Composition
Printer: Maple Press

© 1999, by LIPPINCOTT WILLIAMS & WILKINS
227 East Washington Square
Philadelphia, PA 19106-3780 USA
www.LWW.com

Printed in the USA

Library of Congress Cataloging-in-Publication Data

Constant, Jules, 1922–
    Bedside cardiology / Jules Constant. — 5th ed.
      p.   cm.
    Includes bibliographical references and index.
    ISBN 0-7817-2168-7
    1. Heart—Diseases—Diagnosis. 2. Heart—Sounds. 3. Physical
diagnosis. I. Title.
    [DNLM: 1. Cardiovascular Diseases—diagnosis. 2. Physical
Examination.   WG 141 C757b 1999]
    RC683.C59   1999
    616.1′2075—dc21
    DNLM/DLC
    for Library of Congress   99-21282
                                      CIP

10 9 8 7 6 5 4 3 2 1

To Elizabeth, my wife

Contents

Preface   ix

1   The Evolving Checklist in History Taking   1

2   Cardiac Clues from Physical Appearance   16

3   Arterial Pulses and Pressures   30

4   Jugular Pressure and Pulsations   67

5   Inspection, Palpation, and Auscultation of the Chest   94

6   The Stethoscope   119

7   Diagraming and Grading Heart Sounds and Murmurs (The Auscultogram)   123

8   The First Heart Sound (S_1)   127

9   The Second Heart Sound (S_2)   143

10   The Opening Snap (OS)   171

11   The Third Heart Sound (S_3)   181

12   The Fourth Heart Sound (S_4)   195

13   Ejection Murmurs   208

14   Systolic Regurgitant Murmurs   238

15   Diastolic Murmurs   283

16   Abdominal Murmurs   313

17   Prosthetic Valve Sounds   315

18   Systolic Time Intervals   317

Subject Index   325

Preface

The Fifth Edition of *Bedside Cardiology,* like the previous editions, is designed for those who wish to balance the advances in technology by increasing their skills in diagnosing cardiovascular disorders through history-taking and physical examination. This book also encourages use of phonocardiograms and pulse-tracings for teaching and self-improvement of the reader.

This book attempts to teach and not simply to tell the facts by using the three best methods in the psychology of teaching:

1. Explain the facts as simply as possible.
2. Focus attention by the use of questions and answers (Socratic method).
3. Help the reader to remember the facts by using logical tricks (e.g., analogies and conversion to round numbers).

The Socratic method not only focuses the attention of the reader, but also prevents the author from rambling. In addition, it provides the option of covering up the answer and using the book as a programmed learning approach.

It is important to teach physicians that all technology, such as echocardiography, has false positives and false negatives. Also, it is not always possible to utilize this technology: it may be unavailable due to cost; the patient may not be a good candidate; the technician or reader may not be qualified; equipment may be substandard or in need of repair.

The false positives and false negatives that every technology suffers from must be combined with physical examination to decide what is true and what is false. History and physical examination are cost-effective skills, and can help return the physician's focus to the patient. This allows the physician to have the satisfaction of feeling like a "real doctor" rather than simply an interpreter of laboratory data.

Jules Constant, M.D.

1

The Evolving Checklist in History Taking

ADVANTAGES OF A CHECKLIST

Traditionally, students have learned to take a history by memorizing a standard checklist, and they have been warned that a checklist should not be used in front of a patient. It is my contention that not using a checklist can lead to a poor history.

Many physicians fear that reading questions in front of a patient diminishes the patient's opinion of the interviewer. When the opinions of patients were solicited concerning the reading of questions in front of them, however, it was found that patients either did not recall that a checklist had been used, or, if patients had been to other doctors, they would often claim that it was the first time they had had a thorough history taken.

The final history as written on paper may be very short because no negative findings need be recorded. If no checklist is used, it is necessary to list all negative findings for the reader to know what has been asked. The history can be taken more rapidly with a checklist than without, because you do not hesitate while trying to recall your place, as would be the case with a memorized checklist, especially if the patient rambles. Best of all, on leaving the patient, there is no feeling of insecurity because you fear you may have forgotten to ask something. A good history of a chief complaint can be taken with this checklist because if the patient answers affirmatively in regard to any important symptom, one then can turn to another page in the section of follow-up questions, which covers the differential diagnosis in the form of further questions. Thus, the cardiologic diagnosis can be elicited with the checklist discussed in this chapter.

The checklist proposed here is not to be used as a "check-off" list with yes or no answers, but rather as a "reminder" list. The patient's answers to the reminder list can be written down in an unorganized form on separate sheets of paper and later reorganized under a few headings, such as the following:

1. Name, date, age, address, and telephone number.
2. Orientation (why the patient came or was referred, and who referred the patient).
3. Marital status and occupation.
4. History of the chief complaint or complaints. For example, if the patient has chest pain, write the complete story of the chest pain as obtained from the follow-up questions of the checklist.
5. Chamber enlargement possibilities. This is the place for palpitations.
6. Other etiologies pertinent to the chief complaint. These headings should contain the word *possibilities*. For example, if the patient has known valvular disease, "Rheumatic Heart Disease Possibilities" would be an appropriate heading.

1

Note: 1. Do not record negative answers. The checklist makes them unnecessary.
     2. Do not repeat symptoms under separate headings.
     3. Do not give your opinion regarding the diagnosis or symptoms in the history.

REMINDER LIST HISTORY

If the Patient Has Had Cardiac Surgery

1. Indicate date, place, type of operation, complications, name of surgeon, and effect on cardiac symptoms.
2. Catheterization results?
3. Medications after surgery (e.g., anticoagulants)?

Left Ventricular Failure or High Left Atrial Pressure Possibilities

1. Dyspnea on exertion (DOE) on the level or on climbing either hills or steps? (If yes, see page 7 for follow-up questions.)
2. Orthopnia? (If yes, see page 8.)
3. Paroxysmal nocturnal dyspnea (PND)? (If yes, see page 8.)
4. Dyspnea in pregnancy? (If in first trimester, may be caused by placental product.)
5. Is patient on diuretics, loop or thiazides? Are there muscle cramps or weakness? Were preload or afterload reducers used? Any drugs that could precipitate borderline failure (e.g., beta blockers, calcium blockers, or disopyramide)? Were potassium-retaining agents or supplements used?

Peripheral Venous Congestion or Pseudo Right Heart Failure Possibilities (Traditionally Called Right Ventricular Failure)

See footnote.[1]

1. Peripheral edema, maximum and minimum weight? (If yes, turn to follow-up questions on page 9.)
2. Abdominal swelling? (If before orthopnea, consider tamponade.) (See page 4 for symptoms of tamponade.) If before leg edema, consider constrictive pericarditis. Upper abdominal pain with exercise or bending discomfort? (Suggests hepatomegaly.)
3. Upper abdominal pain with exercise.

Low-output State Possibilities

1. Weakness and fatigue? Only in the morning (depression)? Afternoon nap necessary? On drugs that could cause weakness (e.g., digitalis, diuretics, beta blockers, or tranquilizers)? Psychoneurotic basis (relationship to family, spouse, friend, or work supervisor)? Possible folic acid deficiency (contraceptive pill, diphenylhydantoin, or spironolactone)?

---

[1]Right ventricular failure is a poor term because it has two meanings. It may mean pure right ventricular failure resulting from severe obstruction of right ventricular outflow (as in severe pulmonary hypertension, pulmonary stenosis, or massive pulmonary embolism) or from right ventricular dysfunction (right ventricular infarction, severe tricuspid or pulmonary regurgitation). However, these causes are relatively rare in comparison with the second meaning of right ventricular (RV) failure. When the left ventricle fails, high venous pressure is caused by increased venous tone secondary to increased sympathetic outflow and norepinephrine levels, as well as an increase in volume secondary to salt retention. Peripheral edema is caused by salt retention and high venous pressure, for which a preferable term is peripheral venous congestion.

2. Cold hands or feet? For how long?

3. Excess perspiration? With warm hands, suggests hyperthyroidism; with cold hands, suggests neurocirculatory asthenia (psychoneurosis) or failure (resulting from an impaired ability to dissipate body heat). Recent in an adult and not due to hyperthyroidism or neurosis? (Suggests severe failure.) If pulmonary edema is mild, perspiration may be mainly on the forehead; if moderate, perspiration may spread to the chest; if severe, to the abdomen (2).

4. Insomnia caused by hyperpnea on going to sleep or dozing (Cheyne-Stokes respiration)?[2]

5. Nocturia with polyuria (daytime failure compensated at rest)?

6. Faintness or syncope?

Chamber Enlargement Possibilities

1. Trepopnea? (See page 8 for definition.)

2. Palpitations or awareness of heart beat? (If yes, see page 13.)

3. Told of enlarged heart? If determined from electrocardiogram (ECG), x-ray, echocardiogram, or physical examination, give dates.

Rheumatic Heart Disease Possibilities

History of Rheumatic Fever

Joint pains or chorea (St. Vitus' dance)? Twitches or clumsiness for a few months before age 20? Red, swollen joints or only fever plus murmur as a child? Prophylactic penicillin? Family history of rheumatic fever? Murmur history (school examination, operation, insurance, or military service)? Cardiac catheterization or echo? Were there "growing pains" or nocturnal leg pains (not rheumatic)?

Complications of Rheumatic Heart Disease

1. If mitral stenosis:
   a. Hemoptysis?
   b. Hoarseness? Ortner or cardiovocal syndrome (pressure of a large left atrium on dilated pulmonary artery against recurrent laryngeal nerve (5,23)?
   c. Embolic phenomena (hematuria, pleurisy, unilateral weakness or partial vision loss in one eye caused by calcium emboli from aortic valve)?

2. If aortic stenosis: Exertional dyspnea, syncope, or angina (classic aortic stenosis triad)?

3. If aortic regurgitation: Nocturnal angina or awareness of large pulsations in arms, neck, or chest?

4. **If infective endocarditis**: Severe night sweats or embolic phenomena (back pain or cerebrovascular accident)? Prior dental work or any surgery?

Ischemic Heart Disease Possibilities

1. Chest pains, tightness, pressure, or discomfort? Perspiration on exertion? (If yes, see page 11.)

2. Previous myocardial infarction? Symptoms, hospital course, postinfarction drugs [e.g., beta blockers, aspirin, or angiotensin-converting enzyme (ACE) inhibitors]? Which clot lysing drugs used?

---

[2]The gradually increasing depth of Cheyne-Stokes respiration can cause cerebral stimulation and prevent sleep because it is often precipitated by dozing, but it may also awaken the patient from sleep (9,14). The periods of apnea following the hyperpnea may last from a few seconds to 1 minute.

3. Risk factors
  a. Major: Hypertension, high levels of cholesterol or triglycerides, low levels of high-density lipoprotein (HDL) cholesterol, smoking, family history of infarction at an early age?
  b. Minor: Diabetes, premature menopause, intermittent claudication, gout, high levels of uric acid (8)? Is patient type A (hostile, aggressive, and impatient)? Stressful job or home situation? On diet or taking drugs to decrease lipids? High Lp(a) or homocysteine.

4. Marked postprandial somnolence? (Suggests severe hypertriglyceridemia or insulin resistance.)

Hypertensive Heart Disease Possibilities

Hypertension? (If yes, see page 13.)

High-output Failure Possibilities

1. Anemia: Under treatment? The cardiac output is usually not elevated in anemia until the hemoglobin falls to about 50% of normal. Heavy periods, bleeding, hemorrhoids, or melena? Upper gastrointestinal surgery (B_{12} deficiency)? Sickle cell disease history? Lead contact? Radiation or anticancer drugs?

2. Thyrotoxicosis: Heat intolerance, warm skin, weight loss, polydipsia, polyuria, excess perspiration, frequent stools, restlessness, muscle weakness on climbing, or palpitations?

3. **Beriberi**: Evidence of alcoholism with a poor diet? Bartender job? Fad diets or peripheral neuritis? Cold skin with oliguria (acute "shoshin" beriberi) or warm, wet skin (chronic beriberi) (26)? Long-term use of large doses of diuretics?

Cor Pulmonale Possibilities

1. Chronic obstructive pulmonary disease (COPD): Smoking history? Told of emphysema or has chronic cough with wheezing and sputum? Easier to breathe leaning forward? Pulmonary function tests performed? Coal miner? Abnormal findings on chest roentgenogram? Severe obesity (pickwickian syndrome)?

2. Asthma: Is wheezing helped by bronchodilators? Seasonal dyspnea?

3. Pulmonary emboli: History of long sitting, pregnancy, phlebitis, oral contraceptives? Sudden dyspnea at rest with pleurisy or faintness with cold sweat or hemoptysis? Recent trauma or surgery?

4. Primary pulmonary hypertension: Raynaud's phenomenon (32)?[3] Fixed-output symptoms? Edema before dyspnea?

Pericarditis, Effusion, Constriction, or Tamponade Possibilities

Etiologies

Chest trauma? Postcardiotomy or postmyocardial infarction syndrome (Dressler syndrome) with fever, pleurisy, and polyserositis as long as 2 months after surgery? Chest radiation, uremia, metastatic carcinoma, lymphoma, leukemia, lupus, rheumatoid arthritis, tuberculosis contact, or recent viremia? Drugs: procainamide, hydralazine, or isoniazid?

---

[3]Progressing from blanching to cyanosis to painful redness (reactive hyperemia), Raynaud's phenomenon is occasionally a precursor of a connective tissue disease. Acrocyanosis is a persistent blueness and coldness of the distal part of the extremities.

Symptoms of Pericarditis

1. Chest pain on motion, swallowing, or inspiration.
2. Past history of pericarditis (idiopathic type may be recurrent).
3. Epigastric pain for a few days before chest pain.

Symptoms of Tamponade

1. Dyspnea on exertion, especially if it stops immediately when exertion is stopped.
2. Edema or abdominal swelling beginning before or simultaneously with dyspnea on exercise.

Myocarditis, Endocarditis, and Other Heart Disease Possibilities

1. Recent influenza-like illness with myalgia?
2. **Infective endocarditis**: Drug addiction, fevers, surgical or dental procedures, or recent back pain?
3. Collagen disease: Raynaud's phenomenon, dysphagia, arthritis, or arthralgia?
4. Ankylosing spondylitis: Hip, sciatic, or back pain, especially on awakening or increasing with coughing?
5. Hypophosphatemia: High intake of phosphorus-binding antacids (e.g., aluminum hydroxide)? Acute alcohol excess?
6. Hypertrophic cardiomyopathies: Sudden death in family? Angina or syncope after exercise? Intermittent murmurs? Dyspnea not helped by digitalis?
7. Luetic: Aortic regurgitation or aneurysm? Venereal disease or hoarseness (aneurysm compressing recurrent laryngeal nerve)?
8. Rupture of valve caused by trauma: Traumatic tricuspid regurgitation (may not cause symptoms for up to 3 years after accident) (22)?

Infiltrative Cardiomyopathy Possibilities

1. Hemochromatosis: Diabetic? Skin color changes? Liver failure? Impotence, upper abdominal pain, gynecomastia, or arthritis? Frequent transfusions?
2. Sarcoidosis: Syncope (from atrioventricular block)? Abnormality on chest x-ray, kidney stones, or eye symptoms (uveitis)?
3. Amyloidosis: Postural hypotension, peripheral neuropathy, or skin lesions, especially if pruritic or if they bleed when scratched.
4. Parasitic disease: Trichinosis or Chagas' disease? (Has patient eaten rare meat or been to a foreign country?)
5. Hypothyroidism or myxedema: Voice change, dry skin, cold intolerance, sluggishness, weight gain, constipation, menorrhagia, or decreased hearing? Thyroid tests?

Cardiac Tumor Possibilities

1. Atrial myxoma,[4] embolic phenomena, fevers, arthralgias, skin lesions, paresthesias? Presyncope or syncope with change of posture?
2. **Carcinoid heart disease**: Flushing of face, neck, and front of chest for 10 to 20 minutes? Diarrhea? Asthma? Edema?

---

[4]Atrial myxoma is a tumor of friable tissue on a pedicle attached to the area of the fossa ovalis, twice as likely to occur in the left as in the right atrium. The tumor may obstruct an atrioventricular valve or cause regurgitation. If it becomes calcified, a "wrecking ball" effect may destroy the valve. It acts as an inflammatory agent and can produce fevers and a high sedimentation rate. It may be associated with clubbing and mimic endocarditis or a collagen disease.

Congenital Heart Disease Possibilities

To Be Asked Only If Patient Is an Infant

1. Frequent pneumonias? (Suggests increased pulmonary blood flow.)
2. Excess perspiration? (Sign of failure or of lesion such as left-to-right shunt large enough to cause a propensity to failure.)
3. Mother aware of infant's heartbeat or vibration of a thrill?

To Be Asked Only If Patient Is a Child or Adult

1. Hoarseness? (Suggests large ductus or primary pulmonary hypertension [15].)
2. Mental retardation? (Consider Down syndrome or supravalvular aortic stenosis.)
3. Hypertrophic osteoarthropathy with swelling, pain, warmth, and tenderness of lower extremity? (Consider ductus with Eisenmenger syndrome.)
4. Recurrent bleeding from nose, lips, and mouth with melena and hemoptysis as a result of hereditary hemorrhagic telangiectasis or Rendu-Osler-Weber disease? [Suggests pulmonary arteriovenous (A-V) fistula, especially if patient is cyanotic.]
5. Presyncope or syncope? On exertion? (Suggests aortic stenosis or primary pulmonary hypertension.) With straining or after sleep and with cyanosis? (Suggests tetralogy.) At rest? [Consider epilepsy or complete atrioventricular (AV) block with Stokes-Adams attack.]
6. Squatting? (Suggests tetralogy, pulmonary atresia, or Eisenmenger syndrome.)
7. Headaches, epistaxis, leg fatigue, cold legs, or claudication? (Suggests **coarctation**.)

To Be Asked If Patient Is an Infant, Child, or Adult

1. Murmur at birth? (Suggests stenotic lesion. If delayed a few weeks, suggests left-to-right shunt.)
2. Results of cardiac catheterization?
3. Pregnancy with rubella? (Suggests **persistent ductus**, **ventricular septal defect**, **atrial septal defect**, pulmonary arterial (not valvular) stenosis, or **tetralogy of Fallot**.
4. Normal growth and development? (High birth weight suggests transposition.)
5. Mother's pregnancy: Viral illness? (May produce myocarditis in newborn.) Diabetes? (Suggests transposition.) Age of mother when pregnant? (If in 40s, suggests tetralogy of Fallot.)
6. Family history of congenital heart disease or murmur?
7. Cyanosis? When did it begin? (If from birth, suggests transposition or tetralogy. If delayed until teens or middle age, suggests Eisenmenger syndrome or Ebstein's anomaly.) Does it occur with crying, feeding, or warm bath, or only with syncope? (Suggests tetralogy.) Differential cyanosis and clubbing (fingers pink but toes blue)? (Suggests ductus with Eisenmenger syndrome.) Frequent phlebotomies?
8. Stroke? (Consider embolus from endocardial fibroelastosis, idiopathic cardiomyopathy, paradoxical embolus from the right atrium, or endocarditis. If cyanotic, consider cerebral abscess.)
9. Crying during feeding (the most strenuous effort of a baby)? (Suggests angina resulting from anomalous origin of the left coronary artery.)

FOLLOW-UP QUESTIONS

If Patient Says Yes to Dyspnea on Exertion

Orientation

When was patient last able to perform normal activities comfortably? How far or for how long can the patient walk on the level or on stairs before dyspnea? Walking more slowly? Can patient walk and talk simultaneously? Patient's most strenuous activity in the past few months?

Etiologies

1. Failure
   a. Effect of digitalis, diuretics, salt reduction, or afterload treatment?
   b. Is there orthopnea, PND, cough, or wheeze on exertion? (If suddenly worse, suggests ruptured chordae or aortic cusp, atrial fibrillation, pulmonary embolus, or acute infarction.)
   c. If on digitalis, any gastrointestinal or visual symptoms? Weakness (18), faintness, dizziness, or palpitations?
2. Pulmonary dysfunction
   a. Associated with weight gain?
   b. Wheezing (especially with exertion)? Bronchodilator effects?
   c. COPD? Smoking history?
   d. Sputum? Has the patient had pulmonary function tests or been told of emphysema?
   e. Does the patient exhibit pickwickian syndrome (marked obesity)?
3. Anginal equivalent: DOE lasting 10 to 20 minutes? (One-third of patients with angina have simultaneous dyspnea without heart failure (13,17). With nausea or occasionally with angina? Had Holter monitor? Only profuse perspiration with exertion (27)?
4. Arrhythmia: Palpitations? Begins and ends suddenly? Ever had palpitations or check pulse when short of breath?
5. Anxiety: Nervous breakdown or tranquilizer history? Hyperventilation with paresthesias? Cold perspiration? Palpitations? Days without dyspnea? (Suggests neurocirculatory asthenia.[5])

If Patient Says Yes to Orthopnea

See footnote.[6]

---

[5]Neurocirculatory asthenia is a syndrome occurring is some patients with anxiety neurosis. It consists of shortness of breath, nondescript chest pains, chronic fatigue, palpitations, tachycardias, and other signs of sympathetic overactivity. It has been called DaCosta syndrome (during the American Civil War) (16), soldier's heart (World War II), effort syndrome, neurotic heart syndrome, cardiac neurosis, and vasoregulatory asthenia. If these patients are chronic hyperventilators, their breath-holding time will be less than 20 seconds.

[6]Orthopnea is dyspnea occurring after elevation of the legs and abdomen. It is caused by an increase in left atrial pressure that results when blood from the lower body returns to the heart. This increase of venous return occurs within 20 to 30 seconds.

Orientation

When did it begin? Spontaneous, or patient told by physician to use more pillows?

Etiologies

1. Trepopnea: Horizontal discomfort not resulting from heart failure. Result from feeling large heart against bed when on left side? Result from musculoskeletal pain or dizziness?

> *Note*: The opposite of orthopnea is platypnea (i.e., relief of dyspnea in supine position). It is sometimes called platypnea-orthodexia. It has been seen with severe COPD, pulmonary embolus, and pulmonary A-V fistula and after pneumonectomy. In one case, it was caused by a right-to-left shunt across the intraatrial septum, despite the absence of pulmonary hypertension. Venous blood flowed from the inferior vena cava toward the foramen ovale, either from an abnormally large eustachian valve at the junction of the inferior vena cava and right atrium, or from an anatomic distortion (elongation) of the heart with downward displacement of the right atrium and septum, which caused the foramen ovale to open only if the patient was in the erect position.

2. High left atrial pressure
   a. Does the dyspnea occur whether the patient lies on back, left side, or right side?
   b. Is it relieved by digitalis or diuretics?
   c. Does it begin within half a minute of lying flat?
3. Is there a markedly decreased vital capacity?
   a. Patient not completely free of dyspnea at any chest elevation? (Often seen in severe mitral stenosis.)
   b. Is the patient dyspneic for less than 1 minute in the supine position and does the patient then feel no dyspnea? (Suggests pulmonary hypertension.)

If Patient Says Yes to Paroxysmal Nocturnal Dyspnea

Orientation

When did PND begin? How frequently does it recur?

Etiologies

Left Ventricular Failure

1. How long after the patient is asleep does it occur? (Redistribution of fluid takes 2 to 4 hours to raise left atrial pressure.)
2. Does the patient dangle legs to get relief? (If not, it is *not* PND.)
3. Duration? (It should take 10 to 30 minutes to redistribute fluid back into tissue.)
4. With cough, wheezing, or frothy, pink sputum?
5. Obstructive sleep apnea? History of heavy snoring (21)?

Not from Pulmonary Edema or Left Ventricular Failure

Occurs also during the day? No effect of digitalis, diuretics, and afterload therapy? Patient awakens with palpitations, chronic cough, postnasal drip, or nocturia before shortness of breath noted? Awakens with chest pain or tightness (nocturnal angina)? Awakens during the hyperpneic phase of Cheyne-Stokes respiration, as suggested by frequent awakening and fatigue from lack of sleep (29)?

If Patient Says Yes to Edema

Orientation

When did it begin? Shoes too tight? Extends to knees? Gone in the morning? Effect of digitalis, diuretics, and afterload treatment? Maximum and minimum weights?

Etiologies

1. Cardiac: Helped by cardiac drugs?
2. Stasis or obstructive edema: Began with weight gain or pregnancy? Tight undergarments, varicose veins, or phlebitis? Shirt collar tight and face swollen and flushed? (Suggests superior vena cava obstruction.) Abdominal swelling? (Suggests constriction, tamponade, or ovarian cancer.)
3. Hormonal causes
    a. Premenstrual syndrome: Breast fullness, headache? On estrogens or contraceptive pills?
    b. Aldosteronism: Hypertension, weakness, tetany, paresthesias, or high licorice intake?
    c. Myxedema: Voice change, dry skin, cold intolerance, sluggishness, weight gain, constipation, menorrhagia, or decreased hearing? Thyroid tests?
4. Intermittent idiopathic edema of women: Menstrual disorders?
5. Drug-induced: On vasodilators, nonsteroidal antiinflammatory agents, calcium blockers, or estrogens?
6. Renal: Facial and hand edema? Worse in the morning?
7. Cirrhosis: Alcoholism, hepatitis, or jaundice? Anorexia, fatigue, weakness, ascites, or bleeding from varices? (If polycythemia vera is present, consider hepatic vein thrombosis as cause of ascites [Budd-Chiari syndrome].)
8. Constriction or tamponade: Did edema begin before dyspnea? (Can also occur in severe pulmonary hypertension.)
9. Severe COPD edema caused by the following:
    a. High intraabdominal pressure during inspiration, as well as the normal elevation of intraabdominal pressure with inspiration, and
    b. High carbon dioxide tension, which may dilate afferent renal arterioles more than efferents and result in fluid retention in kidneys (similar to the effect of calcium channel blockers).

If Patient Says Yes to Presyncope, Syncope, or Dizziness

Orientation

When did it begin? Duration and frequency? By dizziness, does the patient mean faintness, loss of balance, lightheadedness, blurred vision, sinking feeling, floating sensation, unsteadiness, swaying, swimming feeling, or vertigo?

Etiologies

1. Potentially fatal
   a. Cardiac syncope: With palpitations? Long QT syndrome (precipitated by quinidine, disopyramide, exercise, fatigue, anxiety, or sudden loud noise)? Preceded by nausea or headache? (A pause as short as 3 seconds can result in syncope in some elderly patients.)
   b. Obstruction to flow: Pulmonary embolism (preceded by lightheadedness with or without dyspnea)? Pleuritic pain, hemoptysis, or cold sweat (12,15)?
   c. Acute infarction: Preceded or followed by chest or arm discomfort, shortness of breath, perspiration, nausea, or faintness with bradycardia (Bezold-Jarisch reflex with posteroinferior infarction)?
2. Epilepsy: How long unconscious? Is mind clear after? Prodrome? Begin with a twitch? Sore tongue, incontinence, or head trauma? Family history? Convulsions witnessed? Had electroencephalogram (EEG) or neurologic examination? Anticonvulsants administered? Bradycardia with faintness or preceded by epigastric discomfort (temporal lobe epilepsy)?
3. Hysterical: Always in the presence of someone else? Paresthesias with dyspnea (hyperventilation)? Ever injured self?
4. Orthostatic: After prolonged bed rest? On diuretics, antihypertensives, nitrates, or dialysis? Autonomic abnormalities, diabetes, nocturnal diarrhea, impotence, peripheral neuritis, or absent sweating? Worse if hot or fatigued? Large varicose veins? Addison's disease: craving for salt, abdominal and back pain, nausea and vomiting?
5. Excess bleeding: Hemorrhoids, melena, menorrhagia, on anticoagulants, trauma? (A ruptured spleen may produce symptoms a week after trauma.) Ulcer history?
6. Carotid insufficiency: Unilateral blindness, weakness, paresthesias, dysarthria, or aphasia for a few minutes or hours?
7. Vasovagal: Preceded by nausea, yawning, or sinking epigastric feeling? Skin wet and pale after? Associated with tight collar, turning head, or hyperextension? (Suggests hypersensitive carotid sinus.) Cough syncope (usually in children with asthma) (1)? With micturition or defecation? Swallow syncope? (Usually results from variable degrees of AV block from balloonlike distension of the esophagus [24], or from sensitive oropharynx in children [7].) Vasovagal syncope results when a relatively empty ventricle contracts vigorously because of initially heightened sympathetic activity. Seven percent of cases have slight convulsions. Does not occur in supine position. The onset of atrial fibrillation may trigger vasovagal syncope.
8. Fixed output or obstruction to flow: Known pulmonary hypertension or stenosis? Syncope after exercise cessation? (Suggests hypertrophic obstructive cardiomyopathy [HOCM]. The increased flow of exercise increases the outflow gradient in valvular aortic stenosis; in HOCM, however, the decrease in preload after stopping and the temporary persistent increase in sympathetic stimulation exaggerate the outflow obstruction. Fixed aortic stenosis syncope occurs during exercise.) Atrial myxoma, fevers, embolic phenomena, or dyspnea with changes of posture?
9. Stokes-Adams attack[7]: Flushed after the attack? Slow pulse noted at the time?
10. "Drop" attacks (sudden loss of postural tone without loss of consciousness): Was pa-

---

[7]A Stokes-Adams attack (also known as Adams-Stokes attack) is an episode of syncope secondary to complete AV block. Any cerebral symptom secondary to complete AV block can probably also be considered a minor Stokes-Adams attack because it may presage syncope and death. Syncope secondary to any other arrhythmia should be referred to as cardiac syncope, not a Stokes-Adams attack.

tient a dead weight when someone tried to raise his or her body? (Pressure on soles of feet restores postural tone.)

11. Subclavian steal: Symptoms of vertebral-basilar insufficiency (occasional syncope) such as vertigo, tinnitus, diplopia, dysarthria, unilateral transient blindness with repeated arm movements? Claudication of arm (10)? (See page 43 for definition of subclavian steal.)

12. Stroke: Unilateral weakness or slurred speech?

13. Sick sinus syndrome: History of slow pulse or palpitations, as in bradycardia-tachycardia syndrome?

14. Metabolic: Hypoglycemia?

15. Glossopharyngeal neuralgia with pain at base of tongue, pharynx, tonsillar region, and ear?

16. Cyanotic heart disease: Fallot's tetralogy.

17. Exercise-induced syncope or sudden death: Hypertrophic cardiomyopathy, anomalous origin of left coronary artery and dissecting aneurysm, aortic stenosis, myocarditis, exercise-induced vasovagal syncope, arrhythmias (Wolff-Parkinson-White syndrome, long QT syndrome, and catecholamine-sensitive supraventricular or ventricular tachycardia).

If Patient Says Yes to Chest Pain or Pressure

Orientation

When did it begin? How often does it recur? Longest and shortest time between episodes?

Note: The secret of history taking, especially for chest pain, is to not let the patient know what answer is expected. If angina is suspected, the physician should ask if exercise relieves the pain. If the patient says that the opposite is true, the likelihood of angina is strengthened.

1. Site: Ask the patient to show you where pain or tightness is. Do not ask the patient to point. (If the patient points, the pain is likely nonanginal. If the pain is classic angina, the patient will lay a fist or hand over the sternum or across the chest.) Is there radiation? Several chest pains?

2. Character: Classic angina is characterized by tightness and pressure, but pain of any character can be angina.

3. Nonanginal pain: Points to site with one finger? Lasts less than 5 seconds or more than 30 minutes? Increases with inspiration, local pressure, or one movement of the arms or chest? Relieved immediately when patient lies down? Seeks relief by walking? (Occasionally occurs with acute infarction.) Radiates down lateral side of forearm to thumb? (Anginal pain radiates down medial aspect to little finger.)

4. What diagnostic tests were used? Was an ECG performed, with and without exercise? What kind of exercise? What were results? Coronary angiography or nuclear tests and results?

Etiologies

1. Coronary obstruction: Precipitated by food, cold air, or anything that increases heart rate or afterload? Occurs mainly after first exercise in morning? With pallor, flatulence, nausea, sweating, or dyspnea? Relieved by drugs that decrease preload, afterload, heart rate, or inotropism? Aortic dissection? (By involvement of the coronary vessels.) (See paragraph 8 in

section on noncoronary causes for questions to ask. *Risk factors*: Diabetes, hypertension, artificial menopause, contraceptive use, smoking, intermittent claudication,[8] family history of coronary disease, low levels of HDL cholesterol, high levels of low-density lipoprotein (LDL) cholesterol, previous infarction or gout. [Ischemic symptoms will develop in about 16% of patients with gout within 8 years (8)].

2. Vasospastic angina (Prinzmetal's angina): At rest, especially at night toward morning? Precipitated by cold air? Good and bad days?

3. Unstable angina: Occurs more frequently with less provocation? Lasts longer? Occurs at rest?

4. Microvascular angina: Normal angiograms but positive exercise tests? [These patients have abnormal exercise radionuclide-ejection fractions or wall motion (4).]

5. Acute infarction (site either is similar to that of patient's chronic angina or is lower but more widespread) (31): With perspiration, faintness, syncope, nausea or vomiting? Hiccups may be specific for inferior infarction. If a second infarction occurs with pain in a different site, it suggests multiple sites of infarction. May pace about to try to get relief (rare with angina).

6. Aortic stenosis: A high-velocity jet through the stenotic valve may induce the Venturi phenomenon, reducing blood flow into the coronary ostia.

Noncoronary Causes

1. Pericarditis: Worse in supine position and with inspiration? Relieved by leaning forward? Elevation of legs increases pain? Increases with swallowing or extension of neck? May be referred by phrenic nerve to left side of neck, shoulder, and arm. May be referred to abdomen, especially in children.

2. Congenital absence of pericardium: Brought on by lying on the left side? Lasts a few seconds or minutes? Relieved by changing position in bed?

3. Esophagitis or spasm: Burning pain on eating or lying down? Acid reflux (water brash)? Relieved by antacids or hot drinks? Hiatal hernia on x-ray? Dysphagia? Nitroglycerin takes at least 3 minutes to relieve pain?

4. Root neuritis: Had herpes zoster or chest injury? Radiates to radial side of the hand? (Suggests herniated cervical disk.) Brought on by walking or arm or head movements and helped by nitroglycerin? (Suggests cervical root compression syndrome. Test by having patient try to touch left shoulder with right hand while turning head to right, and vice versa.)

5. Scalenus anticus or thoracic outlet syndrome: Paresthesias and pain along the ulnar distribution? Worse with head turning, arm abduction, weight lifting, working with hands over the shoulder, or sleeping on side (3,30)?

6. Costochondritis, myositis, or local neuritis: Brought on by local pressure? Tietze syndrome (painful swelling of costal cartilage). Helped by salicylates (20)?

7. Fixed-output syndrome: Known severe aortic or pulmonary stenosis? [Pulmonary hypertension is not thought to produce angina (33).]

8. Aortic dissection (pain similar to that of infarction): If in the back, the aneurysm is probably distal to subclavian. Pain maximal at onset? Radiates to abdomen or legs? Pain tearing or ripping? Presyncope or syncope with pain? Does it begin in epigastrium and radiate to

---

[8]If the obstruction in intermittent claudication is high in the aortoiliac area, the pain may be in the hip or buttock. However, the pain may be felt in unusual sites, such as the thighs or arch of the foot. When the ischemia is caused by thrombosis of the lower aorta (chronic aortoiliac occlusion), impotence and leg weakness may also occur (Leriche syndrome) (19). If the celiac or mesenteric arteries are involved, the pain that occurs after meals is called abdominal angina. Intermittent claudication is not related to the nocturnal leg or foot muscle cramps that occur in bed.

chest? Pain may pulsate with heart beat. Is patient pregnant? Have Marfan syndrome, or coarctation?

9. Mitral valve prolapse syndrome: Pain associated with lightheadedness, fatigue, and palpitations? Ever had echocardiogram?

10. Gout: Mimics coronary pain and lasts from minutes to days (11)?

11. Pulmonary infarction: Intercostal tenderness (Briscoe's sign)? Increases with inspiration, one movement of arm or chest?

If Patient Says Yes to Palpitations

Orientation

When did they begin? Shortest and longest duration, and length of time between episodes?

Types and Rate of Arrhythmias

1. Is beat continuous, or only occasional strong beat? Regular or irregular? (A history of sustained irregular palpitations is fairly specific for atrial fibrillation. However, a history of regular palpitations can be obtained from a patient with either paroxysmal atrial tachycardia or atrial fibrillation.) Ask patient to tap out rate and rhythm. Ever taken own pulse during palpitations? Is ECG abnormal? (Consider Wolff-Parkinson-White syndrome.)

2. Ectopic tachycardia versus sinus tachycardia: Does it begin and end suddenly? Occurs at rest or always with exertion? (Suggests sinus tachycardia.) Any maneuvers to stop it?

3. Do pulsations in neck come and go? (A giant A wave of pulmonary hypertension or tricuspid stenosis disappears with atrial fibrillation. Cannon A waves occur whenever there is AV dissociation or retrograde P waves.)

4. Do any maneuvers or medications stop it?

Etiologies

1. Does patient drink much tea, coffee, cola, or alcohol? On drugs such as digitalis, diuretics, anticholinergics, or cocaine? On tachycardia-producing drugs (hydralazine, anticholinergic ulcer drugs, vasodilators, or decongestants)?

2. Thyroid disease, heat intolerance: See section on high-output failure possibilities, page 4.

3. Pheochromocytoma: With flushing, headaches, or perspiration?

4. Sick sinus syndrome with tachycardia-bradycardia: Is there presyncope, syncope, or slow pulse? Had Holter monitor?

If Patient Says Yes to Hypertension

Orientation

When first told? For how long treated, with what drugs and side effects? Was patient compliant?

Severity

Past blood pressure readings? Had convulsions, strokes, headaches, nocturnal dyspnea, dyspnea on exertion, orthopnea, or epistaxis? Abnormal findings on x-rays and ECG?

Etiologies

1. Essential hypertension: Family history? Onset date? (Essential hypertension usually begins in fourth decade, between ages 30 and 40.)

2. Renal: Kidney infections or stones, back injury, urinary frequency, polyuria, prostatism, gout, or severe diabetes?

3. Coarctation: Cold legs, claudication, or pain in shoulder girdle?

4. Pheochromocytoma: Flushing, pounding headaches, dizziness, perspiration, palpitations, nausea, chest pains, paresthesias, or weight loss? Elevated blood sugar?

5. Eclampsia: Edema, hypertension, albuminuria, or convulsions in pregnancy?

6. Aldosteronism: Episodic or continual weakness, tetany, polyuria (mostly nocturnal) or polydipsia, or headaches? Excessive licorice consumption?

7. Hormonal: On contraceptives? Cushing syndrome? On steroids? Hirsutism, easy bruising, acne, weakness, kidney stones, emotional lability, or depression?

8. Hyperparathyroidism: Peptic ulcer? (Calcium stimulates gastric secretion.) Renal calculi, constipation, lethargy, or polyuria?

NEW YORK HEART ASSOCIATION FUNCTIONAL CLASSIFICATION

This functional classification refers to fatigue, dyspnea, or angina. The original classification is too long to memorize, and a simplified one follows.

Class 1: The patient is asymptomatic, or symptoms occur on extraordinary exertion. (There is no class 0 or classification for a patient with a normal heart.)

Class 2: Symptoms occur on ordinary exertion.

Class 3: Symptoms occur on less-than-ordinary exertion.

Class 4: Symptoms occur at rest or on slight exertion.

The functional classification is easily recalled if one simply remembers the words *ordinary exertion*. For class 1, simply add *extra* to *ordinary*; for class 2, add nothing to *ordinary*; for class 3, add *less than* to *ordinary*.

REFERENCES

1. Aaronson DW, Rovner RN, Patterson R. Cough syncope: case presentation and review. *J Allergy Clin Immunol* 1970;46:359.
2. Aderka D, Pinkhas J. Sweating with pulmonary edema. *Ann Intern Med* 1984;101:402.
3. Adson AW. Surgical treatment for symptoms produced by cervical ribs and the scalenus anticus muscle. *Surg Gynecol Obstet* 1947;85:687.
4. Cannon RO. Diagnosis and management of microvascular angina. *Primary Cardiol* 1990;16:15.
5. Daley R. Massive dilatation of the left atrium. *Br Heart J* 1980;44:724.
6. Darsee JR, Nutter DO. Reversible severe congestive cardiomyopathy in three cases of hypophosphatemia. *Ann Intern Med* 1978;89:867.
7. Engelhardt W, Kotlarek F, von Bermuth G. Deglutition syncope in childhood with complete atrioventricular block. *Am J Cardiol* 1986;58:1113.
8. Fessel WJ. High uric acid as an indicator of cardiovascular disease: independence from obesity. *Am J Med* 1980; 68:3.
9. Findley LJ, Zwillich CW. Cheyne-Stokes breathing during sleep in patients with left ventricular heart failure. *South Med J* 1985;78:11.
10. Folger GM Jr, Shaw KD. Subclavian steal in patients with Blalock-Taussig anastomosis. *Circulation* 1965; 31:241.
11. Frank M, DeVries A, Atsmon A. Gout simulating cardiac pain. *Am J Cardiol* 1960;6:929.
12. Fred HL, Willerson JT, Alexander JK. Neurological manifestations of pulmonary thromboembolism. *Arch Intern Med* 1967;120:33.

13. Hagman M. Relationship between dyspnea and chest pain in ischemic heart disease. *Acta Med Scand* 1981; 644:16.
14. Harrison TR, et al. Congestive heart failure: Cheyne-Stokes respiration as a cause of paroxysmal dyspnea at the onset of sleep. *Arch Intern Med* 1934;54:891.
15. Hornsten TR, Hellerstein HK, Ankeney JL. Patent ductus arteriosus in a 72-year-old woman. *JAMA* 1967; 199:148.
16. Jarcho S. Functional heart disease in the Civil War. *Am J Cardiol* 1959;4:809.
17. Kennedy HL, Underhill SJ. Ischemic ST segment depression and dyspnea. *Am Heart J* 1975;89:544.
18. Lely AH, van Enter CH. Non-cardiac symptoms of digitalis intoxication. *Am Heart J* 1972;83:149.
19. Leriche R, Morel A. The syndrome of thrombotic obliteration of the aortic bifurcation. *Ann Surg* 1958;127:193.
20. Levey GS, Calabro JJ. Tietze's syndrome: report of two cases and review of the literature. *Arthritis Rheum* 1962; 5:261.
21. Malone S, et al. Obstructive sleep apnoea in patients with dilated cardiomyopathy: effects of continuous positive airway pressure. *Lancet* 1991;338:1480.
22. Marvin RF, Schrank JP, Nolan SP. Traumatic tricuspid insufficiency. *Am J Cardiol* 1973;82:723.
23. Morgan AA, Mourant AJ. Left vocal chord paralysis and dysphagia in mitral valve disease. *Br Heart J* 1980; 43:470.
24. Nakagawa S, et al. A case of swallow syncope induced by vagotonic visceral reflex resulting in atrioventricular node suppression. *J Electrocardiol* 1987;20:65.
25. Oster MW, Leslie B. Syncope and pulmonary embolism. *JAMA* 1873;224:630.
26. Pang JA, et al. Shoshin beriberi: an underdiagnosed condition. *Intensive Care Med* 1986;12:380.
27. Pfeifer MP, Hardison JE. Profuse diaphoresis relieved by coronary angioplasty. *Am J Med* 1989;86:338.
28. Powers PP, Read JL, Porter RR. Acute idiopathic pericarditis simulating acute abdominal disease. *JAMA* 1955; 157:224.
29. Rees PJ, Clark TJH. Paroxysmal nocturnal dyspnoea and periodic respiration. *Lancet* 1979;2:1315.
30. Riddell DH, et al. Scalenus anticus symptoms: evaluation and surgical treatment. *Surgery* 1981;47:299.
31. Short D. Diagnosis of slight and subacute coronary attacks in the community. *Br Heart J* 1981;45:299.
32. Walcott G, Burchell HB, Brown AL Jr. Primary pulmonary hypertension. *Am J Med* 1970;49:70.
33. Zimmerman D, Parker BM. The pain of pulmonary hypertension: fact or fancy? *JAMA* 1981;246:2345.

2

Cardiac Clues from Physical Appearance

SKIN

1. How can you distinguish central from peripheral cyanosis clinically?

   ANS.: Central cyanosis is seen in warm as well as cold areas (compare with the tongue of a normal patient). In black patients, cyanosis may be seen in the conjunctivae. Central cyanosis is not usually recognized unless the arterial oxygen saturation is lowered to about 80% (12). Peripheral cyanosis is seen only in cool areas, such as the nail beds, nose, cheeks, earlobes, and outer surface of the lips, where slow flow decreases the amount of hemoglobin in the surface capillaries. If clubbing is present or if the hands are warm, the cyanosis is probably central.

2. How should you test for mild clubbing?

   ANS.: Look for obliteration of the normal angle between the base of the nail and the proximal skin. Obliteration of the "window" produced by placing the dorsal surfaces of the terminal phalanges of the third or fourth fingers against each other is the earliest sign of clubbing. The angle between the nails does not normally extend more than halfway up the nail bed. Clubbing produces a wide and deep angle (10,15).
   Note: No matter how severe the cyanosis, clubbing is rare before 3 months of age (Fig. 1).

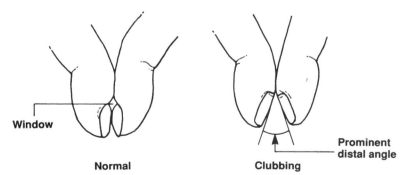

FIG. 1. The small window made by the abutment of a dorsal fingernail of each hand against each other becomes smaller and then disappears with increasing degrees of clubbing.

3. What is differential cyanosis and what is its significance?

    ANS: In differential cyanosis, the fingers are pink but the toes are cyanotic (and usually clubbed). It signifies the presence of a persistent ductus arteriosus (PDA) with a reversed right-to-left shunt caused by pulmonary hypertension (Eisenmenger syndrome). The left hand may also be cyanotic because the ductus may be located at the branching part of the left subclavian artery (Fig. 2).

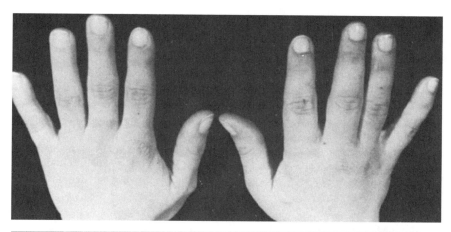

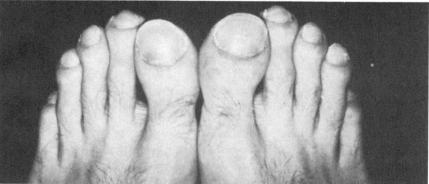

FIG. 2. The feet of this 23-year-old man with a reversed shunt through a patent ductus were cyanotic and clubbed, whereas his hands were normal.

4. What are the skin signs secondary to the small emboli of infective endocarditis?

    ANS: a. Clubbing

        b. Splinter hemorrhages in the nails.

          Note: Most splinter hemorrhages are not embolic and are caused by repeated jarring. Because they are in the nail substance, they move with the nail as it grows and extend to the distal nail edge. Embolic splinters are subungual and usually do not extend to the distal nail edge. Fresh red hemorrhages, especially at the base of the nails, are more important than brown linear streaks near the tips of the fingers.

        c. Osler's nodes: Painful, tender, reddish brown, raised areas, 3 to 15 mm in diameter, on the palms and soles that do not blanch with pressure.

        d. Janeway lesions: Painless, circular or oval, pink-to-tan macules about 5 mm in diameter on the palms and soles that do not blanch with pressure.

5. What cardiac condition is suggested by brownish, muddy pigmentation of the skin and signs of hepatic failure, such as loss of axillary and pubic hair?

   ANS: Hemochromatosis with a cardiomyopathy caused by intracellular deposits in the heart muscle, with secondary interstitial fibrosis.

6. When can amyloid disease with cardiac involvement cause skin lesions? What kind of lesions?

   ANS.: Only if it is primary or if it is secondary to infection. Yellowish brown papules, nodules, or plaques may develop that are often pruritic, with signs of bleeding resulting from scratching.

7. What is livido reticularis? What is its significance?

   ANS.: It is a marbling reticulation or fishnet mottling of the lower trunk, buttocks, and extremities, precipitated or exaggerated by cold or emotion. It occurs in about 20% of patients with lupus erythematosus, periarteritis nodosa, or cryoglobulinemia. If recent in a man over age 50, it suggests cholesterol embolization from an abdominal aortic aneurysm (9). In the palmar aspect of the digits, it suggests acute bacterial endocarditis (16).

   Note: Multiple cholesterol emboli may result in gangrene, skin ulcerations, petechiae, or purple toes.

8. What diagnosis can be made by noting facial flushing following a syncopal attack?

   ANS.: A cardiac arrest or a Stokes-Adams attack (see footnote 7 in Chapter 1). The flush is probably a manifestation of the total-body reactive hyperemia that follows a temporary cessation of circulation.

9. What are the cutaneous manifestations of intestinal **carcinoid** disease? What are the cardiac manifestations?

   ANS.: The face and neck may show various blends of red and purple, often patchy and mottled. A sudden flush may be accompanied by facial and periorbital edema.

10. What conditions besides thyrotoxicosis can affect the heart and cause warmer-than-average skin?

    ANS.: Severe anemia and beer drinkers' acute **beriberi**.

11. What kind of conditions are suggested by cold hands and feet?

    ANS.: a. If the hands and feet are also moist, they suggest anxiety and may explain chest pains, palpitations, and fatigue as seen in neurocirculatory asthenia (DaCosta syndrome). (See page 7.)

    b. If only the feet are cold and the patient has a history of intermittent claudication, peripheral arterial obstruction with poor collateral circulation is suggested.

    c. If cold extremities are relatively recent (a few weeks to a few years), a low-output syndrome is suggested.

    Note: a. The cold hands of the low-output syndrome can become warm when palmar erythema ("liver palms") develops secondary to cardiac cirrhosis.

    b. The smooth, glossy, drum-tight skin on the fingers seen in scleroderma may be associated with myocardial fibrosis or cor pulmonale caused by pulmonary fibrosis.

12. What should you suspect if the fingertips are red?

    ANS.: This is tuft erythema and signifies intermittent right-to-left shunts resulting from pulmonary hypertension and a balanced shunt, usually through an atrial septal defect (ASD).

    Note: A red lunula (resulting from adhesions of the base of the nail, the usually whitish half-moon area, to the underlying connective tissue) is most commonly associated with congestive heart failure. It has been seen also in myocardial infarction and angina. It is best seen in the thumbs (19).

13. What cardiac lesion is associated with multiple lentigines (i.e., multiple pigmented spots that, unlike freckles, begin at about age 6 and do not increase in number with sunlight)?
    ANS.: Mild pulmonary stenosis (PS) or hypertrophic subaortic stenosis (HSS), also known as hypertrophic obstructive cardiomyopathy (HOCM) (6,18).

14. What condition that affects the cardiovascular system is associated with neurofibromatosis?
    ANS.: Pheochromocytoma (occurs in about 5% of cases).

15. How can the distribution of perspiration help to grade the degree of acute pulmonary edema (1)?
    ANS.: Stage I Mild; of forehead.
    Stage II Moderate; on forehead and chest.
    Stage III Severe; on forehead, chest, and abdomen (usually need assisted ventilation).

16. What cardiac lesion is associated with tuberous sclerosis [triad of mental deficiency (not always), epilepsy (80%), and adenoma sebaceum (salmon-colored papules around nose and mouth)]?
    ANS.: Rhabdomyomas of heart.

CONGENITAL AND ACQUIRED FACIES

1. What is the facies of supravalvular aortic stenosis, also known as Williams syndrome?[1]
   ANS.: A broad, high forehead; puffy cheeks; low ears; hypertelorism (eyes set widely apart) with strabismus; an upturned nose with a long filtrum (the vertical groove between nose and mouth); a wide, pouting mouth; dental abnormalities; and a hypoplastic mandible (3,13) (Fig. 3).

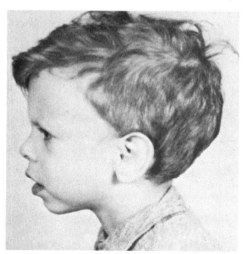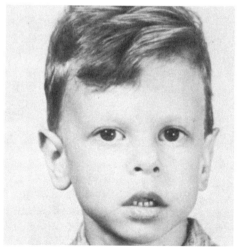

FIG. 3. This boy with severe supravalvular aortic stenosis does not have all the associated facial characteristics (e.g., there is no hypertension or strabismus).

[1]The fetal alcohol syndrome (offspring of heavy maternal drinkers) is associated with a diminished-to-absent philtrum and a thin upper lip.

2. What are the facies of Down syndrome (trisomy 21)? What are the cardiac abnormalities?

   ANS.: A flattened occiput, disproportionately small head, epicanthal folds that give the impression of slanted eyes, a mouth held open by a large protruding tongue, and underdeveloped nasal bones. The most common cardiac abnormalities are various combinations of ASD, ventricular septal defect (VSD), and atrioventricular (AV) valve regurgitation resulting from various degrees of endocardial cushion defects.

3. What is the de Musset sign?

   ANS.: Nodding movements of the head secondary to the ballistic force of severe aortic regurgitation (AR).

   Note: The sign was named after Alfred de Musset, a French poet whose nodding movements were described by his brother in a biography.

4. What is the facies of myxedema? What cardiac abnormalities are expected?

   ANS.: Characteristic features are puffy lids and loss of the outer third of the eyebrows; scanty, dry hair; coarse, dry skin; expressionless face; and an enlarged tongue. These patients have cardiomyopathies resulting from increased interstitial fluid and mucoid infiltration. They also have pericardial effusions, often with a high cholesterol content.

5. What is meant by an earlobe crease, and what is its significance?

   ANS.: This is an oblique or diagonal crease in the earlobe. Ninety percent of patients over age 50 with significant triple-vessel coronary disease have a deep earlobe crease. In one study, a unilateral ear crease was found to be associated with an intermediate degree of coronary obstruction (11). The earlobe crease should be considered a strong and independent risk factor for coronary disease and *not* diagnostic for the presence of coronary disease, for which it is only about 60% sensitive (4).

   A higher correlation has been found between coronary artery disease and the earlobe crease than between coronary artery disease and hypertension, smoking, or diabetes. The earlobe crease is more prevalent in hypertensives (especially those with retinopathy), diabetics, and patients who have had a myocardial infarction than in control populations in the same age groups (4). In diabetics, the diagonal ear crease is significantly more common in those with retinal angiopathy than in those with normal retinal vessels (Fig. 4).

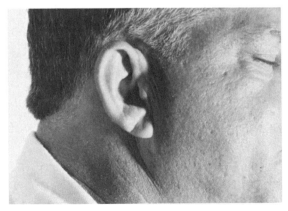

FIG. 4. This 47-year-old man had a deep ear crease bilaterally. Although he had no significant coronary disease, his ratio of total to HDL cholesterol was 8:1 and he had sinus node dysfunction. He was about 50 lbs overweight.

6. What is the malar flush?

    ANS.: Cyanotic cheeks with a slight telangiectasia. It was once thought to be specific for mitral stenosis, pulmonary hypertension, and high venous pressure. It can also be seen, however, in any patient with low cardiac output and high venous pressure. Patients who lead an outdoor life or with myxedema may also have a malar flush. It is sometimes seen in patients with severe PS, those with an ASD and cushingoid moon facies, and persons with the carcinoid syndrome.

    In systemic lupus, the cheeks are also reddened, but a butterfly erythema covers both the cheeks and the bridge of the nose. In these patients, lesions are also found in exposed areas like the scalp, external auditory canal, neck, and upper chest. The heart may be involved in lupus with pericarditis, myocarditis, Libman-Sacks verrucous endocarditis of the mitral or aortic valve, and occasional myocardial infarction resulting from coronary arteritis.

7. Which cardiac abnormalities are suggested by neck webbing?

    ANS.: a. Turner syndrome with coarctation (see footnote 6, page 25).

    b. Noonan syndrome, or Ullrich syndrome with PS, and more rarely hypertrophic cardiomyopathies.

8. What is the facies of some patients with severe pulmonary valve stenosis?

    ANS.: Highly colored "moon" facies, as in Cushing syndrome. This facies is found in about one-third of patients with severe PS. Hypertelorism (eyes set widely apart) is often found in PS with ASD.

9. What is the velocardiofacial syndrome?

    ANS.: These patients have a long face and deep overbite; a cleft soft palate (*velum* means palate); a broad nasal bridge; a VSD, tetralogy of Fallot, prolapse of an aortic cusp, and right-sided aortic arch; and learning disabilities.

EYES

1. How does infective endocarditis affect the eyes?

    ANS.: a. Conjunctival hemorrhage and petechiae are often associated with a white center (caused by a bleeding tendency plus minute emboli). Evert the lids, especially the lower lids, to see these lesions.

    b. Roth's spots (oval or canoe-shaped hemorrhages) near the optic disc with a white (cotton-wool) spot (lymphocytes in nerve layer) in center.

2. Which cardiac condition other than hypertensive heart disease is associated with papilledema?

    ANS.: Hypoxic cor pulmonale[2] with hyperpnea, in which papilledema is caused by high cerebrospinal fluid pressure (resulting from high levels of carbon dioxide) with little elevation of jugular pressure.

3. Which cardiac lesions are part of the rubella syndrome?

    ANS.: A PDA and pulmonary artery (*not* valve) stenosis are the most common cardiac lesions. Other features may include cataracts, deafness, and mental deficiency resulting from microcephaly. The rate of growth may be slow.

4. Which cardiac abnormalities are associated with hypertelorism?

---

[2]Cor pulmonale is RV hypertrophy (**not** RV failure) secondary to a lung abnormality. The pulmonary problem is usually chronic obstructive pulmonary disease (formerly known as emphysema) or arteriolar obstruction caused by emboli or idiopathic (primary) pulmonary hypertension.

ANS.: a. PS, especially in association with ASD. Hypertelorism also occurs in Down syndrome, Noonan syndrome[3], and multiple lentigines syndrome (6).

b. Hurler syndrome[4], or gargoylism, with mitral regurgitation.

c. Supravalvular aortic stenosis.

5. Which kind of corneal arcus is associated with hypercholesterolemia or coronary disease?

ANS.: A thick band that begins inferiorly and is inside the limbus, allowing a thin rim of iris pigment to be seen between the arcus and the sclera.

Note: a. The usual arcus senilis is not necessarily associated with hyperlipidemia or coronary disease. It begins superiorly and extends to the rim or limbus of the iris.

b. An arcus may be absent or diminished on one side if blood flow to that side is reduced by carotid occlusion or previous inflammation (8) (Fig. 5).

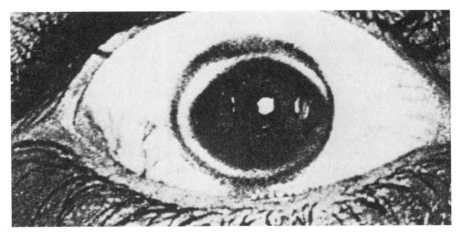

FIG. 5. This type of arcus is a thick band of yellowish material surrounded by peripheral pigment and suggests a high level of serum cholesterol. It is not an arcus senilis, which has little known significance. (Courtesy of Ayerst Laboratories.)

6. Which cardiac lesions are common in patients with the epicanthus of Down syndrome?[5]

ANS.: Endocardial cushion defects, especially of the complete variety.

7. Which cardiac lesions should you suspect in the presence of an Argyll Robertson pupil (a pupil that reacts to accommodation but not to light)?

ANS.: Luetic aortic aneurysm or luetic AR with coronary ostial stenosis.

8. Which cardiac condition besides thyrotoxic heart disease can be associated with exophthalmos?

---

[3]Noonan syndrome comprises the physical characteristics of Turner syndrome, but without any known chromosomal abnormalities. (The condition is known as Ullrich syndrome in Europe.) It has been referred to as male Turner syndrome, a poor term because it ignores the condition in female patients. (See Turner syndrome, page 25, for physical and cardiac characteristics.)

[4]Hurler syndrome is a rare autosomal recessive metabolic disorder in which abnormal glycoproteins are deposited in most of the organs, resulting in dwarfism, mental retardation, and cardiomyopathy. The heart valves may be thickened.

[5]The outstanding findings in Down syndrome (trisomy 21 or mongolism) are mental retardation, hypotonia, medial epicanthus, large (often protruding) fissured tongue, small orbits, a circle of grayish white dots along the outer circumference of the iris that disappear after the first year of life (Brushfield spots), short fingers, a distally displaced axial triradius, and a transverse side-to-side palmar crease (simian crease).

ANS.: Advanced congestive heart failure with high venous pressure and weight loss. The stare is probably a consequence of lid retraction caused by the strong sympathetic tone accompanying low cardiac output and exaggerated by the slight proptosis.

Note: Severe tricuspid regurgitation can even cause systolic pulsation of the eyes. A pulsatile exophthalmos also may be caused by a carotid-cavernous sinus arteriovenous (A-V) fistula, in which case a murmur can be heard over the eyeball.

9. What cardiac lesions should you suspect if you see a tremulous iris (iridodonesis)?

ANS.: Iridodonesis is a tremulous motion of the iris when the gaze is rapidly shifted from one object to another. This sign suggests the Marfan syndrome, in which the iris is not properly supported by the lens because of dislocation or weakness of the suspensory ligaments. The cardiac lesions associated with it are aneurysm of the aorta or pulmonary artery and myxomatous degeneration of the aorta or mitral valve with consequent regurgitation.

Note: In the Marfan syndrome, the lens is dislocated upward. In congenital homocysteinuria, the lens is dislocated downward (look for arterial and venous thrombosis, myocardial infarction, and pulmonary embolism).

10. What are the retinal signs of various degrees of arteriosclerosis (16)?

ANS.: Grade 1 The light reflex is increased in width.

Grade 2 Crossing abnormalities (arteriolovenous nicking and right-angled crossings of the arterioles over the veins).

Grade 3 Copper-wire arterioles (red color is slightly brownish because of thick walls).

Grade 4 Silver-wire arterioles (no red color is seen at all, only a whitish light reflex).

Note: a. The copper-wire sign implies that the light streak has become so wide that it occupies most of the surface of the vessel.

b. Hollenhorst plaques are flakes of cholesterol emboli seen as glinting spots, often seeming larger than the vessels in which they reside.

c. Only the central artery and the branches inside the papilla are arteries and can manifest atheromas. The peripheral "arteries" are really arterioles and can show only intimal thickening, hyaline changes, and luminal narrowing. The fundal "arteries" actually show arteriolar sclerosis (14,16).

d. The widened light reflex seen in grade 1 arteriolar sclerosis is considered to be a normal retinal sign of aging (20).

e. Arteriolovenous nicking is seen as a venous column either tapering or disappearing on both sides of the arteriole.

11. What are the retinal signs of different degrees of hypertension?

ANS.: Grade 1 Generalized attenuation (arteriolovenous ratio of less than 2 : 3 or 3 : 4). Venous engorgement, as with congestive failure, must be ruled out.

Grade 2 Focal constriction or spasm.

Grade 4 Papilledema.

Note: a. Pure attenuation of the arterioles is best seen in toxemia of pregnancy or in young persons with rapid onset of hypertension. Minimal narrowing is most easily seen beyond the first bifurcation, where the arteries actually become arterioles.

b. Corkscrew tortuosity of the retinal arterioles (frequent *u*-turns) may be seen with the hypertension of aortic coarctation, sometimes with retinal hemorrhages.

12. What are "Hollenhorst" bodies?

ANS.: Shiny yellow patches at the bifurcation of a retinal vessel, caused by emboli of atheromatous plaques detached from basilar or carotid arteries.

13. What are angioid streaks? Significance?

    ANS.: Brown or gray lines running perpendicular to the direction of blood vessels. They are most often seen in Ehlers-Danlos syndrome and in pseudoxanthoma elasticum, which affects the skin (pebbly papules), retinae, blood vessels (hypertension and claudication), and heart, the latter mainly by endocardial fibrosis and valvular regurgitation.

14. What is the significance of xanthelasma?

    ANS.: There is no significant correlation between xanthelasma and hypercholesterolemia. Patients with xanthelasma even tend to be protected from atherosclerosis by having higher levels of high-density lipoproteins (HDLs) than the general population (5,17).

15. What three cardiac conditions are associated with blue sclerae?

    ANS.: a. Osteogenesis imperfecta is associated with AR.

    b. The Marfan syndrome is associated with aneurysms of the great vessels and mitral or aortic valve regurgitation.

    c. Ehlers-Danlos syndrome, with its hyperelastic, fragile skin, hyperextensible joints, and kyphoscoliosis, is associated with an ASD, tetralogy of Fallot, or regurgitant valve.

EDEMA

1. How can you demonstrate edema even when it is slight?

    ANS.: Press on the skin over a bony area for 10 seconds with at least three fingers spread slightly apart and feel for valleys between hills after release.

2. What is the significance of "slow" and "fast" edema?

    ANS.: With slow edema, the pitting remains for more than 1 minute, and it is most likely caused by congestion. If, however, the pitting disappears in less than 40 seconds (fast edema), the cause is almost certainly a low albumin level (4).

    Note: The venous pressure and rate of venous flow presumably control the rate of flow of tissue fluid from the legs. Ascites with high intraabdominal pressure can also cause slow edema.

3. What are the usual causes of noncardiac bilateral leg edema besides low albumin?

    ANS.: Premenstrual state (hormonal), tight undergarments, and obesity (obstructed lymphatics).

    Note: Localized nonpitting pretibial edema is related to hyperthyroidism and not to congestive failure. It is pruritic and erythematous in the early stages and may appear years before or after the hyperthyroidism. Myxedema may occasionally cause a generalized nonpitting edema.

4. Where should you check for edema in a patient who is bedridden?

    ANS.: Only presacral edema may be present if the patient has been in bed for some time.

    Note: You can rule out a cardiac cause for the edema by checking the venous pressure. Normal venous pressure is incompatible with a cardiac cause of the edema unless diuretics have been given. Face and hand edema in an ambulant patient tend to rule out a cardiac cause.

5. How is the degree of edema graded?

    ANS.: a. By depth of pitting as grades 1 to 4, meaning slight, moderate, moderately severe, and very severe.

    b. By extent above ankle. Edema may be on lateral and posterior thigh and not anterior thigh.

6. How much body fluid may collect in tissue before pitting occurs?

    ANS.: At least 10 lb (4.5 kg).

7. How can you tell that a distended abdomen is caused by ascites secondary to congestive heart failure (CHF)?

ANS.: a. If the flanks are resonant to percussion, ascites is unlikely and the swelling is probably gaseous distension, which is common in severe CHF.

b. If the ascites is caused by CHF, the liver is almost always enlarged and is often ballotable, giving an impulse similar to that of a fetal head just below the right costal margin.

EXTREMITIES

1. What cardiac lesion is suggested by short stature and cubitus valgus (medial deviation of the extended forearm)?

ANS.: Turner syndrome[6], with coarctation as a common abnormality.

Note: a. Coarctation of the aorta is the most common associated cardiovascular lesion. When a patient with Turner syndrome, especially a male patient, has normal sex chromosomes, hypertelorism with a slight antimongoloid slant to the eyes, ptosis of the upper lids, and exophthalmos, the patient likely has PS and is said to have Noonan syndrome. Hypertrophic cardiomyopathies and PDA have also been associated with Noonan syndrome.

b. When web neck, cubitus varus, short stature, and hypogonadism are found in male subjects, the condition is called Ullrich-Noonan syndrome; PS is the most commonly associated cardiac abnormality (Fig. 6).

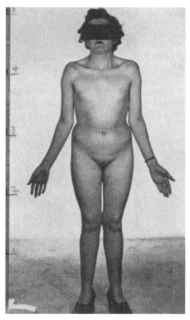

FIG. 6. The patient's height is 5 ft (1.5 m). (From Oram S. Clinical heart disease. Philadelphia: FA Davis Co, 1971.)

---

[6]Turner syndrome is a female phenotype characterized by short stature, receding chin, webbed neck, low hairline over the back of the neck, broad (shield) chest resulting in widely separated nipples, exaggerated carrying angle, sparse axillary and pubic hair, lymphedema of the lower extremities (in infancy), and short fourth metacarpal. It is sometimes simply described as short stature, neck webbing, and sexual infantilism in female subjects with a sex chromosome abnormality (absence of one of the two sex chromosomes).

2. Which abnormalities of the extremities are found with **ASD's**?

    ANS.: a. The thumb may have an extra phalanx ("fingerized thumb"), and it may lie in the same plane as the fingers, so that it is difficult to oppose thumb and fingers.

        b. There may be distal radial and ulnar deformities causing difficulty in supination and pronation.

        Note: If (a) and (b) are both present, the syndrome is known as the Holt-Oram syndrome, and the **ASD** is usually of the secundum type (7). Pectus deformities of the sternum also occur (2).

3. What hand and wrist signs suggest the Marfan syndrome, with its possible cardiac abnormalities of AR or mitral valve prolapse syndrome?

    ANS.: a. Fingers are slender and long ("spider" fingers, or arachnodactyly).

        b. Thumb sign: When a fist is made over a clenched thumb, the thumb should not extend beyond the ulnar side of the hand. [False-positives occur in 1% of white and 3% of black children (Fig. 7).]

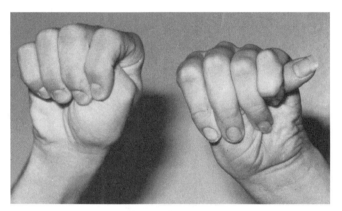

FIG. 7. The normal subject (*left*) is unable to extend his thumb beyond his clenched fingers, as can the patient with Marfan syndrome (*right*), who can do so because of a long thumb and lax joints.

        c. Wrist sign: When the wrist is encircled by the thumb and little finger (with light pressure), the little finger will overlap at least 1 cm in 80% of patients with the Marfan syndrome (21).

        d. The span of the outstretched arm exceeds the height by at least 5 cm (Fig. 8).

        Note: A *forme fruste* (incomplete form) of the Marfan syndrome with kyphoscoliosis, pectus carinatum (pigeon breast), and long extremities may occur in homocystinuria, in which there may be thrombosis of intermediate-sized arteries that causes myocardial infarction.

4. What is the only hand deformity ever correlated with rheumatic heart disease?

    ANS.: Ulnar deviation of the fourth or fifth fingers and flexion at the metacarpophalangeal joints. (This is Jaccoud's arthritis, which is very rare.) The fingers can be moved freely into correct alignment (22).

5. What cardiac lesions are expected in an infant if the fingers are clenched, with the index finger crossing over the third finger?

    ANS.: This is characteristic of trisomy 16-18, in which a VSD or PDA is common. Also associated is double-outlet right ventricle (RV).

    Note: The facies are abnormal (small mouth and jaw).

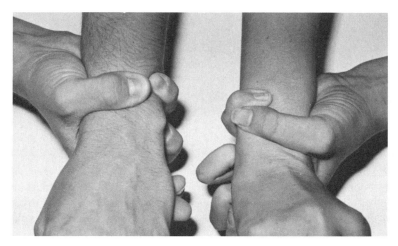

FIG. 8. The normal person (*left*) cannot wrap his thumb and little finger around his wrist because, unlike the patient with Marfan syndrome (*right*), his fingers are not long relative to his wrist.

6. What is the most common cardiac lesion associated with rheumatoid arthritic changes in the extremities?
   ANS.: Pericarditis and even occasional constriction.
7. What skeletal deformities suggest that an ejection murmur is caused by an ASD other than the Holt-Oram syndrome?
   ANS.: a. Any skeletal deformity in the Marfan syndrome suggests not only pulmonary artery or aortic dilatation but also an ASD.
   b. A prominent left precordium suggests not only that the RV was dilated during childhood but also that it was working against a high pressure. This deformity suggests that the ejection murmur is caused by an ASD with hyperkinetic pulmonary hypertension.
   Note: The RV never enlarges to the right, so that the right border of a heart on roentgenogram is either the right atrium or a very large left atrium.
8. Which cardiac lesions are expected with the Ellis-van Creveld syndrome (chondroectodermal dysplasia, an extra finger and often an extra toe, hypoplastic fingernails, and dwarfism)?
   ANS.: About two-thirds of patients have an ASD, usually ostium primum, or VSD, and often a complete endocardial cushion defect or a single atrium. The upper lip of these patients is "tied" down to the alveolar ridge by multiple frenula. It is common among inbreeding populations such as the Amish.
9. Which congenital syndromes involving heart and vascular abnormalities are also characterized by bradydactyly (short fingers) and polydactyly?
   ANS.: Turner syndrome, Down syndrome, Ellis-van Creveld syndrome, and mucopolysaccharidosis are characterized by bradydactyly. Trisomy 13-15 and trisomy 18 are characterized by polydactyly.

CHEST AND RESPIRATION

1. Which cardiac abnormalities are suggested by a pectus excavatum (posterior displacement of the lower sternum)?

ANS.: Aortic or pulmonary artery aneurysms, myxomatous degeneration of the mitral and aortic valves with regurgitation, or ASD.

Note: Three degrees of severity of pectus excavatum have been described as the "saucer," "cup," and "funnel." If the anteroposterior measurement of the adult chest measured with obstetric calipers is about 16 cm, the heart is very likely compressed. If the anteroposterior measurement is less than 11 cm, the entire heart is usually displaced to the left but is not compressed. The apex beat is almost always displaced to the left, even in saucer depressions.

2. What is the significance of a short breath-holding time?

ANS.: It signifies either of the following:

a. Chronic hyperventilation, or

b. Poor psychophysical control of the breathing apparatus. Normal subjects (with legs dangling) can hold their breath for 30 seconds with a little encouragement. Inability to hold it for at least 20 seconds is abnormal and can explain dyspnea on exertion.

Note: Chronic hyperventilation may be caused by either a severe pulmonary problem, which should be obvious, or emotional factors, in which case it could account for nondescript episodes of chest pain, faintness, and syncope.

3. What is a shield chest, and what does it suggest?

ANS.: It is a broad chest with a greater angle than usual between the manubrium and the body of the sternum, as well as widely separated nipples. In a female patient with neck webbing, wide carrying angle, and short stature (under 150 cm) it suggests Turner syndrome and concomitant coarctation. In a male patient, it is called Noonan or Ullrich syndrome and is commonly associated with PS.

4. What should Cheyne-Stokes respiration suggest in a cardiac patient?

ANS.: A very low output at rest. The anoxic respiratory center becomes insensitive to normal tensions of carbon dioxide, and apnea again occurs.

5. What is Ewart's sign of a large pericardial effusion?

ANS.: It is the compression of the lung by an effusion, which causes

a. A patch of marked dullness between the angles of the left scapula and the spine.

b. Tubular (bronchial) breathing and aegophany (also egophany) in the same area as above.

6. How can crackles (formerly called rales) be used to diagnose various pathologic conditions of the lung and heart by means of their situation in the inspiratory phase?

ANS.: Paninspiratory crackles suggest pneumonia or CHF, although when failure is resolving, they become late. Early inspiratory crackles suggest severe chronic obstructive pulmonary disease (COPD), asthma, and chronic bronchitis. Late inspiratory crackles suggest interstitial edema or pulmonary fibrosis. Early-to-mid crackles suggest bronchiectasis.

Note: Much confusion is caused by the misinterpretation of crackles at the lung bases. In practice, most crackles are caused by sputum in the air passages, and the inference that they are caused by heart failure is more often wrong than right, especially if they disappear with several coughs. In the early stages of heart failure, crackles may even be absent.

REFERENCES

1. Aderka D, Pinkhas J. Sweating with pulmonary edema. *Ann Intern Med* 1984;101:402.
2. Antia AU. Familial skeletal cardiovascular syndrome (Holt-Oram) in a polygamous African family. *Br Heart J* 1970;32:241.
3. Beuren AJ, et al. The syndrome of supravalvular aortic stenosis and peripheral pulmonary stenosis. *Am J Cardiol* 1964;13:471.

4. Elliott WJ, Karrison T. Increased all-cause and cardiac morbidity and mortality associated with the diagonal ear-lobe crease: a prospective cohort study. *Am J Med* 1991;91:247.
5. Gomez JA, et al. Apolipoprotein E phenotypes, lipoprotein composition, and xanthelasmas. *Arch Dermatol* 1988;124:1230.
6. Gorlin RJ, Anderson RC, Blaw M. Multiple lentigines syndrome. *Am J Dis Child* 1969;117:652.
7. Holt M, Oram S. Familial heart disease with skeletal malformations. *Br Heart J* 1960;22:236.
8. Kaptein EM. Unilateral corneal arcus without carotid artery stenosis. *JAMA* 1977;283:303.
9. Kazmier FJ, et al. Livedo reticularis and digital infarcts. *Cardiol Comp* 1966;1:56.
10. Lampe RM, Kagan A. Detection of clubbing: Schamroth's sign. *Clin Pediatr* 1983;22:125.
11. Lichstein E, et al. Diagonal earlobe crease and coronary artery sclerosis. *Ann Intern Med* 1976;85:337.
12. Lin YT, Yeh L, Oka Y. Pathophysiology of general cyanosis. *N Y State J Med* 1977;9:1393.
13. Myers AR, Willis PW. Clinical spectrum of supravalvular aortic stenosis. *Arch Intern Med* 1966;118:553.
14. Sapira JD. The two hypertensive retinopathies. *Dis Mon* 1984;30:39.
15. Schamroth L. Clubbing of the fingers: a method of assessment. *S Afr Med J* 1976;50:297.
16. Scheie HG. Evaluation of ophthalmoscopic changes of hypertension and arteriolar sclerosis. *Arch Ophthalmol* 1953;49:117.
17. Schrire V, Beck W, Chesler E. The heart and the eye. *Am Heart J* 1973;85:122.
18. Sommerville J, Bonham-Carter RE. The heart in lentiginosis. *Br Heart J* 1972;34:58.
19. Terry R. Red half-moons in cardiac failure. *Lancet* 1954;2:842.
20. van Buchem FSP, et al. Hypertension and changes of the fundus oculi. *Acta Med Scand* 1964;176:539.
21. Walker BA, Murdoch JL. The wrist sign. *Arch Intern Med* 1970;126:276.
22. Zvaifler NJ. Chronic postrheumatic fever (Jaccoud's) arthritis. *N Engl J Med* 1962;267:10.

3

Arterial Pulses and Pressures

METHOD OF ARM PALPATION

1. Why, besides speeding up the palpation of the pulses, is palpating both brachial and radial arteries simultaneously an efficient method of palpating the arm pulses?

    ANS.: It allows you to estimate the systolic blood pressure without a stethoscope or cuff (described later in this chapter) (Fig. 1).

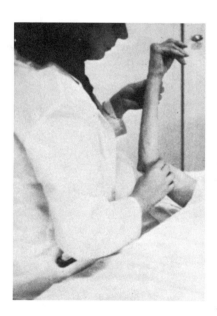

FIG. 1. Simultaneous palpation of the radials and brachials speeds up the process and reminds you to palpate the brachials, where you can easily appreciate rates of rise, the bisferiens pulse, pulse volume, and the hardened vessels of medial sclerosis.

    Note: a. If a radial pulse is missing, it is probably due to arterial occlusive disease, as in the thoracic outlet syndrome, or due to a brachial cutdown used for cardiac catheterization.

        b. In the young patient, the brachial artery may be hidden under the biceps. In the older patient, brachial tortuosity displaces the artery medially away from the biceps.

2. What questions must you answer as you palpate a peripheral pulse?

    ANS.: a. Is the rate of rise slow, normal, or fast?

b. Is there a shoulder on the upstroke or a midsystolic dip, shudder, or thrill?
c. Is the pulse volume or pressure small, normal, or large?
d. Is the vessel hard; i.e., does it roll too easily under the finger?
e. What is the blood pressure? (For the method of estimating blood pressure by palpation, see p. 43.)

RATES OF RISE AND PULSE VOLUME

Normal Rates of Rise

1. How can you recognize a normal rate of rise and volume of a carotid or brachial pulse?
   ANS.: It feels like a gentle tap against the fingertips.
   > *Note*: a. In subjects over age 45, the tap is often followed by a slower rise, producing a shoulder. This is called an anacrotic shoulder (*ana* means "up," *crotic* means "beat"). The initial tap is caused by a rapid rise to a peak known as the percussion wave. The slower rise following it is called a *tidal wave*. The tidal wave is a result of waves reflected from areas where arteries divide. A fusion of reflected and percussion waves form the tidal wave. The shoulder following the percussion wave produces a total sensation of a "tap and push."
   > b. Because pulse rises become more rapid as you palpate more peripherally, a shoulder may disappear by the time the pulse reaches the brachials or may even disappear high in the neck in comparison with low in the neck (57) (Fig. 2).

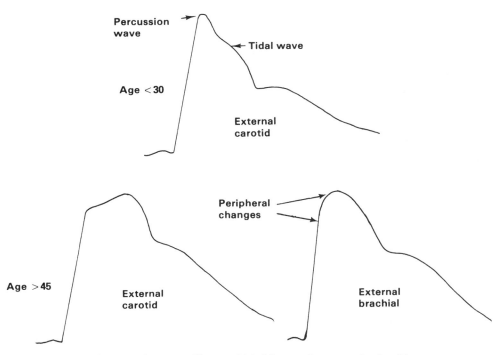

FIG. 2. The normal percussion wave (first peak) is felt as a sharp tap. In the older age groups an anacrotic shoulder occurs, resulting in a late tidal wave, which is felt as a further outward motion after the initial tap. More peripherally, the shoulder to a high tidal wave disappears.

c. The percussion wave is associated with flow rates and occurs during the peak velocity of flow; the tidal wave is controlled more by pressure and occurs at peak aortic pressures (62). With aging, the velocity of ejection may decrease, thus lowering the percussion wave. If the peripheral resistance rises, the tidal wave becomes higher relative to the percussion wave, as after the administration of a vasopressor agent or with the decreased aortic distensibility of advancing age (42) (Fig. 3).

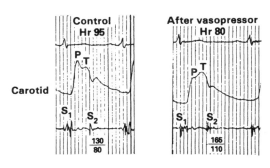

FIG. 3. After an artificial rise in blood pressure, the tidal wave (T) becomes higher than the percussion wave (P), just as in older age groups and in hypertension.

2. What have you ruled out by feeling a normal rate of rise and normal pulse pressure in a carotid pulse?
   ANS.: There is not likely to be an important fixed-orifice obstruction; that is, there is no significant valvular, supravalvular, or discrete subvalvular aortic stenosis (see p. 34; see also note on p. 33 for an exception to this interpretation of a normal rate of rise). There is also no moderate to severe aortic regurgitation (AR) because such significant AR would have an increased pulse pressure. The exception to this can be found in the patient with severe depression of myocardial function (see p. 38).

Slow Rates of Rise

1. What is the sensation to the fingers when there is a slow rate of rise? Why?
   ANS.: The first indication that the rise is slow is the absence of a tap. Then you may notice that the sensation is one of a caressing lift, a gentle push, or a nudge. If you feel a tap followed by a push, then you may be feeling an anacrotic shoulder followed by a late, slow-rising tidal wave (Fig. 4).

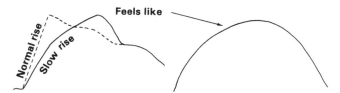

FIG. 4. The normal rise is a tap; the slow rise is a caress.

Note: If you elicit a tap, then check to see if the pulse continues to rise after it. A moderately slow delayed rise after the initial tap can be missed and called normal. This is probably the most common cause of calling a slow rise normal (66).

2. What is the significance of a slow rate of rise in the carotid pulse?
ANS.: It tells you that there is probably aortic stenosis (AS) due to a fixed obstruction to aortic flow.
Note: The slowly rising pulse of AS has been called an anacrotic pulse, plateau pulse, and pulsus parvus. Since the literal meaning of **anacrotic pulse** is so different from the usage meaning, the term is best avoided. **Anacrotic shoulder** and **anacrotic notch** are useful terms to retain because they refer to a shoulder or notch on the upstroke (Fig. 5).

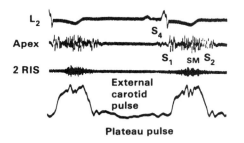

FIG. 5. If an almost normal tap is followed by a sustained thrill, this is the plateau pulse of AS. (L2 = lead 2; 2 RIS = microphone in second right interspace.)

Severity of Aortic Stenosis by Rate of Rise

1. How does the increased rate of rise as you palpate a peripheral artery, such as the brachial, affect an anacrotic shoulder or slow rise of mild AS?
ANS.: The shoulder or slow rise in the carotid may become a normal rate of rise in the brachials. However, if myocardial function is decreased, the slow rise of even mild AS may be transmitted to the brachials (Fig. 6).

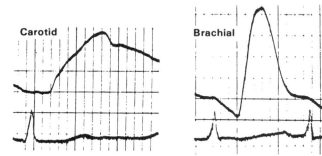

FIG. 6. Carotid and brachial pulse contours in a patient with mild AS. By the time the pulse wave reached the brachials, it had become normal.

2. What does a slow rise of the carotid pulse (absent percussion wave) tell you about the degree of aortic gradient?
ANS.: In the presence of a fairly normal myocardium, the gradient is probably over 50 mm Hg.
Note: With the rigid aorta of severe **arteriosclerosis** in the elderly there may be a normal rate of rise in the carotids despite significant AS. This phenomenon is presumably due to the inability of a stiff aorta to expand slowly.

3. Why does supravalvular AS have both rate of rise and blood pressure (blood pressure) greater (by about 20 mm Hg) on the right carotid and subclavian than on the left?

   ANS.: Because there is streaming of the jet straight up along the ascending aorta toward the innominate, right carotid, and right subclavian arteries (Fig. 7).

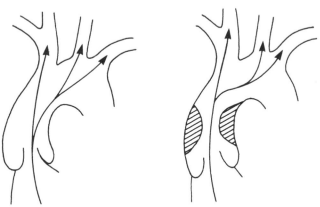

FIG. 7. Supravalvular obstruction causes the blood in the aorta to take a relatively sharp turn before it can exit through the left carotid and subclavian arteries.

4. How can simultaneous palpation of the apex beat and carotid pulse diagnose the presence of severe aortic stenosis?

   ANS.: In one study, a lag between the onset of the apical pulse followed by the carotid impulse predicted a valve area of less than 1 square cm (severe aortic stenosis) with a sensitivity of 95% and specificity of 100%.

Rapid Rates of Rise (Brisk Pulse) with Normal Pulse Pressures

1. When will a large volume ejected from the left ventricle (LV) have a normal pulse pressure?

   ANS.: If there are two outlet orifices for ejection, as in mitral regurgitation (MR) or ventricular septal defect (VSD).

2. Why is the pulse rise brisk in MR and VSD volume overloads?

   ANS.: The period of ejection into the aorta (ejection time) is not longer than normal in MR or VSD; that is, the LV does not take longer than normal to eject its forward stroke volume into the aorta. Because the LV is actually moving a greater volume in a normal or even reduced ejection time, it must be moving both the forward and regurgitant streams at a very rapid rate. The LV accomplishes this rapid ejection by means of the stretched myocardium at the end of diastole (Starling effect) (Fig. 8).

3. Why is there a brisk rate of rise with hypertrophic subaortic stenosis (HSS) (also known as hypertrophic obstructive cardiomyopathy [HOCM])?

   ANS.: In HOCM there is no obstruction until the outflow tract contracts and approximates the thickened septum to a mitral leaflet. Because of a catecholamine effect on the hypertrophied muscle, the LV ejects as much as 80% of its blood before the obstruction occurs. The rate of rise in HOCM is among the fastest in cardiology (Fig. 9).

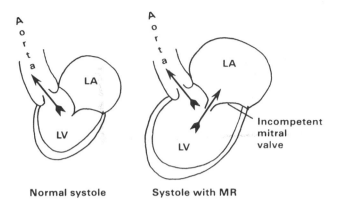

Normal systole   Systole with MR

FIG. 8. Note that the *arrows* representing ejection into the aorta are equal; that is, the forward stroke volume in MR is not reduced unless the MR is very severe or there is cardiac damage.

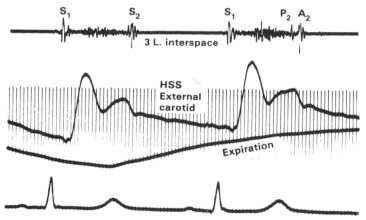

FIG. 9. This is a phonocardiogram and pulse tracing from a 34-year-old woman with HSS. The outflow gradient was 70 mm Hg. Some mitral regurgitation was present. There was an S3 on auscultation and a large LV on x-ray. Note the rapid rate of rise to a high-percussion wave and the midsystolic dip that produce the "pointed-finger" carotid pulse contour.

4. What is the Brockenbrough effect?

ANS.: In normal subjects the postextrasystolic pulse pressure after a long pause is larger than normal. In HOCM it appears to stay the same due to the increase in obstruction from the Starling effect, the postextrasystolic potentiation effect (see p. 211), and the decrease in afterload, all of which cause an increase in contractility (Fig. 10).

Note: a. In constrictive pericarditis there is also no change in systolic pressure after a long diastole due to a premature ventricular contraction (PVC). This is because ventricular filling with constrictive pericarditis occurs rapidly in early diastole, is abruptly halted by the rigid, unyielding pericardium, and cannot increase during the pause of a long diastole (30).

b. A midsystolic dip in the aortic pressure pulse of some patients with HOCM tends to create a double beating or bisferiens effect. This dip

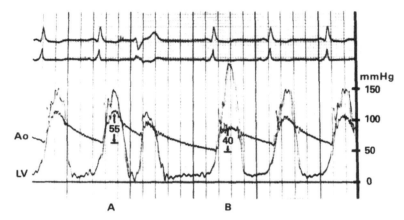

FIG. 10. The Brockenbrough effect is seen in the postextrasystolic beat B, because the pulse pressure decreased to 40 mm Hg from 55 mm Hg during normal sinus rhythm A.

may be due to a Bernoulli effect caused by the high velocity flow through the narrowed outflow tract.

Rapid Rates of Rise with Increased Pulse Pressure

1. What conditions should be considered if there is a rapid rate of rise and a large pulse volume (the bounding pulse)?

   ANS.: The most rapidly rising bounding pulses are found in AR, persistent ductus arteriosus (PDA), coarctation, thyrotoxicosis, pregnancy, and severe anemia. AR is by far the most common cause of a bounding pulse.

   More rarely, a large arteriovenous fistula or a single great vessel arising from the heart (e.g., a persistent truncus or the large aorta in pulmonary atresia) may also cause a large pulse volume and rapid rise (Fig. 11).

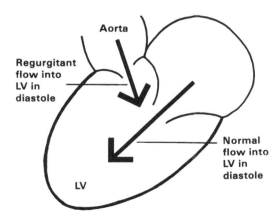

FIG. 11. This illustration represents ventricular diastole in a patient with aortic regurgitation. The reason for the large volume in diastole in AR is obvious, since the LV fills from two sources. As long as the LV is healthy, it ejects the usual 60% to 75% of its increased end-diastolic volume; that is, its ejection fraction remains normal. Thus, the aorta receives a large stroke volume with each systole.

Note: The pulse of AR is bounding because of the ejection of a large volume (from two sources) and because the diastolic pressure is low. Also, stretching the LV creates the rapid rise.

2. What causes the low diastolic pressure in AR?

    ANS.: The lower diastolic pressure in AR is only partly due to backflow into the LV dur-
    ing systole. It is mostly due to the reflex decrease in peripheral resistance caused
    by the large stroke volume stretching the carotid and aortic sinuses. Although
    gross AR generally has a diastolic pressure of about 50 mm Hg or less, if the pa-
    tient goes into heart failure, the resultant reflex increase in peripheral resistance
    caused by low output may raise the diastolic pressure to normal values.

3. How can you exaggerate the rapid rate of rise of AR?

    ANS.: By raising the patient's arm high or by having the patient stand up (21). (In sub-
    jects without AR, standing produces a decrease in the rate of rise.)

    Note: In patients with AR, the increased rate of rise of the pulse on standing does
    not mean that more AR occurs on standing. The expected increase in pe-
    ripheral resistance on standing should increase the amount of AR, but this
    effect is attenuated by the decreased venous return, resulting in no signifi-
    cant change in the quantity of AR.

    The increased rate of rise of the brachial pulse on standing is related to
    the fact that the supine AR patient has more peripheral vasodilation caused
    by a decrease in sympathetic tone. Therefore, the lower than normal sym-
    pathetic tone in the supine position changes to an exaggerated increase in
    sympathetic tone on standing because of the need for enough peripheral
    vasoconstriction to maintain pressure. It is presumably the increased level
    of catecholamines or sympathetic outflow that causes a more rapid rate of
    rise of the peripheral pulses.

4. What are some of the names given to the pulse in AR other than "bounding"?

    ANS.: Corrigan pulse, water-hammer[1] pulse, and collapsing pulse.

    Note: The term **Corrigan pulse** refers only to a visibly bounding pulse, not to
    what you feel; the term **water-hammer pulse** requires that you remember
    the name of an obsolete toy, and the term **collapsing pulse** omits the rate
    of rise (13). Therefore, it may be best to call this a **bounding pulse,** or sim-
    ply a rapidly rising or slapping pulse with a large volume.

5. Why is there a large volume in the LV in PDA, creating a rapid rise and large pulse pres-
    sure?

    ANS.: The LV receives both the blood shunted from the aorta to the pulmonary artery and
    the normal volume of pulmonary venous blood.

6. Why may severe AR sometimes not produce a large-volume pulse pressure?

    ANS.: In sudden, severe AR, the stroke volume may be low or normal or only slightly in-
    creased because

    a. The high diastolic pressure in the LV may close the mitral valve in mid-diastole,
    which limits filling from the left atrium, and

    b. The LV resists dilatation when it is suddenly presented with a regurgitant volume,
    probably because the pericardium resists acute stretching.

    Note: The pulse pressure is larger than normal in almost all patients with sudden,
    severe AR, but the systolic pressure is not usually higher than normal. The
    diastolic pressure tends to be reduced to between 40 and 60 mm Hg, and
    this is what increases the pulse pressure. In chronic AR, the systolic pres-
    sure increases because of the large forward stroke volume.

---

[1]A water-hammer was a Victorian toy. It was a tube in which a vacuum was produced and contained water that
dropped like a rock when the tube was inverted.

Note: If myocardial function is severely depressed by long-standing severe AR, the heart may reach an irreversible (inoperable) stage in which none of the peripheral arterial signs of severe AR are present.

7. What traditionally characteristic signs of severe AR can be picked up by auscultation of the femoral arteries?

ANS.: a. Traube's "pistol-shot" femorals. This is the loud sound heard when the stethoscope is placed over the rapidly rising large-volume pulsations of the femoral artery.

Note: Venous pistol-shot sounds have been described as the loud systolic sounds heard over a femoral vein in the presence of severe tricuspid regurgitation (27).

b. Duroziez double murmur. This is

1. The systolic murmur of excessive forward flow produced by placing the stethoscope chestpiece on the femoral artery and gradually compressing the artery proximal to the stethoscope with your finger, plus

2. The diastolic murmur produced by gradually compressing the artery distal to the stethoscope. This murmur is due to backflow as the blood in all the large arteries flows backward toward the aorta in diastole.

Note: a. A double sound over the groin can be heard when a strong atrial contraction occurs. The first sound is from the femoral vein and the second is from the femoral artery (2).

b. These signs are of more historical than practical interest, because usually no more information is gained than that acquired from palpating the pulses and taking the blood pressure.

8. When can the right carotid pulse volume be so unilaterally increased as to suggest a pulsating aneurysm?

ANS.: When the right carotid becomes elongated and loops back sharply on itself (kinked carotid). (Usually occurs in hypertensive women over age 50.)

PULSUS BISFERIENS

1. What is meant by a bisferiens pulse?

ANS.: *Bis* means twice and *feriens* means beating. Therefore, a bisferiens pulse is a twice-beating pulse. Actually it is a double-peaked arterial pulse, so there is a midsystolic dip in systole. See Fig. 12.

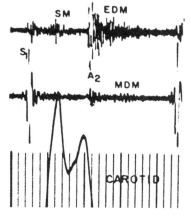

FIG. 12. Bisferiens pulse in a patient with severe AR. (EDM = early diastolic murmur of AR at left sternal border; MDM = mid-diastolic murmur at apex [Austin Flint murmur].)

2. What is the physiologic significance of a bisferiens pulse?

ANS.: It is always associated with the ejection of a rapid jet of blood through the aortic valve. At the peak of flow, a Bernoulli effect (suction effect of rapid flow over a surface) on the walls of the ascending aorta causes a sudden decrease in lateral pressure on the inner aspect of the wall (Fig. 13).

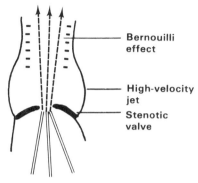

Bernouilli
effect

High-velocity
jet

Stenotic
valve

AS + AR

FIG. 13. The fall in lateral-wall pressure during peak velocity requires a high velocity of ejection. This implies the presence of a relatively healthy myocardium.

3. What causes the most marked bisferiens pulse?

ANS.: A combination of moderate AS and severe AR (75).

Note: a. **Carotid shudder** is a term that was used to describe the very short vibration effect that occurs when a patient with combined AS and AR had a double systolic outward movement (15). It is now known as a bisferiens pulse. A bisferiens pulse is not present if myocardial contractility is depressed (28). About one-third of patients with severe AR have a carotid thrill instead of a bisferiens pulse (1).

b. The finding of a unilateral bisferiens pulse is highly suggestive of a dissection. This has been palpated in the left femoral artery where the right femoral artery did not show this.

c. In some patients, the two peaks not only are palpable but may be audible as double Korotkoff sounds heard as the blood pressure cuff is deflated.

4. When can AS cause a bisferiens pulse in the absence of AR?

ANS.: Severe HOCM can have a bisferiens pulse because in this condition there is initially no obstruction to outflow. When obstruction occurs in midsystole, as the mitral valve approximates the hypertrophied septum, there is a sudden dip in the pulse as the flow virtually ceases (confirmed by Doppler studies). This is often followed by a secondary rise as the LV overcomes the obstruction (see Fig. 9).

Note: Pure AR can also cause a bisferiens pulse, especially if the AR is severe (Fig. 12).

THE PALPABLE DICROTIC WAVE

1. What is the dicrotic wave?

ANS.: This is the small wave that follows the dicrotic notch in an external carotid pressure tracing.

> *Note:* The dicrotic notch is the post-tidal wave dip that occurs on a carotid pulse tracing at the time of aortic valve closure. The same notch in an aortic pressure tracing is called the **incisura**.

2. When does a dicrotic wave become palpable?

ANS.: When there is a very low output; a soft, elastic aorta; and a high peripheral resistance. The most common causes of a palpable dicrotic wave are

   a. Severe congestive failure, usually secondary to a dilated cardiomyopathy.

   b. Tamponade (46).

   c. The low output state following open heart surgery, especially after aortic valve replacement for AR (4,50).

   > *Note*: a. A low stroke volume is important for the production of a palpable dicrotic wave; therefore, it is more likely to appear or to become accentuated after a sudden short diastole, after the weaker beats of a pulsus alternans, in the straining phase of a Valsalva maneuver or the inspiratory phase of respiration, or when there is a heart rate of over 90 beats per minute.
   >
   > b. Soft, elastic blood vessels seem to be necessary to make a dicrotic wave palpable as shown by the rarity of the palpable dicrotic wave when blood pressure is over 140 mm Hg and in subjects over age 40.
   >
   > c. A dicrotic pulse after open heart surgery for AR correlates with continued LV dilatation and decreased left ventricular function.
   >
   > d. An excessive dicrotic wave in a carotid tracing is present if about 50% or more of the pulse pressure occurs from the dicrotic notch to the peak of the dicrotic wave (16) (Fig. 14).

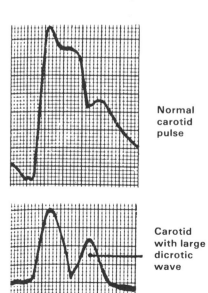

Normal carotid pulse

Carotid with large dicrotic wave

Short ejection time

FIG. 14. At first glance, a large dicrotic wave gives the appearance of a bisferiens pulse because of the short ejection time seen in all patients with severe heart failure; the large dicrotic wave is usually seen only in such patients.

PALPATION OF PERIPHERAL LEG PULSES

1. What can you learn about the heart from palpating the popliteal arteries?

   ANS.: Vascular disease of the lower extremities is highly correlated with the presence of coronary disease.

   > *Note*: Obstructive disease of the carotids with an arterial murmur in the neck is also highly correlated with coronary atherosclerosis.

2. What is the most important aid in palpating the popliteal pulses?

   ANS.: You must not try to feel a popliteal blood vessel; instead, try to feel a small area of diffuse transmitted pulsation. It does not feel like a carotid or brachial artery.

3. How do you examine for faint popliteal and pedal pulses?

   ANS.: With the patient supine, place the fingers of both hands in the popliteal space with the palms of your hands in complete contact with the patient's skin, including the anterolateral aspect of the knee (Fig. 15). (Air over one part of the palm with skin over another part of the palm may prevent the detection of a faint pulsatile kinesthetic sensation in one area.)

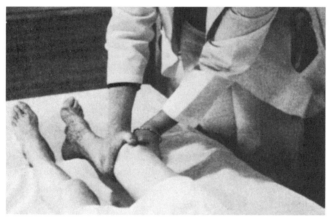

FIG. 15. It will not be necessary to place the patient in the prone position if you remember that the key to popliteal palpation is to feel for an area of transmitted pulsation.

   a. Relax the muscles around the popliteal area by bouncing the knee up and down a few times.

   b. Squeeze with the entire hand (i.e., with the thumbs as well as the fingers), so that the sensation is equal all through the hand. Usually firm pressure is necessary to feel the movements due to popliteal pulsations.

   c. Slight dorsiflexion of the foot to stretch the popliteal artery may help.

   d. To bring out a faint posterior tibial pulse, dorsiflex the foot to various degrees with one hand as you palpate with the other. A tendon passes diagonally over the dorsalis pedis, and the extensor retinaculum of the ankle crosses perpendicularly over it. Plantar flexion may tighten these overlying structures and obliterate the pulse. Dorsiflexion separates them from the artery beneath.

   > *Note*: There are many normal variations of foot pulses. The dorsalis pedis may not be palpable in the usual line between the great toe and the index toe, or it may be absent in as many as 10% of normal subjects (29). Normal

adult subjects may have a palpable posterior tibial or dorsalis pedis only on one side. For this reason it is important to document the foot pulses as a baseline for future follow-up in case peripheral vascular problems develop.

ABDOMINAL AORTIC ANEURYSMS (AAA)

1. Which patients should be routinely screened for AAA?
   ANS.: Patients with increased risk, especially over age 50 with hypertension or coronary disease history.
2. When should abdominal pulsations suggest an aortic aneurysm?
   ANS.: Pulsations of the normal aorta do not usually extend below the umbilicus even in these individuals.
3. How can palpation be used to screen for AAA?
   ANS.: Attempt to "roll" the aorta under the fingertips to find the lateral margins and estimate the diameter. Next, note the separation of the index fingers with each systole with an index finger placed on each side of the aorta. If the pulsating area is more than 2.5 cm in width after allowing for skin thickness, a pulsatile mass should be considered to be present. (Abdominal or femoral bruits are of no help.) In a thin abdomen, almost all AAA can be detected. By ultrasound an AAA is a dilatation of more than 1.5 times the diameter of the proximal aorta.

BLOOD PRESSURE

1. How do the heart and blood vessels control arterial systolic and diastolic pressure levels?
   ANS.: Systolic blood pressure is controlled by the stroke volume of the heart and the stiffness of the arterial vessels that receive the stroke volume. Diastolic blood pressure is controlled primarily by peripheral resistance, but also by the duration of diastolic run-off into the periphery and by the elasticity of the aorta.
   > *Note*: a. A compliant aorta with good elastic diastolic recoil is necessary to maintain a high diastolic pressure. This implies that the patient with a high peripheral resistance *can have a normal diastolic pressure* if the aorta is stiff with atherosclerosis and loss of elastic tissue!
   >   b. In most patients with systolic hypertension the stiff brachial vessels can cause a falsely high diastolic pressure by as much as 15 mm Hg by cuff when compared with direct intraarterial pressure; that is, the diastolic pressure is most often normal when measured directly intraarterially (72).
2. What are normal systolic and diastolic blood pressures in adults, infants, and children?
   ANS.: In the adult, the upper limit of normal blood pressure is about 140/90 mm Hg. In infants and children, you may use the rule that by age 1 the systolic pressure is about 90 mm Hg and increases by 5 mm Hg about every 3 years, so that by age 13 or 14 it has reached the adult level of 120 mm Hg.
   A rough rule of thumb, then, would be that the systolic blood pressure in a child would be roughly

$$90 + (\text{age} \times 5)/3$$

The diastolic pressure tends to be about 60 ± 10 mm Hg in infants and children of all ages.

3. Why does severe AS usually not cause a lower blood pressure than normal despite a low output?

ANS.: As the stroke volume falls, peripheral resistance rises and keeps the blood pressure normal. In very severe AS, however, a decrease in systolic blood pressure may occur as the patient progresses toward cardiac failure.

> *Note*: The highest blood pressure I could find reported in severe valvular AS was 280/140 mm Hg (75).

4. How does AR affect blood pressure?

ANS.: The increased stroke volume causes a higher systolic pressure than normal, whereas the decreased peripheral resistance causes a lower diastolic pressure than normal. However, in young subjects with soft blood vessels, even severe AR may not raise the systolic blood pressure to more than about 140 mm Hg. In older patients with stiff vessels, even moderate AR may raise the systolic pressure as high as 180 mm Hg. In hypertensive patients, the increased peripheral resistance can produce a normal or even high diastolic pressure despite severe AR.

Blood Pressure Differences in the Arms

1. What should you suspect if the blood pressure is higher in one arm than in the other?

ANS.: a. Arterial obstructive disease may be present, either atherosclerotic or embolic, or it may be due to a thoracic outlet syndrome such as a cervical rib.

b. It may be an artifact due to the lack of simultaneous recording.

c. If it is higher on the right, it may be due to supravalvular AS, which directs its jet preferentially up the innominate artery. A difference in carotid pulsation volume, as well as the presence of a murmur of AS, gives additional information. (See p. 19 for the facies of supravalvular AS.)

2. In what percentage of patients is there a difference of 10 mm Hg or more in *systolic* blood pressure between the arms, if the pressure in both arms is taken separately or simultaneously?

ANS.: If the blood pressure is taken separately, 25% of patients will have a difference in blood pressure pressure of at least 10 mm Hg (and a difference in diastolic blood pressure of 5 mm Hg). If it is taken simultaneously, only 5% will have such a difference (24,70). The greatest differences are in hypertensive patients.

> *Note*: If the history suggests vertebral-basilar insufficiency and the blood pressure is lower in one arm than the other, a subclavian steal[2] should be suspected.

blood pressure With and Without a Cuff

1. How can you take a systolic blood pressure by palpation alone, that is, without a blood pressure cuff or stethoscope?

ANS.: While simultaneously palpating the brachial and radial arteries, apply slight, moderate, and marked pressure on the brachial artery in an attempt to obliterate the radial pulse. If only slight pressure on the brachial artery is required to obliterate the radial pulse, the systolic pressure is probably 120 mm Hg or less. If moderate pressure is needed, the systolic pressure is probably between 120 and 160 mm Hg. If marked pressure is required, the blood pressure is probably more than 160 mm Hg.

> *Note*: The radial artery should be palpated with enough pressure to give a maximum pulse pressure. If you push the brachial artery to one side, no amount of

---

[2]**Subclavian steal** refers to the use of a vertebral artery as collateral circulation to feed a subclavian artery beyond an obstruction (usually on the left). Blood from a vertebral artery flows retrogradely into the distal subclavian, thus "stealing" blood from the brain. (See checklist on p. 11 for symptoms.)

pressure on the brachial artery obliterates the radial pulse. Comparing the pulse in both arms helps to prevent a false reading.

If the pulse pressure in the radials is too small, you will obliterate the radial pulse sensation too easily and may get a false impression of a normal or low blood pressure.

2. How can you take a blood pressure reading by cuff (sphygmomanometer) and palpation alone (i.e., without auscultation)?

ANS.: With the thumb on the brachial artery, just under the distal edge of the cuff, you can palpate the systolic pressure as the cuff is deflated and the pulse returns. As the cuff is further deflated toward diastole, the brachial pulse becomes increasingly more slapping and hyperdynamic, until it suddenly changes to a more normal rate of rise. This point of change correlates well with the diastolic pressure at about the time of muffling (54).

Note: a. The diastolic point is difficult to appreciate at the radial pulse.

b. It is useful to obtain the diastolic pressure by palpation alone in subjects in shock and in those without a sharp disappearance or muffling point, as occurs in AR, when the Korotkoff sounds may be heard down to zero.

Korotkoff Sounds

1. What generates the Korotkoff sounds?

ANS.: They are produced by the pulsations of the artery under a partially constricting blood pressure cuff (described by the Russian physician N. S. Korotkoff in 1905). Arterial wall oscillations have been shown to be associated with major components of the sounds (68).

Note: a. Five phases of Korotkoff sounds are conventionally recognized:

Phase 1. Onset of tapping sounds.

Phase 2. At a pressure of about 10 to 15 mm lower, a murmur may be heard after the tap.

Phase 3. Reappearance of only the tapping sound.

Phase 4. The higher frequencies are then attenuated and the tap is eliminated, leaving only the murmur (44). This is the muffling phase.

Phase 5. Disappearance of all sounds.

b. If the heart sounds are very loud, they may be transmitted by bone conduction to the brachial area (e.g., after vigorous exercise). Korotkoff sounds are *not* transmitted heart sounds.

2. What can make the Korotkoff sounds difficult to hear?

ANS.: A slow rate of rise in the pulse wave, as in AS, poor blood flow to the limbs, or a small pulse pressure.

3. How can inaudible blood pressure sounds in a limb be made audible, or soft ones made louder?

ANS.: a. Have the subject open and close his or her fist about 10 times, either before or during cuff inflation. If the popliteal or foot blood pressure is being taken, have the subject flex and extend the ankle. This increases flow and dilates the forearm or leg blood vessels. Thus, it may increase the gradient of volume and pressure between the proximal and distal cuff blood vessels. This degree of mild exercising of the hand or foot does not alter the blood pressure reading.

b. Inflate the cuff quickly. This minimizes the quantity of venous blood trapped in the forearm during the low occlusion pressures, which act as a venous tourniquet during inflation before arterial occlusion pressure is reached. Obstructing venous flow increases the tissue pressure distal to the cuff, thus decreasing the flow gradient for the arterial blood passing under the cuff.

c. If the sounds are still soft, then elevate the arm before you inflate the cuff. This empties the arteries beyond the cuff, thus increasing the flow gradient.

Note: A patient recording his or her own blood pressure often gets a slightly higher blood pressure reading than another person taking it a few minutes before or later (9). This can occur if the patient squeezes the sphygmomanometer bulb with the hand of the arm that is cuffed. This makes the Korotkoff sounds louder, resulting in a truer systolic pressure than if another person took the blood pressure.

Chestpiece Placement and Choice

1. Where are Korotkoff sounds loudest? In the center of the cuff? At the edge of the cuff? A few centimeters distal to the cuff edge?

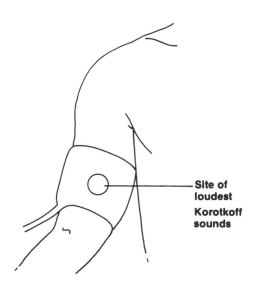

Site of loudest Korotkoff sounds

FIG. 16. Since a stethoscope chest piece cannot be placed completely under a cuff, the best compromise is to slip as much as possible of the diaphragm chest piece under the distal edge of the cuff.

ANS.: In the center of the cuff (Fig. 16).

2. Are Korotkoff sounds dominantly low or high frequency?
ANS.: Low.

3. If Korotkoff sounds are dominantly low frequency, why is it better to use the diaphragm chestpiece, which is designed for high frequencies?
ANS.: a. A bell chestpiece cannot get as close to the center of the cuff as can a diaphragm because a piece of the diaphragm can be inserted under the cuff.

b. A good air seal is difficult to obtain with a large-diameter bell on the round arm surface. If you use firm pressure to get a good air seal with the bell, you can get a falsely low diastolic pressure, because you create turbulence with excessive pressure (39). The lightest pressure possible should be used for an accurate diastolic pressure.

Note: a. Even if no Korotkoff sounds at all are heard at the edge of the cuff (as in patients in shock), they can be heard if a diaphragm is placed deeply under the cuff (77).

b. In shock the high frequencies tend to disappear, so that the bell may be better than the diaphragm for the soft Korotkoff sounds (43).

Diastolic Pressure Recording

1. What is the true diastolic pressure, the point of muffling, or the disappearance of the Korotkoff sounds?

ANS.: In 1939, the American Heart Association (AHA) and the Cardiology Society of Great Britain recommended phase 4 (muffling). In 1951, an AHA committee recommended phase 5 (disappearance). (This was also Korotkoff's recommendation.) In 1967, an AHA committee recommended that both phases 4 and 5 be recorded whenever possible.

Comparative studies have shown that muffling occurs at a point about 10 mm Hg higher than the diastolic pressure obtained by direct intraarterial needle (19,40). When the rate of rise of the brachials is rapid and large in volume, as in hyperkinetic states such as AR, those Korotkoff sounds that depend mostly on flow are replaced, often imperceptibly, by the sounds of mechanical slapping of the arterial walls against the stethoscope chestpiece. Therefore, Korotkoff sounds may be heard even down to zero, which is obviously not the true diastolic pressure. In AR, muffling is probably closer to the true intraarterial diastolic pressure. In any condition in which the disappearance point is more than 10 mm Hg lower than the muffling phase, muffling should be taken as the more accurate pressure reading. Recording both the muffling and the disappearance points aids in communication, thus blood pressure might read 140/70–40 mm Hg.

2. What are the other advantages of taking the disappearance point rather than the muffling phase as the diastolic pressure?

ANS.: a. It is easier to agree on where the disappearance point is than where muffling is. The muffling phase has often been controversial because some people take a sudden change from loud tapping to quieter tapping, and others take full muffling as the diastolic point (60).

b. Because the disappearance point will give a slightly lower diastolic pressure, you are less likely to overtreat on the basis of a questionable blood pressure elevation.

c. Repeatedly clenching the fists can eliminate the muffling phase altogether, suggesting its unreliability (59).

Note: The idea that muffling denotes diastolic pressure was introduced by Erlanger in 1921, in an experiment in which blood from the heart was pumped into an exposed segment of artery enclosed in an air compression chamber (19). As the pressure in the chamber was reduced, the Korotkoff sounds muffled just as the artery first became full and round throughout the pulse cycle. Low-frequency muffled sounds (phase 4 of Korotkoff sounds) continued for a further short period of decompression.

Sources of Error in Taking Blood Pressure

Equipment

1. Why should a mercury manometer always be used in preference to an aneroid (rotating needle) type?

ANS.: About one-third of hospital aneroid manometers are inaccurate by about 10 mm

Hg when tested against a mercury manometer. The error can be in the low, middle, or upper pressure range (53).

2. What is the effect of an overly narrow or an overly large cuff on the blood pressure reading?

ANS.: A too narrow cuff may require excessive inflation pressure to occlude the brachial artery, and the systolic pressure readings may be as much as 50 mm Hg too high (usually only about 10 mm Hg too high), and the diastolic pressure about 5 mm Hg too high (5). A overly large cuff in adults rarely underestimates the blood pressure by more than 5 mm Hg systolic or diastolic.

3. What is the advantage of decreasing the inflation pressure slowly when one is first beginning to deflate the cuff?

ANS.: Spasm of the artery occurs on initial compression. Also, the patient may be anxious and apprehensive on feeling the discomfort of the pressure, causing the blood pressure to be too high. Slow initial deflation allows spasm and anxiety to disappear by the time the blood flow occurs under the cuff.

Note: 1. Slow initial deflation allows the detection of pulsus alternans (see p. 51).

2. After the first detection of Korotkoff sounds has established the presence or absence of pulsus alternans, further slow deflation will cause forearm congestion and will soften the Korotkoff sounds so that the disappearance point may be falsely high.

4. How can you overcome the small cuff problem if a large cuff is not available for a fat arm?

ANS.: a. Place the cuff on the forearm and either auscultate or use a Doppler probe over the radial artery.

b. Use the formula

$$32 - (1.05 \times \text{arm circumference in cm})$$

for systolic pressure. If the number is positive, add it to the recorded pressure. If the number is negative, subtract it.

Note: The error will be less if the cuff is slightly larger than recommended than if the cuff is slightly smaller. In children, a cuff width that is more than 40% of the arm's circumference may give a systolic/diastolic blood pressure not more than 5 mm over that which would be obtained with a 40% cuff/arm circumference ratio.

5. How can you determine accurately if the cuff is the correct width for the limb?

ANS.: For most adult arms it must be at least 20% wider than the diameter of the arm (multiply the diameter of the limb by 1.2). The cuff width according to the preceding formula should be at least 40% of the arm circumference.

One study showed that as long as the width of the cuff is at least 12 cm and the length of the bladder encompasses at least one-half the circumference of the arm, the reading will be reliable even for a fat arm when compared with intraarterial pressure. This requires that the center of the rubber bladder be placed over the brachial artery. Larger or longer cuffs were found to be no more accurate for the fat arm (10).

Note: a. Several studies have shown that the ideal pneumatic bag bladder pressure is transmitted with the least delay to the underlying artery when the rubber bag completely encircles the arm (31). Some studies have shown that there are no falsely low readings when unusually wide cuffs are used in the adult and that the width may even be more than half the arm

circumference. In the thin arm of a child, however, you should expect at
least a 5% underestimation of the blood pressure if too large a cuff is
used (20).

b. Maximum accuracy in pediatric age groups requires cuffs of several
sizes. From birth to age 1, a cuff that is 2.5 cm in width should be available. For ages 1 to 4, a 5-cm cuff is usually needed. For ages 4 to 8, a
9-cm cuff may be needed to achieve a width that is almost half the circumference of the arm.

Systolic Pressure and the Auscultatory Gap

1. Why is it usually taught that you should first inflate the cuff until you feel the radial pulse
disappear?
ANS.: It is said that this will
   a. Prevent inflating the cuff higher than necessary.
   b. Prevent confusion caused by the auscultatory gap.
2. What is meant by the auscultatory gap?
ANS.: It is the silence caused by the disappearance of Korotkoff sounds after the first appearance of the true systolic pressure and the reappearance of pressure some 10 to
20 mm Hg lower.
3. Why is it unnecessary to feel the radial pulse disappear first before applying the stethoscope?
ANS.: a. An auscultatory gap requires venous distention of the forearm and concomitant
low flow. If you routinely have the patient clench his or her fist 10 times and inflate the cuff rapidly, you prevent the auscultatory gap, and the extra time required to feel the radial pulse for this purpose is eliminated. This is another way
of saying that the Korotkoff sounds may be faint when the tissue pressure is high
distal to the cuff (55,58).
   b. It is just as easy to inflate the cuff until the Korotkoff sounds disappear as it is
   to inflate the cuff until the radial pulse disappears.
   Note: The kind of pulse contour necessary before a reduced blood flow can produce an auscultatory gap is usually one with an anacrotic shoulder, as in
   subjects with AS or in elderly subjects with sclerotic aortas or hypertension.

Avoiding Technical Errors in Finding Systolic Pressure

1. How high should you inflate the cuff?
ANS.: It is not necessary to inflate the cuff more than 20 mm Hg above systolic pressure.
Unnecessarily higher inflation may cause discomfort and arterial spasm that can
elevate the blood pressure falsely. A higher inflation also takes longer to deflate to
systolic pressure. In adults you can immediately raise the cuff pressure to 140 mm
Hg and listen for Korotkoff sounds. If Korotkoff sounds are present, then inflate
another 10 mm Hg and keep doing this until the Korotkoff sounds disappear. In
children it is probably better to inflate immediately only to 120 mm Hg. Thus, you
never inflate to more than 10 or 20 mm Hg higher than necessary.
2. How slowly should you deflate the cuff?
ANS.: Not more than 5 or 10 mm Hg per second, especially when beginning to deflate.
This prevents deflation through the first Korotkoff sounds or through a pulsus alternans (5- to 10-mm Hg difference in blood pressure in alternate beats; see p. 51

under Pulsus Alternans). Slow deflation also prevents development of a negative pressure above the mercury column.

3. Where should the brachial artery be in relation to heart level when taking blood pressure?

   ANS.: The brachial artery should be at near heart level (i.e., at about the fourth interspace). Otherwise gravity adds its pressure to the brachial artery pressure. If the artery is at xiphoid level, both systolic and diastolic pressures are about 5 mm Hg too high; if at sternal angle level, it may be about 5 mm Hg too low (47).

   Note: If the arm is held out unsupported for about a minute, isometric contraction effects may cause the diastolic pressure to increase by about 5 mm Hg (64).

4. What errors occur if the rubber part of the cuff balloons beyond its covering or if the cuff is so loose that central ballooning occurs?

   ANS.: Both conditions require excessive cuff pressure to compress the artery, and the reading is falsely high (49).

5. How does exercise affect intraarterial versus auscultatory blood pressure?

   ANS.: During and after exercise intraarterial blood pressure is usually higher than cuff blood pressure, especially diastolic, which may be as much as 30 mm Hg higher (25).

Doppler Method of Taking Blood Pressure

1. When is it especially useful to take blood pressure by a Doppler probe rather than by stethoscope?

   ANS.: a. In infants.
   b. In legs, especially when there is arterial occlusive disease, coarctation, or a low output state.
   c. In patients in shock states.
   d. During cardiopulmonary resuscitation to test for effectiveness of blood flow.

   Note: The blood pressure obtained by a Doppler probe can be accepted as nearly the same as that obtained by stethoscope, but only a systolic pressure can be obtained (69).

Reproducibility and Accuracy of Blood Pressure Recording

1. Why should we round off blood pressure readings to the nearest 5 or zero digit rather than the nearest 2?

   ANS.: It is more scientific because pressure readings in the same patient fluctuate too much between different physicians and under different circumstances to make the last figure significant to the nearest 2 (31,60). The National Bureau of Standards has set a figure of ± 3 mm Hg as the limit of reproducibility for sphygmomanometers. Also, blood pressures change by at least 2 mm Hg spontaneously from moment to moment and may vary by as much as 30 mm Hg systolic and 20 mm Hg diastolic when continuous recordings are made during 24 hours. The 24-hour variability is greatest among hypertensives (34).

   Note: Most examiners record blood pressures to the nearest 2 because (a) manometers are graduated in increments of 2; (b) it gives them a sense of increased accuracy; and (c) a definition of hypertension for treatment or insurance purposes is often based on 140/90 mm Hg as being the limit of upper normal, so that 140/92 mm Hg would require treatment or a change in insurance rating. Most physicians would not record a blood pressure as 141/89 mm Hg, because they know that blood pressure is not accurate or reproducible to the nearest 1; yet they do not hesitate to record 142/88 mm Hg as if blood pressure were accurate and reproducible to the nearest 2.

2. What are some factors that can change blood pressure beyond 2 mm Hg if the blood pressure is taken by the same physician at two different times?

ANS.: a. If the blood pressure is read during inspiration on one day and expiration on another, the readings on expiration will be slightly higher.

b. If blood pressures are read with the antecubital fossa at the level of the fourth parasternal interspace on one day and the xiphoid on another, the blood pressure will be about 5 mm Hg higher in the xiphoid area level.

c. If the room is cold on one occasion and warm on another, or if the noise level is higher one time than another, the blood pressure will be slightly higher under the cooler or noisier conditions.

d. If the patient is under stress on one day and not on another, the readings may differ.

e. It is impossible to obtain the same blood pressure on two occasions if the patient is in atrial fibrillation (8).

f. If a second blood pressure is taken after examining the heart and lungs, the reading before the heart and lung examination may be higher by as much as 30 mm Hg if the patient was anxious.

g. Because of the patient's circadian rhythm, the patient's blood pressure will be different at different times of the day. Although most patients have a lower blood pressure in the morning than in the late afternoon by as much as 20 mm Hg, individual differences exist.

3. What are some of the factors that can change blood pressure beyond 2 mm Hg in the same patient because two different examiners have taken the blood pressure?

ANS.: a. If one physician uses muffling and the other uses disappearance for the diastolic pressure, the readings will be different by as much as 10 mm Hg.

b. If one physician presses the chestpiece harder than the other, the diastolic reading may be lower, especially if the brachial artery is soft, as in young subjects.

c. If one physician takes the reading with the patient's arm unsupported and the other has the patient rest the arm on a table, the reading may be 5 mm higher in the former than in the latter.

d. If one physician uses an aneroid manometer and the other uses a mercury manometer, the reading may be higher or lower by at least 5 mm Hg.

e. If one physician applies the cuff more loosely than the other, there may be a difference of as much as 10 mm Hg.

f. If one physician routinely inflates the cuff to almost 200 mm Hg and the other to about only 20 mm Hg above systolic pressure, the discomfort caused by the first physician will cause a higher systolic pressure.

g. If one physician uses a relatively small cuff on a fat arm, and the other uses a large cuff, there may be as much as a 50-mm Hg difference in pressure.

h. If one physician's appearance and manner are threatening and the other has a more pleasant and benign personality, the patient's blood pressure may be higher by at least 5 mm Hg when taken by the former.

i. If one physician takes the blood pressure with the patient sitting in a comfortable chair and the other with the patient sitting on an examining table with the legs dangling, the former will obtain a lower reading.

4. What are some factors that can change blood pressure beyond 2 mm Hg due to the presence of soft Korotkoff sounds?

ANS.: a. The hearing acuity of physicians differs.

b. The physician who has the patient open and close his or her fist a few times to increase blood flow may hear soft Korotkoff sounds at a higher pressure than the physician who does not do this.

   c. The physician who inflates the cuff more rapidly, thus decreasing venous congestion in the forearm, may hear the first Korotkoff sounds at a higher reading.

   d. The physician who places the chestpiece partly under the cuff will hear the faint first Korotkoff sounds sooner than one who places it 1 or 2 cm below the cuff.

5. What are some of the advantages of being scientific and recording the blood pressure to the nearest 5 or 10?

   ANS.: a. It is easier to remember and record three rather than six numbers between each 10 mm Hg (e.g., 120, 125, and 130 rather than 120, 122, 124, 126, 128, and 130).

   b. Estimation to the nearest 5 mm Hg is faster because the slight fluctuations of blood pressure that occur from moment to moment make it difficult and time-consuming to try to determine the pressures to the nearest 2 mm Hg.

PSEUDOHYPERTENSION

1. What is meant by pseudohypertension?

   ANS.: Pseudohypertension refers to a misleadingly high systolic, diastolic, or mean blood pressure measured with a cuff compared with the pressure measured directly by an intraarterial needle.

2. What is the effect of calcified brachial arteries ("pipestem" brachials) on blood pressure taken by cuff?

   ANS.: Medial sclerosis of the brachial arteries (Mönckeberg arteriosclerosis) may be severe enough to strongly resist compression by a blood pressure cuff. This could give a falsely high systolic pressure of more than 300 mm Hg despite an intraarterial needle blood pressure of only 130 mm Hg (65).

   Note: Studies that use femoral or radial intraarterial pressure to prove that hard brachial arteries, as in elderly patients, produce a falsely elevated blood pressure by cuff may themselves produce falsely low intraarterial pressure because of the effect of standing waves (65).

3. When should you suspect pseudohypertension?

   ANS.: The suspicion of pseudohypertension is based on the following findings. The patient is elderly and has

   a. A blood pressure that is elevated disproportionately to the clinical findings (i.e., no ECG evidence of LV hypertrophy, no cardiomegaly on x-ray or physical examination, and no hypertensive retinopathy).

   b. A palpable radial artery after the radial pulse has been eliminated by inflation of the cuff above systolic pressure. This is a variation of Osler's maneuver in which he compressed the radial artery with the index finger and felt for a palpable artery beyond the site of compression.

   c. An Osler positive test is only reliable in patients with severe hypertension off hypertensive medication.

PULSUS ALTERNANS

1. What is meant by pulsus alternans?

   ANS.: This is an alternating fluctuation in pulse pressure (i.e., in every other beat, the blood pressure is lower) (Fig. 17).

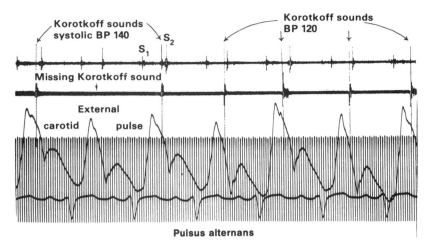

Pulsus alternans

FIG. 17. The heart sounds are shown in the top line. The next line was taken with a microphone over the brachial artery distal to a blood pressure cuff. Note the doubling of the number of Korotkoff sounds when the cuff was deflated from 140 to 120 mm Hg.

2. What is the significance of pulsus alternans?
   ANS.: a. It is usually associated with myocardial damage of the type that is either severe enough to cause gross failure or, more rarely, mild but associated with a chronic increase in afterload as in hypertension or AS.
   b. Even more rarely, it may be secondary to ectopic tachycardias even in a normal heart. It has also occurred during an episode of angina with severe anterior descending proximal obstruction.
   Note: When the alternans is associated with heart failure, the diagnosis of the failure is usually so apparent (marked dyspnea, edema, high venous pressure, cardiomegaly, tachycardia, and S_3 gallop) that the presence of alternans is of no additional help in diagnosis. However, in the absence of failure, even the slightest alternans can tell you important new information by suggesting the presence of some myocardial fibrosis or infarction.
3. What is more likely to make a pulsus alternans, a low or high filling pressure?[3]
   ANS.: A low filling pressure, because this decreases the stretch or Starling effect on the ventricle and therefore causes a decrease in cardiac function (45).
   Note: a. In a patient with failure given a diuretic, the appearance of a pulsus alternans (that was not present before the diuresis) may be used as a sign that you have decreased the patient's cardiac output and may be aggravating a low output syndrome.
   b. In examining a new patient for the presence of hypertension, the blood pressure should be taken with the patient sitting, because sitting may provoke alternans when it is absent supine.
   c. Exercise (3 minutes of straight leg raising) can bring out a pulsus alternans in patients with no apparent sign of myocardial dysfunction, either clinically or by physical examination at rest.
4. What beside exercise can start a short run of pulsus alternans in a patient who either has been or is in heart failure?

---

[3]Filling pressure is also equivalent to preload, venous pressure, and atrial or ventricular pressures at the end of diastole.

ANS.: A sudden increase in venous return, as with a deep inspiration or after a PVC in the postextrasystolic cycle (36,37).

   Note: There is no significance to the disappearance of pulsus alternans at rest in a patient who has been or is in heart failure, because pulsus alternans may disappear with either improvement or worsening of the heart failure (61).

5. How much difference in pulse pressure is detectable by finger palpation?

   ANS.: Usually at least a 20-mm Hg difference must be present between beats (35). Because there is usually less than a 10-mm Hg difference between the beats in pulsus alternans, a blood pressure cuff is usually required to detect it.

   Note: 1. Palpation of the radial pulse may be used. The technique involves two-finger palpation of the artery. By increasing the pressure with the proximal finger, the weaker beats can be eliminated under the distal finger while the stronger ones are preserved, thus effectively halving the pulse rate for the distal finger.

   2. Alternans tends to become more marked as the pulse wave moves peripherally. Therefore, the radials and femorals may show it better than the carotids or brachials.

6. What is the cause of pulsus alternans?

   ANS.: Two theories are widely held.

   a. It is due to a sudden critical change in diastolic filling period (67).

   b. It is due to an alteration in the number of cardiac fibers contributing to each systole.

   Note: a. Pulsus alternans has been reported in the pulmonary circulation and has been recorded in pulmonary embolism, primary pulmonary hypertension, and acute myocardial infarction (11,17,63).

   b. When an S_4 is present, it is louder before the weak beats (36).

7. Is electrical alternans (alternating differences in QRS configuration) associated with pulsus alternans?

   ANS.: Pulsus alternans occurs in only about 10% of patients with electrical alternans. (Electrical alternans is most frequently associated with large pericardial effusions.)

SUMMARY OF HOW TO TAKE ARM blood pressure BY LISTENING FOR KOROTKOFF SOUNDS

1. Ask the patient to extend his or her arm with the palm upward. This clarifies the position of the brachial artery.

2. Be sure that the center of the cuff bladder is over the brachial artery, and if you must use an aneroid manometer, make sure that the indicator needle is to the zero area on the dial before inflating the cuff.

3. Place the diaphragm of your stethoscope partly under the cuff, directly over the brachial artery, and press lightly.

4. Ask the patient to open and close the fist about 10 times.

5. With the arm at heart level, raise the cuff pressure by inflating as quickly as possible to 140 mm Hg for an adult and to 120 mm Hg for a child, and listen for Korotkoff sounds. If they are present, pump the cuff up another 20 mm Hg. Repeat the listening and pumping until no Korotkoff sounds are heard.

6. If the Korotkoff sounds are still very soft, raise the arm before inflating the cuff.

7. Deflate the cuff at a rate of about 5 mm Hg per heartbeat or per second until the first Korotkoff sounds of the systolic blood pressure are heard. Record it to the nearest 5 or 10 mm Hg.

8. Listen for pulsus alternans. This requires slow cuff deflation when the first Korotkoff sound is detected.

9. Deflate the cuff further until muffling is heard. Then deflate further until the Korotkoff sounds disappear. If the difference between the muffling point and the disappearance point is less than 10 mm Hg, report the disappearance point as the diastolic pressure. If, however, the difference is greater than 10 mm Hg, report both numbers (to the nearest 5 or 10 mm Hg).
10. If the arm is so fat that the cuff width or bladder length is less than 40% of the arm circumference, use a thigh cuff. If no thigh cuff is available, use an arm cuff over the radial artery.

BLOOD PRESSURE AND PULSES IN THE LEGS

Normal Pressures

1. How does the blood pressure in the legs compare with that in the arms?
   ANS.: It depends on the cuff size used and on whether the pressure is measured by an intraarterial needle or by Korotkoff sounds. With a proper-sized cuff over the thigh, the popliteal systolic pressure should be either the same or as much as 20 mm Hg higher than in the arms. If the systolic pressure in the legs is lower than in the arms, occlusive disease anywhere beyond the origin of the subclavian arteries should be suspected (76).
   Note: a. If an intraarterial manometer in the femoral artery is used to measure leg pressures, the systolic and diastolic pressures in the legs are usually the same as those in the arms (51).
   b. The blood pressure reading can tell you that the cuff is too small for the thigh because with a proper-sized cuff, even though the blood pressure may normally be higher in the leg, the diastolic pressure tends to remain the same as in the arm. Thus, if the diastolic pressure is higher in the leg than in the arm, the cuff is probably too small.
2. Where is the most reliable place to auscultate for blood pressure in the legs?
   ANS.: Over the popliteal artery, with a large cuff on the thigh (Fig. 18).

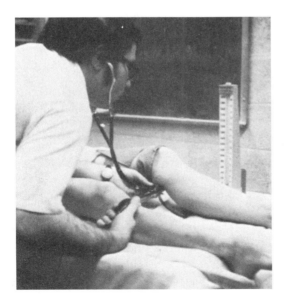

FIG. 18. The usual commercial leg cuff, such as that shown here, must be rolled diagonally around the thigh to keep the edges snug against the skin. The systolic blood pressure in the legs should not be more than 20 mm Hg higher than that in the arms, nor should it be lower.

Note: a. In severe AS, the slow rate of rise may make it impossible to hear Korotkoff sounds in the popliteals because the audibility of the sounds depends partly on the rate of rise.

      b. Compressing the thigh with a blood pressure cuff can cause enough discomfort to cause a false elevation of pressure. When accurate comparison with the brachials is necessary, as in patients with suspected coarctation or aortic regurgitation, the arm and thigh measurements should be done by two persons simultaneously.

      c. To take blood pressure in the lower legs, place an ordinary arm cuff just above the malleolus without including the protuberance of the malleolus. Use a small (pediatric) bell to auscultate the posterior tibial artery. If no Korotkoff sounds are audible, auscultate or palpate the dorsalis pedis instead. If no Korotkoff sounds are present over any foot artery, the Doppler method of taking blood pressure can be used (see p. 49) (Fig. 19).

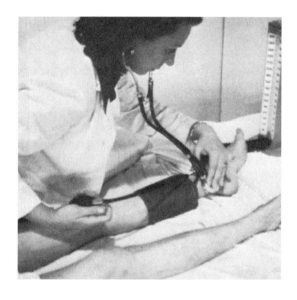

FIG. 19. A convenient method of taking a leg pressure if you do not have a thigh cuff. A pediatric bell should be used to achieve an easy air seal behind the medial malleolus.

3. What are the advantages and disadvantages of using the foot for taking blood pressure in a lower limb?

    ANS.: Although no special size or shape of cuff is necessary and it is more comfortable for the patient (about one in three patients complain of pain with the thigh cuff), no Korotkoff's sounds can be elicited over the posterior tibial or dorsalis pedis in about 10% of patients. Also, marked peripheral constriction, as in a cold room, may cause the blood pressure to be as much as 50 mm Hg lower in the foot than in the arm. Foot pressures, as with popliteal pressures, are normally higher than arm pressures at all ages and with or without hypertension (12).

4. How is blood pressure taken in an infant?

    ANS.: a. By the flush method. The limb is raised until it is blanched (some bind the forearm with a bandage to empty it of blood first). Then the cuff is inflated. The first distal flush as the cuff is deflated is read as the *mean* pressure.

      b. By Doppler ultrasound and a cuff about 3.5 cm wide.

Leg Blood Pressure in Aortic Regurgitation

1. How does AR affect the blood pressure in the legs in comparison with that in the arms? What is this sign of AR called?

   ANS.: AR exaggerates the tendency for the leg systolic pressure to be higher than that in the arms. If the difference is greater than normal, it is known as a positive Hill sign (26).

   Note: a. One theory attempting to explain why the cuff systolic pressure in AR is higher in the legs than in the arms is that reflected waves from the periphery summate with forward waves. These summated waves are known as standing waves. Hyperkinetic hearts can make larger standing waves.

   b. Femoral intraarterial pressure measurements have not always shown a positive Hill sign in AR (52). In a dog, if a catheter is withdrawn from the arch of the aorta to the lower extremities, the iliac pressure is seen to be 30 mm Hg higher than that in the proximal part of the aorta, and the femoral artery pressure is lower than that in the iliacs. Therefore, if femoral arterial catheter pressures are compared with brachial pressures, no Hill sign may be found.

2. How can the Hill sign be used to grade the severity of AR?

   ANS.: In mild AR the difference is up to 30 mm Hg; that is, the difference may be in the normal range. In moderate AR the difference is 30 to 40 mm Hg; in severe AR the difference is more than 60 mm Hg. A difference of between 40 to 60 mm Hg may represent either moderate or severe AR (18).

   Note: A falsely absent or low Hill sign may be produced by

   a. Congestive heart failure, presumably because of the poor stroke volume. The degree of positivity of a Hill sign may depend in part on the strength of myocardial contraction.

   b. Significant AS. Mild AS does not eliminate the normal brachial/popliteal gradient.

Leg Pulses and Blood Pressure in Coarctation of the Aorta

1. When should you suspect coarctation of the aorta?

   ANS.: In any patient with hypertension.

2. What are the characteristics of the pulses proximal to and beyond an aortic coarctation?

   ANS.: The proximal pulses (i.e., the carotid and brachial pulses) are large, bounding, fast-rising pulses. The parts of the body beyond the coarctation (i.e., usually beyond the left subclavian artery) receive blood through enlarged collaterals that do not transmit the percussion wave well. Therefore, not only do the lower-extremity pulses have a low pulse pressure, but their rate of rise is also slow and they have a late peak (i.e., the pulse wave is almost purely a tidal wave).

   Note: a. In infants and children with coarctation, the diastolic pressure in the brachials is normal despite a higher than normal systolic pressure.

   b. Because of the decreased initial flow rate through the femorals, their percussion wave is so low that only the tidal wave is felt. In the radials, however, the usual percussion wave is easily felt, and the velocity of flow and pulse pressure are increased due to their position proximal to the coarctation. The relative delay in the femoral peak is called the **radial-femoral lag** (Fig. 20).

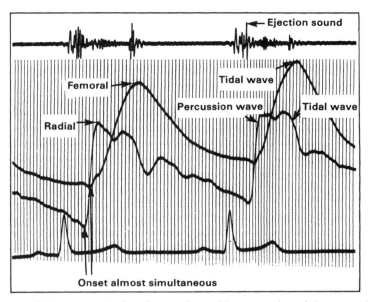

FIG. 20. Intraarterial pressure tracings in a patient with coarctation of the aorta show that the onsets of the femoral and radial pulses remain almost simultaneous. In coarctation, a delay in the femoral pulse is felt on palpating both arteries simultaneously because the percussion wave distal to an obstruction is obliterated by an anacrotic shoulder, which is imperceptible. Thus, only the later tidal wave is felt in the femoral artery, whereas the earlier percussion wave is felt in the unobstructed radial artery.

3. What may make it difficult to compare peaks in the femoral and radial arteries? How can this difficulty be overcome?

    ANS.: They have different pulse pressures, and the finger on the radial may be too far from the finger on the femoral. Femorals are best found with the legs slightly abducted and the foot externally rotated.

    Place the patient's wrist over the femoral artery, so that your fingers on the radial and femoral are on top of one another. Vary the compression force until both pulse pressures feel equal. Then use the lightest possible pressure, so that you can compare peaks (Fig. 21).

4. When may the femoral pulse be easily palpable in **coarctation**?

    ANS.: It is especially important to test for femoral pulse peak delay in suspected coarctation when coexistent AR is present (as may occur with a bicuspid valve) because with AR, all peripheral pulses become more bounding, so that the femoral pulses may have normal volume despite coarctation.

    Note: a. As many as 50% of patients with coarctation may have a bicuspid aortic valve, which is commonly regurgitant.

    b. Kinking of the aortic arch without any pressure gradient across the kinked segment (pseudocoarctation) can also delay the femoral pulse peak when compared with the radials (73). Experimental progressive constriction of the aorta in animals produces a delayed femoral peak when the aorta is constricted to 40% of its cross-sectional area, whereas a significant gradient does not develop until the aorta is narrowed to 30% of its original area (73).

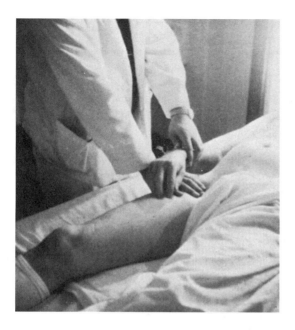

FIG. 21. By placing the patient's wrist over the femoral artery as you palpate both, you can best perceive the obvious delay of the femoral pulse peak over that of the arm. In using the radials rather than the brachials to test for differences between the arm and leg, you take advantage of the increased rapidity of pulse rise as you palpate more peripherally down the arm.

   c. Supravalvular AS can also cause a radial-femoral lag (38). Only a delay between the *right* radial and the femoral occurs because the left radial is also delayed.

   d. The blood pressure may not be elevated in the arms in coarctation in patients in whom there is significant AS plus a PDA (33), or if severe MR is present (74).

   e. You must always palpate the abdomen of a patient with suspected coarctation. If a strong aortic pulsation in the epigastrium suddenly disappears lower down, an abdominal aortic coarctation should be suspected.

PULSUS PARADOXUS

1. What is meant by *pulsus paradoxus*?
   ANS.: This is a fall of 8 mm Hg or more in systolic blood pressure on normal inspiration, usually due to tamponade. An inspiratory fall of less than 8 mm Hg may be physiologic.

Normal Effect of Respiration on Blood Pressure

1. Does the systolic blood pressure normally increase or decrease with inspiration? Why?
   ANS.: It decreases because
      a. Lung capacity increases with inspiration and the pulmonary vascular bed expands; therefore, less blood flows from the lung into the heart.
      b. Intrathoracic pressure decreases with inspiration. Because the aorta is an intrathoracic organ, its pressure also drops.
2. If the systolic pressure normally decreases with inspiration, what is paradoxical about a pulsus paradoxus?

ANS.: Nothing. It is simply an exaggeration of a normal phenomenon.

Note: a. The term **paradoxus** came into use with Kussmaul who, in the late 1800s, described a marked drop in, or even loss of, blood pressure on inspiration in patients with constrictive pericarditis (32). He decided to call it a "pulsus paradoxus" because he noticed that the apex beat did not change in any way despite the loss of radial pulse with inspiration. Kussmaul also thought it was paradoxical that although the peripheral pulse seemed at first to be irregular, it actually came and went regularly.

b. A more descriptive term than **pulsus paradoxus** is **marked inspiratory fall in blood pressure**.

3. How much systolic pressure is usually lost during normal and deep inspiration?

ANS.: During normal inspiration, 2 to 5 mm Hg of systolic pressure is lost. The normal inspiratory fall in systolic pressure seems to increase with higher systolic pressures. With deep inspiration up to 15 mm Hg is lost.

Note: The auscultatory equivalent of pulsus paradoxus is the prompt wide splitting of the second sound due to the early A_2 resulting from the decreased volume in the left ventricle on inspiration. The split is often for only one or two beats.

How to Elicit a Pathologic Inspiratory Fall in Blood Pressure

1. With what depth of respiration is the test done?

ANS.: Not more than a moderate depth of inspiration. If the patient is breathing too shallowly, tell him or her to breathe "just a little more deeply, but not too deeply," only enough for you to see the chest movements out of the corner of your eye while watching the manometer.

2. On moderate inspiration and expiration, what is a positive paradoxus (i.e., how much blood pressure fall on inspiration is definitely abnormal)?

ANS.: A fall of 10 mm Hg or more is generally agreed on in the literature. With practice, however, experience shows that an inspiratory fall of about 6 mm Hg is the upper limit of normal. Some of the probable reasons for believing that between 8 to 10 mm Hg could be normal are errors such as the following.

a. The subject is asked to breathe too deeply or even to hold his or her breath on inspiration and expiration.

b. The physician may fail to realize that as he or she is lowering the cuff pressure below the level of the first Korotkoff's sound on expiration, the blood pressure itself if often falling. Therefore, after the physician hears the Korotkoff's sounds both on inspiration and expiration for the first time, he or she fails to reinflate the cuff to see if the systolic pressure has actually dropped while he or she was performing the test. One need not reinflate the cuff from the zero point but merely from the point where the sounds were heard on both inspiration and expiration.

c. A fall of as little as 6 mm Hg could be a significant loss of systolic pressure and actually mean tamponade if the pulse pressure were markedly reduced, for example, to 20 mm Hg. If the blood pressure were 110/90 mm Hg, for instance, a 5-mm Hg decrease with inspiration could occur with tamponade (3).

Note: If you always test for pulsus paradoxus while taking a patient's blood pressure for the first time, you will get enough practice to make your results more reliable. Also, in this way, you automatically pick up pulsus alternans or pulsus bisferiens.

Mechanism of Inspiratory Fall in Tamponade or Constriction

1. Why is there a more marked drop in stroke volume on inspiration in tamponade than in normal subjects?

   ANS.: Because much less blood enters the left atrium on inspiration than in normal subjects. In tamponade, on inspiration, the left ventricular and left atrial pressure does not drop as far as does the intrathoracic pressure. Thus, on inspiration the pressure in the left atrium may exceed the pressure in the pulmonary veins and blood may even flow backward into the lungs.

2. Why does left atrial and left ventricular pressure not drop proportionately to intrathoracic pressure in the presence of tamponade?

   ANS.: The following is one plausible explanation. With inspiration, the filling pressure and volume of the right ventricle are increased, thus stretching the pericardium and increasing its intrapericardial pressure. The increased intrapericardial pressure is transmitted to the left atrium (which is covered with pericardium), raising its pressure during inspiration (14). Septal bowing into the LV on inspiration also contributes to the decrease of LV volume on inspiration.

Causes of False-Positive and False-Negative Tests for the Inspiratory Fall in Blood Pressure

1. Why do some asthmatic patients seem to have a marked inspiratory fall in blood pressure?

   ANS.: If expiration raises the intrathoracic pressure too high as a result of bronchospasm (similar to a Valsalva maneuver), inspiration, by contrast, seems to lower the systolic pressure excessively. Actually, it is usually an expiratory rise in pressure, not an inspiratory fall. There are patients with emphysema, however, who also have some *inspiratory* obstruction that causes an exaggerated inspiratory fall of intrathoracic pressure (similar to a Müller maneuver).

   Note: a. It is surprising how severe chronic emphysema can be with only a slight expiratory rise in blood pressure, suggesting that the degree of emphysema does not always correlate with the degree of bronchospasm.

   b. The pulse of tamponade may differ from the pulse of a patient with bronchospasm because in bronchospasm the pulse pressure often remains the same on inspiration and expiration. This occurs because cardiac output is only slightly affected by the phasic changes in intrathoracic pressure. In tamponade, on the other hand, the pulse pressure (as well as the systolic pressure) decreases on inspiration because the cardiac output drops markedly on inspiration. Consequently, although the tamponade pulsus paradoxus may occasionally be palpable, the pulsus paradoxus due to bronchospasm alone is not.

   c. The diastolic pressure in tamponade changes very little, whereas in bronchospasm it varies as much as does systolic pressure. An occasional patient with bronchospasm has an exaggerated decrease in stroke volume on inspiration. This is thought to be due to the bulging of the ventricular septum into the LV caused by the Müller maneuver.

   d. The degree of pulsus paradoxus correlates with the severity of an asthmatic attack. A drop of up to 20 mm Hg of blood pressure on inspiration is found in moderate degrees of asthma. A fall of more than 20 mm Hg is a sign of a severe attack (71).

2. Which patients have the greatest inspiratory fall in systolic pressure, those with constriction or those with tamponade?

   ANS.: Only with tamponade are inspiratory drops of 10 mm Hg or more found during quiet breathing (56). In chronic constrictive pericarditis, a pulsus paradoxus is actually uncommon unless it is subacute with some fluid still present (effusive-constrictive). By effusive-constrictive pericarditis is meant a combination of tamponade and constriction, due to pericardial fluid under increased pressure associated with constriction of the heart by the visceral pericardium (epicardium).

> *Note*: In the effusive-constrictive type of pericarditis, a tense effusion adds pressure to a constricting visceral pericardium, which still causes constriction even after complete pericardiocentesis. When the relatively small effusion is present, there is likely to be a marked pulsus paradoxus, just as in pure tamponade (22).

3. Why may congestive heart failure with marked cardiomegaly by itself sometimes cause a falsely exaggerated inspiratory fall in blood pressure?

   ANS.: It may be partly due to a cardiomegaly so great that it stretches even the normal pericardium to its maximum, causing inspiration to create such pressure on the outer cardiac walls that it makes the pericardium behave like a noncompliant restrictive band.

4. What conditions that are neither cardiac nor bronchospastic can cause a marked inspiratory fall in blood pressure?

   ANS.: a. Extreme obesity, which may cause excessive compression of the inferior vena cava at the thoracic inlet on inspiration.

   b. Pregnancy, presumably because the large uterus obstructs the free forward flow of blood in the inferior vena cava during inspiration.

   c. Compression on inspiration of one subclavian artery by a fibrous band of anterior scalenus muscle in thoracic outlet syndromes may account for the occasional unilateral paradoxus effect.

   d. Acute pulmonary embolism, usually with a cardiomyopathy.

   e. Shock.

   > *Note*: Shock can cause a marked inspiratory fall in blood pressure only if it is associated with hypovolemia. This occurs presumably because the depletion of the venous reservoir will cause less blood than normal to be ejected into the lungs on inspiration. Because the pulmonary reservoir is underfilled and has a low mean pressure, an excess amount of pulmonary blood is withheld from the LV on inspiration, thus markedly decreasing the left ventricular output and blood pressure.

   f. Obstruction to the superior vena cava, because this decreases the normal inspiratory increase in return of blood to the right atrium.

5. What is the cause of the marked inspiratory fall in blood pressure seen in some patients with a large acute pulmonary embolism?

   ANS.: Since it is associated with a decrease in pulse pressure during inspiration, there are several possibilities.

   a. An acutely dilated RV on inspiration may encroach on the LV in diastole and reduce the LV stroke volume, as in a reversed Bernheim effect.[4]

   b. The lungs are so empty that there may be excessive pooling in the lungs on inspiration.

6. When will there be no significant inspiratory fall in blood pressure despite marked tamponade?

---

[4]Bernheim effect is characterized by encroachment on the RV cavity by the interventricular septum, which is bowed to the right by a dilated LV, as described by the pathologist Bernheim in 1915. The enlargement of the LV in diastole prevents diastolic filling of the RV but does not interfere with right ventricular outflow; that is, it is not a kind of infundibular outflow obstruction but an obstruction to inflow. Such a large LV is usually due to severe, chronic mitral regurgitation.

ANS.: a. If AR is present, the LV can fill from the aorta during inspiration. Therefore, if dissection of the aortic root causes both AR and tamponade, do not expect a pulsus paradoxus.

   b. In patients with a large atrial septal defect (ASD) the normal increase in systemic venous return on inspiration is balanced by a decrease in left-to-right shunt, so that the right ventricular volume changes very little during inspiration.

   c. In patients with isolated right heart tamponade (usually patients with chronic renal failure).

   d. If the left ventricular diastolic pressure is very high.

   Note: Hypertrophic subaortic stenosis has been reported to cause a reversed pulsus paradoxus. The reason for this is unknown (41).

CAPILLARY PULSATION

1. How do you elicit capillary pulsation (Quincke sign)? What is the mechanism?

   ANS.: Compress the skin of the face or hands with a glass slide, or exert slight pressure on the nailbeds and watch for intermittent flushing. You can also transilluminate the nailbed by holding a flashlight against the pad of the patient's finger while shading the finger with your other hand.

   The mechanism is the transmission of the arterial pulse through dilated capillaries to the subpapillary venous plexus. It is found in any condition that causes capillary dilatation, such as hot weather, a hot bath, fever, anemia, pregnancy, or hyperthyroidism.

   It is also found in any cardiac condition that causes a large pulse pressure, such as AR, systolic hypertension, or marked bradycardia, as in complete atrioventricular block.

   Note: a. When severe, all the preceding cardiac conditions can cause such a marked capillary pulsation that it can be seen merely by inspecting the palms, cheeks, or forehead, without compressing the skin.

   b. Capillary pulsation disappears, even in severe AR, if heart failure intervenes, because of the peripheral constriction that occurs with failure.

EVALUATING CARDIAC FUNCTION BY BLOOD PRESSURE RESPONSE TO A VALSALVA MANEUVER

Normal Valsalva Hemodynamics

1. What happens to the blood pressure immediately on performing a Valsalva strain? Why?

   ANS.: During the strain, the blood pressure rises by an amount equal to the increase in intrathoracic pressure.

2. What happens to the blood pressure, pulse pressure, and heart rate while the strain is maintained for 10 seconds?

   ANS.: The blood pressure and pulse pressure decrease and the heart rate increases because the increased intrathoracic pressure obstructs venous return and progressively decreases ventricular volume (by about 50%) (7). The reflex sympathetic outflow due to the decreased stroke volume and blood pressure causes tachycardia.

3. What happens to the blood pressure, pulse rate, and heart rate on release of the strain?

   ANS.: For a few beats the blood pressure falls because there are a few seconds of decreased flow from relatively empty pulmonary vessels. Then the blood pressure overshoots to above control levels, and the pulse pressure increases because the increased sympathetic outflow (which persists for at least 5 to 10 seconds after the release of the strain) increases peripheral resistance. Added to this is the temporary increase in venous return to the heart of blood that had been dammed up by the increased intrathoracic pressure. This flow reaches the LV after a few seconds and causes an increase in LV stroke volume. The resultant increase in pressure on the carotid sinus, in turn, causes a reflex bradycardia.

Valsalva Effect in Patients with Decreased Function

1. What is the blood pressure response to a Valsalva strain if the ejection fraction is normal (i.e., 70 ± 10% by angiography, or 60 ± 10% by radionuclide methods)?
   ANS.: If the cuff pressure is held at 25 mm Hg above systolic pressure during the strain, a few Korotkoff sounds heard at the beginning of the strain reflect the increased intrathoracic pressure. Then the Korotkoff sounds disappear as the blood pressure falls due to the decrease in venous return. Post-Valsalva, the Korotkoff sounds reappear due to an overshoot of at least 25 mm Hg if the ejection fraction is normal. If no overshoot is obtained, repeat the test, this time holding the cuff pressure at 15 mm Hg above the control pressure. If there is an overshoot to 15 mm Hg, the ejection fraction may be low normal or it may be slightly reduced (79).
2. What kind of blood pressure response to the Valsalva maneuver occurs with a markedly reduced ejection fraction?
   ANS.: During the entire strain the blood pressure stays up, as indicated by the persistence of the Korotkoff sounds, and after the Valsalva maneuver there is no overshoot or bradycardia. This is known as a square wave response and is partly due to the excess lung blood volume in the congested lungs that continues to empty into the LV during the entire 10 seconds of strain, thus maintaining the left ventricular stroke volume (33) (Fig. 22).

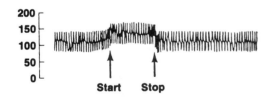

FIG. 22. **The square wave response is present when there is no fall in blood pressure during and no rise in blood pressure after a Valsalva strain. This usually indicates an ejection fraction of 20 ± 10%.**

   Note: The square wave response tells you that the ejection fraction is about 30 ± 10% by angiogram (20 ± 10% by radionuclide methods) and that the end-diastolic pressure in the LV is abnormally high, even as high as 40 mm Hg (78).
3. What happens to the blood pressure response to the Valsalva maneuver if the ejection fraction is reduced to 50 ± 10% by angiography (40 ± 10% by nuclear methods) and has a near normal ejection fraction only with the help of a high end-diastolic pressure?
   ANS.: The blood pressure and pulse pressure decrease during the strain, but there is no poststrain overshoot (78). This is presumably due to the excess sympathetic tone to which hearts with reduced ejection fractions are subject. Any excess pre-Valsalva sympathetic stimulation (e.g., norepinephrine infusion) prevents the overshoot (78). Therefore, the strain does not stimulate enough further sympathetic drive to produce an overshoot after the release of the strain.

Note: In patients with coronary disease who have had a previous infarction and have a decreased ejection fraction, the excess sympathetic stimulation is seen in the compensatory hyperactivity of the noninfarcted muscle as well as in shortening of the QS_2 relative to the QT interval[5] (seen even in patients with coronary disease and no old infarction) (6).

4. What can produce an absence of overshoot despite a normal heart?

ANS.: a. Any cause of autonomic imbalance, such as the use of beta blockers (48).

    b. Decreased blood volume.

    c. Hypertension due to a lessening of baroreflex sensitivity.

    d. A moderate or large ASD.

    Note: A Valsalva maneuver in a patient with an ASD results in less tachycardia and may even produce a square wave response if the ASD is large (23).

5. How can you help the patient perform a Valsalva if he or she cannot comprehend your instructions or cooperate enough to carry out the maneuver?

ANS.: a. Press on the abdomen with one hand and ask the patient to push your hand away with the abdomen. If this does not work, then

    b. Have the patient blow up an aneroid manometer to 40 mm Hg through a rubber tube connection. A 20-gauge needle inserted into the rubber tube ensures that continuous expiration through an open glottis is moving the manometer needle and prevents the needle from moving if only intraoral pressure is raised.

    Note: Another way to use blood pressure to tell if the patient has low cardiac output is to divide the difference between systolic and diastolic blood pressure by the systolic blood pressure. This is known as the proportional pulse pressure. If the difference between systolic and diastolic blood pressure is 25% or less of the systolic pressure, then a severe decrease in cardiac output is probable, and if it is between 25% and 40%, at least a moderate fall in cardiac output is probable.

REFERENCES

1. Alpert JS, Vieweg WVR, Hagan AD. Incidence and morphology of carotid shudders in aortic valve disease. *Am Heart J* 1976;92:435.
2. Alzamora-Castro V, Battilana G. The double femoral sound. *Am J Cardiol* 1960;5:764.
3. Antman EM, Cargill V, Grossman W. Low-pressure cardiac tamponade. *Ann Intern Med* 1979;91:403.
4. Barner HB, William VL, Kaiser GC. Dicrotic pulse after open heart operation. *Circulation* 1970;42:993.
5. Berliner K, et al. Blood pressure measurements in obese persons. *Am J Cardiol* 1961;8:10.
6. Boudoulas H, et al. Effect of increased adrenergic activity on the relationship between electrical and mechanical systole. *Circulation* 1981;64:28.
7. Brooker JZ, et al. Alterations in left ventricular volumes induced by Valsalva manoeuvre. *Br Heart J* 1974; 36:713.
8. Buchbinder WC, Sugarman H. Arterial blood pressure in cases of auricular fibrillation measured directly. *Arch Intern Med* 1940;66:625.
9. Burch GE. On recording your own blood pressure. *Am Heart J* 1975;89:813.
10. Burch GE, Shewey L. Sphygmomanometric cuff size and blood pressure recordings. *JAMA* 1973;225:1215.
11. Calick A, Berger S. Pulmonary arterial pulsus alternans associated with pulmonary embolism. *Chest* 1973; 64:663.
12. Carter SA. Effect of age, cardiovascular disease and vasomotor changes on transmission of arterial pressure waves through the lower extremities. *Angiology* 1970;29:601.
13. Corrigan DJ. Permanent patency of the mouth of the aortic valves. *Edinb Med Surg J* 1832;37:225.
14. Dornhorst AC, Howard P, Leathart GL. Pulsus paradoxus. *Lancet* 1952;1:746.

---

[5]A QS_2 should be 26 ± 13 msec greater than the QT. A reversal is noted in patients with excessive sympathetic stimulation, as in pheochromocytoma.

15. Evans W, Lewes D. The carotid shudder. *Br Heart J* 1945;7:171.
16. Ewy GA, et al. The dicrotic arterial pulse. *Circulation* 1969;39:655.
17. Ferrer ME, et al. Cardiocirculatory studies in pulsus alternans of the systemic and pulmonary circulation. *Circulation* 1956;14:163.
18. Frank MJ, et al. The clinical evaluation of aortic regurgitation. *Arch Intern Med* 1965;116:357.
19. Freis ED, Kyle MC. Computer analysis of carotid and brachial pulse waves. *Am J Cardiol* 1968;22:691.
20. Geddes LA, Whistler SJ. The error in indirect blood pressure measurement with the incorrect size cuff. *Am Heart J* 1978;96:4.
21. Gould L, Lyon AF. Postural changes in the brachial artery first derivative in the normal and pathologic state. *Dis Chest* 1968;53:476.
22. Hancock EW. Subacute effusive-constrictive pericarditis. *Circulation* 1971;43:183.
23. Hancock EW, et al. Valsalva's maneuver in atrial septal defect. *Am Heart J* 1963;65:50.
24. Harrison EG Jr, et al. Bilateral indirect and direct arterial pressures. *Circulation* 1960;22:419.
25. Henschel A, et al. Simultaneous direct and indirect blood pressure in man. *J Appl Physiol* 1954;6:509.
26. Hill L, Rowlands RA. Systolic blood pressure in change of posture and in aortic regurgitation. *Heart* 1911–1912; 3:219.
27. Hultgren HN. Venous pistol shot sounds. *Am J Cardiol* 1962;10:667.
28. Ikram H, et al. The haemodynamic implications of the bisferiens pulse. *Br Heart J* 1964;26:452.
29. Ison JW. Palpation of the dorsalis pedis pulse. *JAMA* 1968;206:2745.
30. Kaul U, et al. Characteristic postextrasystolic ventricular pressure response in constrictive pericarditis. *Am Heart J* 1981;102:461.
31. King GE. Taking the blood pressure. *JAMA* 1969;209:1902.
32. Kussmaul A. Ueber schweilige Mediastinopericarditis und den paradoxen Puls. *Klin Wochenschr* 1873;10:443.
33. Little JA, et al. Coarctation of the aorta with aortic stenosis and patent ductus. *Am J Cardiol* 1963;12:570.
34. Littler WA, et al. The variability of arterial pressure. *Am Heart J* 1978;95:180.
35. Littmann D. Alternation of the heart. *Circulation* 1963;27:280.
36. Littmann D. Cardiac alternation. *Am J Cardiol* 1964;14:420.
37. Liu CK, Luisada AA. Halving of the pulse due to severe alternans (pulsus bisectus). *Am Heart J* 1955;50:927.
38. Logan WF. Familial supravalvular aortic stenosis. *Br Heart J* 1965;27:547.
39. Londe S, Kutzner TS. Auscultatory blood pressure measurement: Effect of pressure on the head of the stethoscope. *West J Med* 1984;141:193.
40. London SR, London RE. Critique of indirect diastolic end-point. *Arch Intern Med* 1967;119:39.
41. MacGregor GA. Spontaneous capillary pulsation in complete heart block. *Br Heart J* 1959;21:225.
42. Masuda Y, et al. Carotid pulse wave contour in normal and diseases. *J Cardiol* 1976;6:725.
43. Maurer AH, Noordergraaf A. Korotkoff sound filtering for automated three-phase measurement of blood pressure. *Am Heart J* 1976;91:584.
44. McCutcheon EP, Rushmer RF. Korotkoff sounds: An experimental critique. *Cir Res* 1967;20:149.
45. McIntosh HD. Discordant pulsus alternans. *Circulation* 1960;26:214.
46. Meadows WR, et al. Dicrotism in heart disease. *Am Heart J* 1971;82:596.
47. Mitchell PL, et al. Effect of vertical displacement of the arm on indirect blood pressure measurement. *N Engl J Med* 1964;271:72.
48. Nishimura RA, Tajik AJ. The Valsalva maneuver and response revisited. *Mayo Clin Proc* 1986;61:211.
49. Nuessle WF. The importance of a tight blood pressure cuff. *Am Heart J* 1956;52:905.
50. Orchard RC, Craige E. Dicrotic pulse after open heart surgery. *Circulation* 1980;62:1107.
51. Pascarelli EF, Bertrand CA. A comparison of blood pressures in the arms and legs. *N Engl J Med* 1964;270:693.
52. Pascarelli EF, Bertrand CA. A comparison of arm and leg blood pressures in aortic insufficiency. *Br Med J* 1965; 2:73.
53. Perlman LV, et al. Accuracy of sphygmomanometers in hospital practice. *Arch Intern Med* 1970;125:1000.
54. Putt AM. A comparison of blood pressure readings by auscultation and palpation. *Nurs Res* 1966;15:311.
55. Ragan C, Bordley J. The accuracy of clinical measurements of arterial blood pressure. *Bull Johns Hopkins Hosp* 1941;69:504.
56. Reddy PS, et al. Cardiac tamponade: Hemodynamic observations in man. *Circulation* 1978;58:265.
57. Robinson B. The carotid pulse. *Br Heart J* 1963;25:61.
58. Rodbard S, Ciesielski J. Auscultatory gap and pulse upstroke. *Am Heart J* 1959;58:221.
59. Rodbard S, Margolis J. The auscultatory gap. *Circulation* 1957;15:850.
60. Rose G. Standardisation of observers in blood-pressure measurement. *Lancet* 1965;1:673.
61. Ryan JM, et al. Experiences with pulsus alternans. *Circulation* 1956;14:1099.
62. Sabbah HN, et al. Effect of turbulent blood flow on systolic pressure contour. *Am J Cardiol* 1980;45:1139.
63. Scoblionko DP, Lozner EC. Pulsus alternans. *Cardiovasc Rev Rep* 1981;2:581.
64. Silverberg DS, et al. The unsupported arm: A cause of falsely elevated blood pressure. *Br Med J* 1977;2:1331.
65. Spence JD, et al. Direct, indirect, and mean blood pressures in hypertensive patients. *Clin Invest Med* 1980; 2:165.
66. Spodick DH, et al. Rate of rise of the carotid pulse. *Am J Cardiol* 1982;49:159.
67. Spodick DH, St. Pierre JR. Pulsus alternans. *Am Heart J* 1970;80:766.
68. Steinfeld L, et al. Updating sphygmomanometry. *Am J Cardiol* 1974;33:107.

69. Tahir AH, Adriani J. Usefulness of ultrasonic technique of blood pressure determination. *Anesth Analg* 1973; 52:699.
70. Toole JF. Bilateral simultaneous sphygmomanometry: A new diagnostic test for subclavian steal syndrome. *Circulation* 1966;10:35.
71. Vaisrub S. Pulsus paradoxus of the airways. *JAMA* 1975;232:1041.
72. Varden S, et al. Systolic hypertension: Direct and indirect blood pressure measurements. *Arch Intern Med* 1983; 143:935.
73. Wang K, et al. Delayed systolic peak of the femoral pulse from kinking of the aortic arch. *Am J Cardiol* 1974; 33:286.
74. Wigle ED, Auger P. Coarctation of the aorta associated with severe mitral insufficiency. *Am J Cardiol* 1968; 21:190.
75. Wood P. Aortic stenosis. *Am J Cardiol* 1958;1:553. (Classic article)
76. Yao ST, et al. Ankle systolic pressure measurements in arterial disease affecting the lower extremities. *Br J Surg* 1969;56:676.
77. Zahir M, Gould L. A new method for measurement of blood pressure in clinical shock. *Am Heart J* 1970;79:572.
78. Zerna MJ, et al. Left ventricular dysfunction (Bedside Valsalva manoeuvre.) *Br Heart J* 1980;44:560.
79. Zema MJ, et al. Detection of left ventricular dysfunction in ambulatory patients. *Am J Med* 1983;75:241.

4

Jugular Pressure and Pulsations

VENOUS PRESSURE BY JUGULAR INSPECTION

1. With which chambers of the heart are the jugular veins in continuity in systole and in diastole?

    ANS.: In systole the jugular veins are in continuity only with the right atrium because the tricuspid valve is closed. In diastole, when the tricuspid valve is open, the jugulars are in continuity with both the right atrium and the right ventricle (RV). Therefore, examination of the jugulars may reveal the contour and pressure in the right atrium and the RV without the need for catheterization) (Fig. 1).

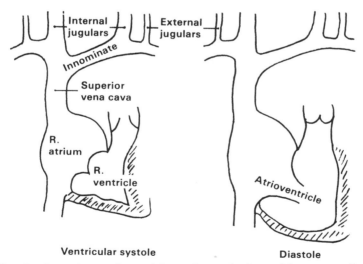

FIG. 1. In diastole, the atrium and ventricle are in continuity and become an "atrioventricle." Note also that the internal jugulars are in a more direct line with the superior vena cava than the external jugulars.

2. Are there venous valves between the jugulars and the superior vena cava?

    ANS.: Yes. The external jugular valves can often be demonstrated by occluding the external jugulars with a finger, preventing venous flow from the head. Valves between the superior vena cava and the internal jugulars have been demonstrated when the intrathoracic pressure is raised, as in coughing or chest compression (10).

The valves usually become incompetent in the presence of tricuspid regurgitation (TR). Doppler studies show no retrograde flow even in the presence of high venous pressure unless there is TR.

Note: a. The venous valves do not interfere with the use of the jugulars as a manometer for the measurement of venous pressure (i.e., as reflectors of right atrioventricular events). Elevated internal jugular venous pressures can apparently be transmitted through the venous valves, which presumably are open during both systole (descent of base of ventricle effect) and diastole (opening of tricuspid valve effect).

    If the venous valves of the arms are destroyed by phlebitis, as in chronic heroin users, the normal jugular pulsations are transmitted to the arm veins. Any vein in the body may transmit jugular pulsations if there is marked elevation of venous pressure or volume of pulsations as in severe TR. Varicose veins in the leg are especially likely to pulsate in the presence of severe TR because their valves are incompetent.

3. Why are the internal jugular veins a more accurate manometer than the externals?

   ANS.: a. The internal jugulars are in direct line with the superior vena cava and right atrium. The external jugulars communicate with the superior vena cava only after two near 90-degree-angle turns: where the external jugular enters the subclavian and where the subclavian enters the superior vena cava. It is difficult to communicate pressure accurately through two sharp turns (6).

   b. The external jugulars are occasionally either absent or too thready to be visible to the naked eye, especially in obese females.

   c. If the external jugulars are narrow in diameter but visible under normal conditions, they may become so constricted with heart failure or shock due to increased sympathetic stimulation and norepinephrine that they become invisible.

4. When do internal jugulars become visible?

   ANS.: Only in the presence of severe TR.

5. If the internal jugulars are usually invisible, how can they be used as a manometer to measure venous pressure?

   ANS.: The pulsations of the internal jugulars are transmitted to the skin of the neck. The top level of the skin's pulsations is taken as the venous pressure. Thus, the jugular is used as a "pulsation manometer."

   Note: a. Normally, the pressure in the right jugulars is either slightly greater than or the same as that in the left jugulars. In some arteriosclerotic patients the left jugular pressure may be falsely elevated due to compression of the innominate vein between the sternum, anteriorly, and the large tortuous arteries arising from a high unfolded aortic arch, posteriorly (33). (An aortic aneurysm may also be the cause of innominate vein compression, but this is rare.) Taking a deep breath decreases manubrial compression against the innominate vein and helps to exclude this left jugular compression artifact.

   b. A persistent left superior vena cava that drains into the coronary sinus causes a slightly higher pressure in the left jugulars than that in the right, possibly due to a relatively greater emptying resistance (16). A persistent left superior vena cava is especially likely in the presence of an atrial septal defect (ASD) (12).

HOW TO USE THE INTERNAL JUGULAR MANOMETER

1. What reference level may be used as zero? Why?

    ANS.: The sternal angle, or angle of Louis (pronounced Looee), which is about 5 cm above the center of the right atrium in the supine position and 10 cm above the center of the right atrium at a 30- to 90-degree chest elevation (30).

    Note: One of the difficulties in judging the top level of jugular pulsations is that they tend to diminish toward the upper level; that is, the top level of pulsation is very much like a fulcrum of movement. Determining the top level of venous pressure really means looking for the fulcrum of internal jugular movement) (Fig. 2).

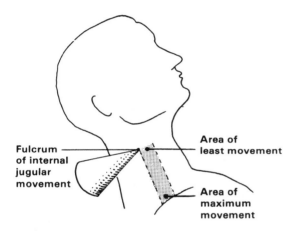

FIG. 2. The top level of pulsations is really an area of subtle disappearance. The accuracy is probably within about 0.5 cm.

2. What upper limits of normal have been suggested for jugular pulsations in (a) the supine and (b) the 45-degree position, using the sternal angle as the zero reference level?

    ANS.: a. In the supine position, the upper limit is 2 cm.

    b. At 45 degrees, the upper limit is 4.5 cm (Fig. 3). (It is easy to remember 4.5 cm at 45 degrees.)

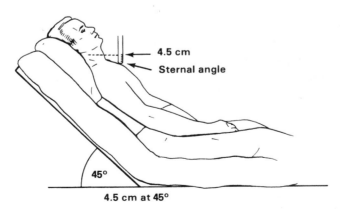

FIG. 3. Venous pressure can be estimated by observing the upper level of internal jugular pulsations above the sternal angle. If it is over 4.5 cm at 45 degrees, it indicates an elevated right atrial pressure.

Note: a. The top level of internal jugular pulsations reflects central venous pressure with sufficient accuracy to be clinically useful. If you find a normal or low venous pressure when you suspect a low cardiac output, inquire about the ingestion of diuretics. X-ray studies with cadavers have shown that the sternal angle is about 5 cm above the right atrium when horizontal, and about 10 cm above the right atrium with the chest tilted 45 degrees or more. However, this information is of no practical value because if at 45 degrees the upper normal above the sternal angle is 4.5 cm and you add 10 cm, the upper normal venous pressure becomes 14.5 cm, which is about three times what is found by a catheter in the right atrium.

b. If the venous pressure is very high so that the top level of pulsations cannot be seen at 45 degrees, the patient may even have to hang legs over the side of the bed to allow jugular pulsations to be perceived.

METHOD OF OBTAINING ACCURATE VENOUS PRESSURE MEASUREMENT

1. How can you detect jugular pulsations that are difficult to perceive?

   ANS.: a. Shine a light tangentially from behind or in front of the neck to throw a jugular shadow (Fig. 4).

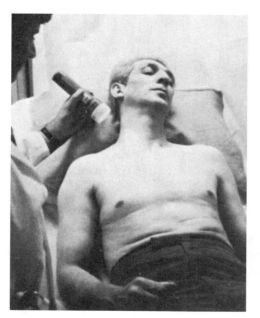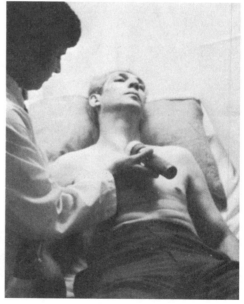

FIG. 4. Jugular movements may be very subtle. Any slight movement of the hand holding the light can produce as much artifactual movement as movement from the jugulars themselves. Therefore, you must support your hand on either the pillow behind or the chest in front.

b. The most accurate way of finding the top level of pulsations is to examine the silhouette of the neck. When you are examining the right side of the neck, you must lean over to the left side of the patient to obtain a view of the silhouette of the skin overlying the right internal jugular (Fig. 5).

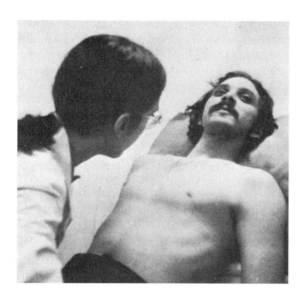

FIG. 5. Leaning over to the left side of the patient to view an outline of the neck against the pillow will show you more subtle motion than could be seen even with an oblique light. Therefore, the true upper level of motion is best seen from this viewpoint.

    c. If the internal jugular pressure is high, the earlobes often pulsate. Unfortunately, a strong carotid pulse pressure can also cause slight earlobe pulsations.

    d. Inspiration may make jugular pulsations easier to see because the RV has more blood volume on inspiration and contracts with more energy (Fig. 6).

    e. Held respiration often eliminates jugular pulsations altogether, probably because of the slight Valsalva effect.

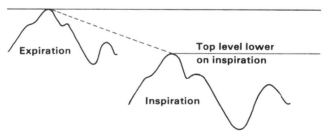

FIG. 6. Note the higher absolute level but smaller amplitude of pulsations on expiration. With bronchospasm, jugular pulsations with normal pressures may only be visible above the clavicle during expiration due to the effect of straining, which elevates intrathoracic pressure with each expiration.

3. How can you obtain an accurate number in centimeters for a venous pressure?

    ANS.: Mark the upper level of jugular pulsations during inspiration with a felt-tipped pen. Place a tongue depressor marked off in centimeters vertically on the sternal angle. The rounded ends make a tongue depressor the most comfortable measuring stick. A carpenter's level gives the most accurate vertical level. If no ruler is available, you can use the thickness of your fingers for a rough estimate. The second interphalangeal joint is generally about 2 cm thick. Measure your own joint for further use. Another method is to place a closed fist on the sternal angle and use each finger breadth as a 2-cm gauge (Fig. 7).

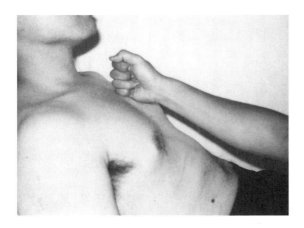

FIG. 7. Since the diameter of each finger is about 2 cm, a fist placed on the sternal angle is the equivalent of a ruler marked off in 2-cm subdivisions.

DIFFERENTIATING JUGULAR FROM CAROTID PULSATIONS

1. How can you tell an internal jugular from a carotid pulsation by palpation?
    ANS.: Normal internal jugulars are not palpable. If the venous pressure is very high, you will occasionally feel an easily compressible, gentle undulation.
        Note: a. Supraclavicular pressure can eliminate jugular, but never carotid, pulsations. There is, however, a caution here. When internal jugular pulsations are very high and strong, they are not eliminated by low supraclavicular compression. You must instead apply pressure at least halfway up the neck to eliminate these high-pressure jugular movements (Fig. 8).

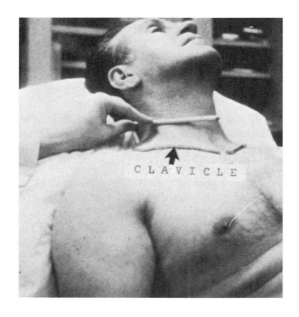

FIG. 8. A very strong jugular pulsation with a high venous pressure in not eliminated by pressure just above the clavicle, probably because the sternomastoid tendons prevent adequate pressure against the vein.

b. A sudden abdominal compression thrust makes the jugulars momentarily more visible but has no effect on carotids.

2. How can the contour of jugular movements help differentiate them from carotids?

ANS.: If the largest, fastest movement is inward, that is, a collapse, then it is a jugular pulsation. The largest, fastest carotid movements are outward.

THE ABDOMINAL COMPRESSION TEST (HEPATOJUGULAR REFLUX)

1. How can you tell that a venous pressure below the upper limits of normal is actually relatively high for a particular person?

ANS.: Abdominal compression causes and maintains a rise of at least 1 cm in the top level of pulsations only if the venous pressure is relatively high. The greater the rise with abdominal compression, the higher the venous pressure. This is called the **hepatojugular reflux** (*not* "reflex").

Note: The effect of abdominal compression is more important than the absolute jugular pressure in determining whether or not the venous pressure is normal or relatively high.

2. What happens to the top level of jugular pulsations if abdominal compression is applied to a patient without heart failure?

ANS.: In the normal patient the jugular pulsation level either remains the same or falls. This is because pressure on the abdomen obstructs femoral venous return almost as effectively as venous tourniquets on the thighs.

Note: One bonus derived from testing for jugular pressure with abdominal compression is the possible discovery of a low vital capacity. Abdominal compression that causes an increase in dyspnea or the use of accessory muscles of respiration implies that the patient's vital capacity is so reduced that he or she cannot tolerate any further decrease produced by pushing up on the diaphragm.

3. What is wrong with the term **hepatojugular reflux?**

ANS.: The term was first applied in 1885, when it was thought not only that pressure on the large liver was an essential part of the test but also that the procedure was a test only for tricuspid regurgitation (28). Actually, the effect can be achieved with a normal-sized liver and with compression on any part of the abdomen, although pressure on the right upper quadrant produces the greatest response. If the right upper quadrant is tender, do not hesitate to compress other areas instead.

The term **hepatojugular reflux** must be retained because it is so widely known that it is useful for indexing and referencing.

4. Why does abdominal compression cause a sustained rise in pressure in a patient with congestive failure?

ANS.: In patients with peripheral venous congestion (high venous pressure and peripheral edema) there is increased venous tone and volume that counteracts the thigh tourniquet effect (36,38). The increase in tone and volume also affects the walls of the right atrium and ventricle. Pushing up on the right atrium and RV, which has decreased compliance, makes it difficult for these chambers to receive blood from the superior vena cava without an increase in pressure (13).

Note: a. The increased venous tone in heart failure is due to sympathetic outflow along the autonomic nerves and increased catecholamines in the blood, both of which are caused by the low cardiac output. Increased venous tone or tension in heart failure has been proved by plethysmography, in which volume and pressure in an encased limb are used to solve for tension by using Laplace's law: Pressure is proportional to tension/volume. There is also an inherent stiffness of the venous system in congestive heart failure that is not related to sympathetic tone.

b. Increased venous tone has been found in all patients with so-called right ventricular failure (31); that is, peripheral venous congestion (increased venous pressure and peripheral edema due to inadequate cardiac output). (See p. 2 for explanation of RV failure terminology.) If diuretics have normalized the absolute height of venous pressure, abdominal compression may still demonstrate the increased tone.

c. The increased venous tone and volume due to the fall in cardiac output may be called an increase in "tone-volume." A tone-volume increase can be produced by left ventricular dysfunction with an increase in wedge pressure of 15 mm Hg or more, or by pure right ventricular dysfunction (as in right ventricular infarction) with a normal wedge pressure (9). The abdominal compression test is a test for increase in tone-volume, irrespective of the cause.

d. The term **positive abdominal compression test** is preferable when describing the results of abdominal pressure. The term **abdominal jugular test** has also been proposed, but for teaching purposes the word **compression** is more specific.

e. If a patient's normal venous pressure is 1 cm above the sternal angle at 45 degrees, it may rise to only 3 cm; that is, a 2-cm increase may occur when failure takes place. This may be higher than normal for this patient but within normal limits for venous pressure. Also, look for an enlarged liver. When a high venous pressure has fallen to normal because of treatment, it may take time before the liver returns to normal.

5. What are the common causes, besides severe loss of vital capacity, of noncardiac rise in the height of jugular pulsations with abdominal compression?

ANS.: a. Inability to tolerate the upward movement of the diaphragm when pressure on the abdomen raises the diaphragm in patients with severe loss of vital capacity (24).

b. Increased blood volume (14).

c. Increased sympathetic stimulation due to such causes as nervousness, pain, or an acute infarct.

d. Abdominal compression often exaggerates the amplitude of the jugular pulsations without actually raising the upper levels. By revealing the true upper level of pulsations, abdominal compression can give a false impression of a rise in venous pressure.

Note: An obstruction of the superior vena cava below the azygos vein is a rare cause of a positive abdominal compression effect (Fig. 9).

6. How should you compress the abdomen to prevent false elevations due to sympathetic outflow?

ANS.: a. Compress with warm hands or with a garment or sheet between your hand and the abdomen.

b. Spread the fingers apart so that there is as little local pressure as possible (Fig. 10).

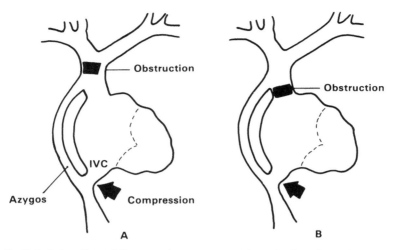

FIG. 9. A: Partial obstruction of the superior vena cava above its junction with the azygos elevates jugular venous pressure. Abdominal compression does not elevate it further because the displaced abdominal blood can reach the area below the obstruction. B: Obstruction, partial or complete, below the junction of the azygos with the superior vena cava also elevates venous pressure, and abdominal compression prevents the jugular blood from emptying freely into the azygos, thus further elevating the jugular pressure.

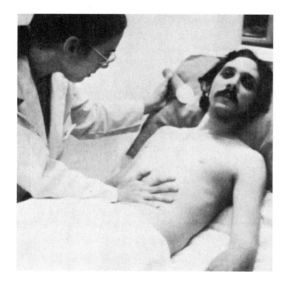

FIG. 10. Spreading the fingers allows you to distribute pressure over a large area, so that more pressure can be applied without producing discomfort. Sometimes only marked abdominal pressure raises jugular pulsations enough to show that they are abnormal.

    c. Start by pressing gently, and gradually increase the pressure to just below the point of discomfort.

    d. Warn the patient that it spoils the test if you produce discomfort.

    e. An abrupt change in jugular pressure is easier to recognize than a gradual change. Therefore, it is sometimes easier to see that the venous pressure has risen by looking for a fall in the level of pulsations when the abdominal pressure is suddenly released (9).

Note: If done properly, the maximum elevation in jugular venous pressure occurs within a few seconds and does not increase with compression longer than 10 seconds (9).

7. What is the Kussmaul sign?

ANS.: Historically, it is the rise in the height of jugular pulsations during inspiration in patients with chronic constrictive pericarditis. However, it is found in only a minority of patients with constrictive pericarditis, and it often occurs with peripheral venous congestion from any cause (19).

    Note: a. Inspiration raises the intraabdominal pressure and can produce an effect like that of abdominal compression (37). Therefore, in any patient with high venous pressure, inspiration may cause a further pressure increase.

        b. This sign should alert you to the presence of RV infarction in a patient with acute inferior infarction and no sign of left ventricular (LV) failure because it will be present in the majority of such patients (1).

8. When can the top level of internal jugular pulsations not be the true venous pressure?

ANS.: In severe TR where the high pressure in the jugular is really transmitted RV pressure. A more accurate measure of venous tone and volume in the presence of severe TR would be the top level of external jugular pulsations.

JUGULAR PULSE CONTOURS

Normal Jugular Pulse Contours

1. What is the difference between the jugular and right atrial pulse contours?

ANS.: None, for all practical purposes, except when jugular pulse tracings pick up carotid artifacts. Therefore, the right atrial contours are explained first because it is right atrial events that produce the jugular contours (Fig. 11).

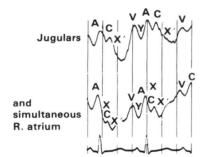

FIG. 11. The atrial and jugular waves are very similar. The crests are A, C, and V; the descents are X, X', and Y.

    Note: The normal right atrial contours consist of A, C, V, and H waves. However, it is also important to explain the descents, which should be called X, X prime (X'), and Y.

The A Wave and X Descent

1. When the P wave of the ECG occurs, what atrial events result? What are their names?

ANS.: The right atrium contracts and produces a rise in right atrial pressures. (Rises in atrial pressures are not named.)

A review of the literature on jugular contours shows that about half the writers on the subject do not actually name the atrial diastolic descent as a separate entity, and those that do name it call it the X descent (4). The rise and fall produces a wave universally known as the A wave (Fig. 12).

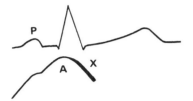

FIG. 12. Atrial relaxation produces the drop in pressure known as the X descent.

The C Wave and X' Descent

1. What atrial event is initiated by the QRS?
   ANS.: The QRS results in RV contraction that pushes up the tricuspid valve and raises the right atrial pressure slightly.
2. Does the RV contract by approximation of its free wall to the septum? Does the apex move up toward the base?
   ANS.: During systole the septum does not move toward the free wall of the RV nor does the apex move up (15). Normal RV ejection is due to two movements: (a) the base moves downward and (b) the free wall moves inward toward the septum (Fig. 13).

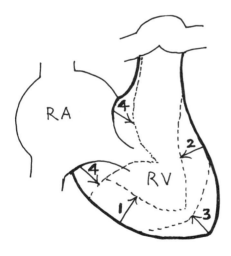

FIG. 13. The broken lines represent the four possible inward movements of the RV that could eject its blood. However, only number 4 and number 1 movements are normally used to eject blood from the RV.

Note: LV ejection differs from RV ejection in that the septum and free wall move toward each other. In the RV the septum and free wall move in the same direction so that the RV depends much more on the descent of the base and the inward movement of the free wall.

3. Why does right atrial pressure fall when the floor of the atrium (base of ventricle) is pulled down during systole? What is this fall called?
   ANS.: Since the walls of the atrium are attached to surrounding structures by their tributary veins, atrial pressure must fall. This produces the major movement of the

jugular pulse known as the X' descent. (This also results in a small wave known as the C wave; see Fig. 14.)

Note: The fall in intrapericardial pressure due to the shrinking heart during systole is transmitted to the right atrium and contributes to the X' descent. Very few cardiologists name this descent, and most who do name it call it X; that is, they give it the same name as that given to atrial relaxation, thus leading to great confusion (4) (Fig. 14).

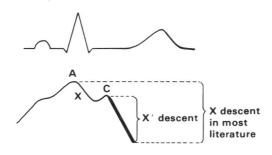

FIG. 14. The jugular pulse descent during systole should not be called X, as it is by most authors, because the X descent is due to atrial relaxation, whereas the jugular systolic descent is due mostly to the pulling down of the base of the ventricle during systole. As shown in the pulse wave diagram, the diastolic X descent precedes the major systolic jugular descent, which is now termed the X' descent.

4. What are the advantages of using the term *X'* for the systolic jugular descent?

   ANS.: a. It is a compromise with those who have always used an X to represent the descent of the base.

   b. No other name has been given to it by anyone who wanted to distinguish it from the X of atrial diastole. The term *X'* was first used by Mackenzie in 1907, in what was apparently the first attempt to distinguish the atrial diastolic X descent from the systolic descent. Mackenzie showed a tracing with a delay in ventricular contraction due to first-degree atrioventricular (AV) block. The systolic jugular descent was so obviously *not* due to atrial diastole, which showed its descent long before, that Mackenzie felt obliged to give a different name to the descent during systole, calling it X' (20). He correctly ascribed X' to a drawing down of the floor of the atrium by the RV contraction.

The V Wave and Y Descent

1. When does RV contraction become too weak to continue pulling down the base? How does this affect the right atrial pressure?

   ANS.: The phase of reduced ejection occurs in midsystole. This attenuates the descent of the base and allows the filling of the right atrium from the venae cavae to raise right atrial pressure (Fig. 15).

2. What ends the rise in right atrial pressure and then allows the pressure to fall, thus making a wave?

   ANS.: RV relaxation allows RV pressures to fall below right atrial pressures, thus opening the tricuspid valve (at the end of isovolumic relaxation). The wave and descent produced by the filling of the right atrium during ventricular systole, followed by diastolic emptying, are the V wave and Y descent (Fig. 16).

   Note: a. The Y descent is rapid because it reflects the rapid expansion phase of the RV.

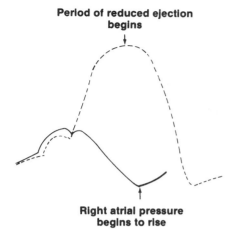

**Period of reduced ejection
begins**

**Right atrial pressure
begins to rise**

FIG. 15. The right atrial pressure rises during the last third of ventricular systole, when right ventricular contraction weakens and the descent of the base is diminished.

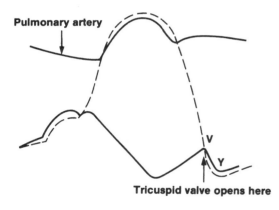

Pulmonary artery

V

Y

Tricuspid valve opens here

FIG. 16. The atrial (and jugular) wave is built up during systole while the tricuspid valve is closed.

  b. When the tricuspid valve is open, the right atrium and ventricle form a common pressure chamber that may be called an "atrioventricle."

3. What happens to RV expansion after the end of the Y descent?
 ANS.: A slow diastolic expansion phase occurs and the pressure in the atrioventricle rises slowly as blood pours into the RV. The wave so produced is called the diastasis, or H wave.
  Note: a. It is crucial to remember that the V wave is a systolic event, occurring while the tricuspid valve is closed (Fig. 17).
   b. The nadirs at the bottom of the X and Y descents are the X and Y troughs. They have no significance except that some textbooks, unfortunately, do not name descents at all and simply assign the letters *X* and *Y* to the troughs.

4. When is forward flow through the superior vena cava and right atrium greatest in the normal heart, during ventricular systole or diastole?
 ANS.: Venal caval forward flow is normally greater during ventricular systole than during diastole (32). This is reflected by the fact that the X′ descent is normally deeper than the Y descent.

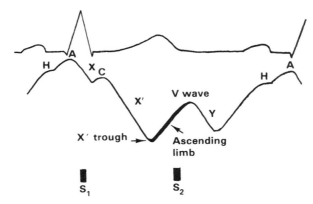

FIG. 17. The jugular V wave is built up during systole, and its height reflects the rate of filling and the elasticity of the right atrium. Between the bottom of the Y descent (Y trough) and beginning of the A wave is the period of relatively slow filling of the "atrioventricle," or diastasis period. The wave built up during diastasis is the H wave. The H wave height also reflects the stiffness of the right atrium.

Contour Recognition

1. Can you see a C wave by inspection of jugular neck pulsations?
   ANS.: No, it is too small. The large C wave seen in some jugular pulse tracings is due to carotid artifact because the pulse wave sensor used to record jugulars cannot separate out the impulse of a carotid movement occurring at about the same time as the tricuspid valve closure C wave. The C wave was originally thought to be entirely due to the carotid pulse; thus, the letter *C* was used for *carotid* (20). If the carotid arterial component is subtracted electronically from the jugular tracing, the C wave becomes diminutive or disappears (25).

2. Why are the V wave and Y descents often not visible or very low in amplitude in most adults?
   ANS.: Because the right atrium is a very compliant or distensible chamber; that is, the right atrium is too distensible to allow its pressure to rise much when the tricuspid valve is closed.

3. If a C wave, V wave, and Y descent are not seen in most adults, what should you look for on an adult jugular?
   ANS.: You should expect to see a single systolic descent consisting only of a small X plus a large X′ (Fig. 18).

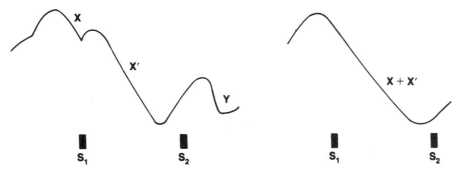

FIG. 18. On the left is a normal jugular pulse tracing. On the right is the jugular pulse usually seen by the naked eye in the normal adult; that is, one descent, the X-plus-X′ but mainly the X′.

Timing Normal Jugular Movements

1. Why is it easier to decipher jugular movements by observing descents or inward collapsing movements, rather than ascents or outward movements?

   ANS.: Because it is easier to perceive large fast movements (X′ and Y descents) than the slower rises (H wave) or the shallower rise of the V wave.

2. How can you recognize an X′ or Y descent by using your stethoscope?

   ANS.: The descent of the base, which causes the X′ descent, is a systolic event. Therefore, it must end at the end of systole, which is marked by the second heart sound (S_2). With your stethoscope, you can time the dominant jugular descent or collapse to see if it appears to fall onto the S_2. If it does, it is a dominant X′, and the wave preceding it must be an A wave (if the patient is in sinus rhythm). If, on the other hand, the dominant descent does not fall onto the S_2, it must be a Y descent and the preceding wave must be a V wave (see Fig. 24).

   Note: If the Y descent is larger than the X′ descent, then a dominant V wave is present, which is always abnormal.

3. How can you recognize jugular descents by palpating peripheral pulses?

   ANS.: Palpate the radial pulse while observing jugular descents. Since both the radial pulse and the X′ descent are systolic, the radial pulse occurs simultaneously with the X′ descent.

   Note: A carotid pulse occurs slightly before the jugular systolic collapse.

4. How does the jugular pulse in a young person differ from that in an adult?

   ANS.: It is normal for the Y descent to be easier to see in a young person than in an adult, presumably because the circulation time is slightly faster in young people than in adults, and the child's right atrium is relatively small for the volume it receives. This tends to raise a higher pressure in the right atrium and make a slightly larger V wave and Y descent in children than in adults.

Making Jugular Movements More Visible

1. Which jugulars should you examine for contours, the internal or the external jugulars? Why?

   ANS.: Because they have the freest communication with the right atrium, the internals are best examined for contours. Occasionally, however, the external jugulars show the only easily analyzable movement.

2. Why should you place the patient in the supine position to examine for jugular contours?

   ANS.: In the supine position, more blood returns to the right atrium. Furthermore, when the chest is raised, the jugulars can disappear below the clavicles.

   Note: If jugular movement is too small to be easily timed, increase the venous return by elevating the subject's legs and have the subject take deeper breaths. Deep inspiration can draw more blood into the right atrium. Placing the patient in the left lateral position between 50 and 75 degrees often makes the amplitude of the descents more visible and therefore easier to time.

Summary of Differences Between Jugular and Carotid Pulsations

1. The carotid pulse has only one descent or collapse; the jugular often has two, the X′ and the Y.

2. The carotid descent is slow, whereas the jugular X′ descent is rapid; if the fastest and greatest movement is a collapse or descent, it is a jugular pulse.

3. Firm pressure just above the clavicle obliterates all but the highest-pressure jugular pulsations but does not affect carotid pulsations.
4. Inspiration may exaggerate jugular pulsations but, if anything, diminish carotid pulsations.
5. Sitting up makes the carotids appear higher in the neck, but the jugulars appear lower in the neck.
6. The carotid, if visible, is always easily palpable with firm pressure. The normal jugular is rarely palpable with firm pressure.
7. The X′ descent ends at the S_2 and is simultaneous with the radial pulse, whereas the carotid descent appears to begin with the S_2 and precedes the radial pulse.
8. Sudden abdominal compression makes the jugulars momentarily more visible but has no effect on the carotids.

Summary of How to Recognize Normal Jugulars

1. With the patient supine, palpate the radial pulse. If the jugular descent occurs simultaneously with the radial pulse, a dominant X′ descent is present.
2. Listen to the heart sounds and time the descents. If the nadir (bottom) of the descent falls onto the S_2, the dominant descent is an X′.
3. If you are still uncertain because of an irregular rhythm, you can confirm your impression by looking at the peaks of the jugular outward movements. If the dominant peak is simultaneous with the S_1, there is a dominant A wave, which is one of the characteristics of a normal contour.

ABNORMAL JUGULAR CONTOURS

The Giant A Wave

1. How high is abnormally high for an A wave?
   ANS.: Over 4.5 cm above the sternal angle with the chest at 45 degrees.

   Note: An A wave that is higher than normal due to too strong an atrial contraction is called a giant A wave.
2. What can cause a giant A wave?
   ANS.: a. Obstruction at the tricuspid valve due to either tricuspid stenosis or right atrial tumor, such as a right atrial myxoma.

   b. A noncompliant or stiff RV due to either pulmonary outflow obstruction, as with pulmonary stenosis, or pulmonary hypertension.

   Note: a. When the RV has a pressure load to overcome, it becomes thicker and less compliant than normal. Because in diastole the atrium and ventricle are in continuity, the pressure in this atrioventricle rises very rapidly as it fills with blood. The stretch of the atrium produces a Starling effect and a powerful atrial contraction, which, in turn, stretches the ventricle before it contracts.

   b. There may seem to be only an A wave in the jugular pulse in severe pulmonary stenosis (PS) because RV systole may be so prolonged that the V wave is also prolonged. If there is a slight tachycardia or a first-degree AV block, the atrium contracts at the time of the V wave peak, and the giant A wave may begin to rise almost as soon as the late peak of the wave is reached.

c. A giant A wave can produce a presystolic sound if you auscultate over the jugulars (7). This loud knocking sound may be accentuated by inspiration.

d. The right ventricle does not fail in Fallot's tetralogy despite the serious right ventricular outlet obstruction, presumably because the ventricular septal defect acts as a relief mechanism. Therefore, the atrium is not called on for help and a giant A wave is not expected (Fig. 19).

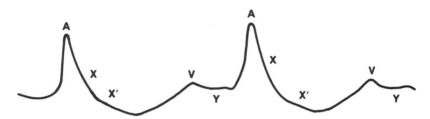

FIG. 19. Tricuspid stenosis. This jugular pulse tracing from a patient with tricuspid stenosis shows a very slow Y descent due to difficulty in emptying the right atrium in diastole. The X′ descent (descent of the base) is also slow, probably because of a poor right ventricular contraction caused by an underfilled right ventricle. Clinically, you could see that this patient had a giant A wave because the top level of the jugular pulsation was high. It was 6 cm from the sternal angle with the chest at 45-degree elevation. (Upper normal is 4.5 cm.)

3. What else besides a strong atrial contraction increases the amplitude of the A wave?
   ANS.: An atrial contraction during ventricular systole. If the atrium contracts when the tricuspid valve is closed, it transmits its pressure backward to form a large A wave called a cannon wave. Cannon waves may occur either in the presence of AV dissociation or when there is an early P wave (e.g., as with a premature atrial depolarization or junctional pacemaker).
   Note: Cannon waves are usually difficult to see unless the atrial contraction is very strong, such as when there is loss of compliance (increased stiffness) of the RV, which occurs in pulmonary hypertension. Because they are easily recorded, cannon waves were probably given their name from the appearance of the recordings rather than from the appearance of the slight variations in jugular pulsation amplitude seen in the neck (Fig. 20).
4. How can the jugular A wave suggest hypertrophic subaortic stenosis (HSS, or hypertrophic obstructive cardiomyopathy [HOCM]) in a patient with an aortic ejection murmur?
   ANS.: If the jugulars show a giant A wave, RV outflow obstruction due to an excessively thick septum is suggested.

Abnormalities of the X′ Descent

1. What can cause a smaller than normal or even absent X′ descent?
   ANS.: a. A poor RV contraction, as in RV infarction, heart failure from any cause, or when there is no presystolic Starling effect stretch, as in atrial fibrillation or flutter.
   b. Tricuspid regurgitation. The X′ descent is encroached on in proportion to the degree of regurgitation.

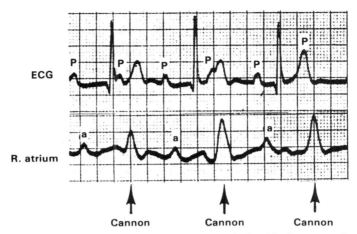

FIG. 20. Note that in this patient with complete atrioventricular block, every other P wave happens to fall on a T wave; that is, it occurs during ventricular systole when the tricuspid valve is closed. Thus, there is a cannon A wave with every other P wave.

      c. Buildup of the V wave earlier than usual, as with loss of capacitance of the right atrium (e.g., when filled by tumor [right atrial myxoma], or with loss of compliance of the right atrium due to hypertrophy as in tricuspid stenosis [TS], or stiffening by sutures in the right atrium after open heart surgery).

      d. Loss of pericardium. For instance, if the surgeon fails to close the pericardium after open heart surgery or if there is congenital absence of the pericardium (22).

         Note: The X' descent (i.e., the fall in atrial pressure during ventricular systole) depends on the presence of a relatively fixed atrial wall, which in turn depends on a relatively fixed pericardial attachment to the surrounding tissue. When the pericardium is disturbed by open heart surgery (21,22) or if it is congenitally absent, there are presumably variable degrees of loss of wall fixation. Therefore, when the floor of the atrium is pulled down (descent of the base during systole), the entire atrium is pulled down so that the fall in pressure inside the atrium may be attenuated or even eliminated. It has been shown that if the X' is diminished enough to equal the Y descent, then this relatively small X' is only an expected result of surgery disturbing the pericardium (23). However, if the X' is smaller than the Y descent after surgery, you should expect decreased RV systolic function (29) (Fig. 21).

      e. A Bernheim effect (see footnote on p. 61) in severe mitral regurgitation.

  2. What can increase the amplitude of the X' descent?

     ANS.: a. Increased volume in the right ventricle as in atrial septal defect, pulmonary regurgitation, and anomalous pulmonary venous connection.

      b. Pericardial tamponade. In tamponade, systolic function is normal, but filling is restricted so that the only time blood can enter the right atrium is during systole. Restriction of filling occurs during both early rapid filling phase and slow filling phase. Therefore, there may be no Y descent.

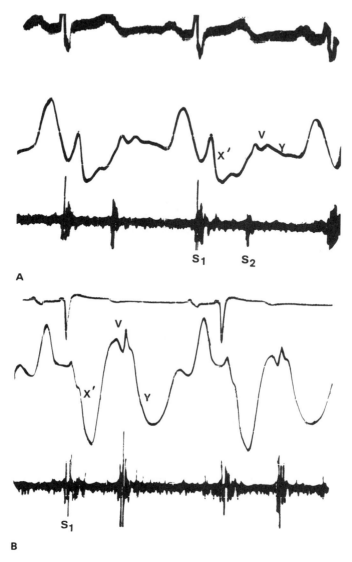

FIG. 21. A: The preoperative jugular tracing with a dominant X-plus-X′ descent. (By inspection the C wave was not visible.) B: The jugular tracing after bypass surgery. Note the prominent Y descent.

Abnormalities of the V Wave and Y Descent

1. What can cause a higher than normal jugular V wave (recognized by seeing a relatively deep Y descent)?

   ANS.: a. Tricuspid regurgitation.

   Note: It is logical to call the atrial wave caused by TR a V wave, even though it is the result of a different mechanism than the usual V wave, because other sources besides the usual venae cavae blood often contribute to the V wave (e.g., in ASD) but we still call it a V wave.

b. Rapid or excessive right atrial filling while the tricuspid valve is closed, as in ASD or hypervolemia.

c. A high venous pressure or high right atrial and ventricular diastolic pressure, as in congestive heart failure or pulmonary hypertension with a high RV diastolic pressure, because then the V wave builds up from a higher base level (29).

d. Loss of compliance of the right atrium, resulting from constrictive pericarditis or from the inflexibility of sutures used in heart surgery.

e. Loss of pericardial attachments to surrounding tissue. (See question 1, p. 84, for complete explanation.)

Note: A relatively high V wave even if not absolutely high may occur in any condition that produces a smaller than normal X′ descent. Thus, the Y descent will tend to equal the X′ descent. For example, a severe pectus that restricts right atrial filling (11), loss of firm suspension of the right atrium to the surrounding structures after surgery, congenital absence of the pericardium, and atrial fibrillation produces a relatively deep Y descent. Much more rarely, a calcified pericardium around the atrium without constriction of the ventricles, a right atrial myxoma, and severe mitral regurgitation (MR), which may push the septum against the right atrium during ventricular systole, can all produce a relatively high V wave.

2. What can cause a relatively high V wave due to rapid atrial filling besides TR and ASD?

ANS.: a. Rapid circulation times, such as those occurring with exercise, anemia, anxiety states, and hyperthyroidism.

b. Anomalous pulmonary venous drainage into the right atrium.

Note: a. A patent foramen ovale may be stretched by severe MR or a large left-to-right shunt such as persistent ductus arteriosus or ventricular septal defect (VSD), thus producing an atrial left-to-right shunt that can enlarge the right atrial V wave (26).

b. In ASD the large volume ejected by the RV causes a deep X′ descent. The large V wave as well as the deep X-plus-X′ produce a characteristic jugular pulse, with both deep X-plus-X′ and deep Y descents (i.e., a prominent A wave and a relatively high V wave). (See Fig. 22.)

c. In children and young adults a moderately deep Y descent is commonly present (with the X′ still dominant). This may be because in the young, the circulation time may be slightly more rapid than in most adults. Thus, when the AV valves close in systole, there is more rapid filling of the atrium than in the adult.

d. After coronary bypass surgery, the amplitude of the X′ may be less than or equal to the Y descent. If the Y descent is deeper than the X′, the right ventricular ejection fraction is likely to be less than 40%.

e. About 60% of children and 20% of adults with ASD have deeper Y than X′ descents; that is, relatively few adults with ASD have the V wave as large or larger than the A wave (27).

3. How does the progression of pulmonary hypertension affect the X′ and Y descent?

ANS.: As pulmonary hypertension develops, the first abnormality may be difficult to note because the X′ is greater than the Y, as in normals. But now the A wave is exaggerated and you may see a slight flicker in the neck near the clavicle before the X′.

The Y is more easily seen than in the normal adults. In the next stage the X′ equals the Y with an exaggerated A. With severe pulmonary hypertension and tricuspid regurgitation developing, the X′ becomes smaller than the Y or there may be only a Y if there is marked tricuspid regurgitation (Fig. 22).

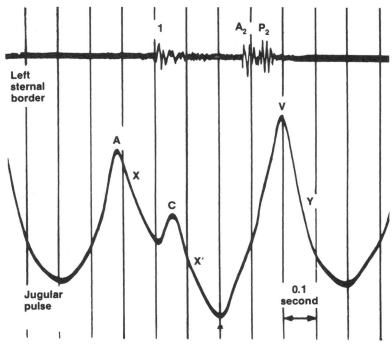

FIG. 22. Shown is a jugular pulse tracing from a patient with an atrial septal defect. Since the eye cannot see the C wave, it appears to be only a large double descent with the systolic descent (X plus X′) appearing larger than the Y descent.

4. Why will double filling of the right atrium by TR not produce deep X′ and Y descents as it does with ASD?

   ANS.: In TR, the tendency to increase the descent of the base is counteracted by the regurgitant stream. Therefore, with increasing amounts of TR, the X′ descent becomes more and more shallow and the Y descent increasingly deep (Fig. 23).

   Note: a. The single large regurgitant CV wave of severe TR resembles the large carotid pulse wave of severe AR and is often confused with this pulsation.

   b. A high venous pressure with TR may cause a large pulsating liver. Systolic expansion of the liver can be identified by placing the right hand upon the right upper quadrant while the left hand is applied posteriorly below the rib cage.

   c. In the presence of severe TR disproportionate systolic filling of the right internal jugular vein which is in direct line with the superior vena cava

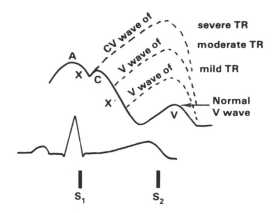

FIG. 23. As the degree of TR increases, the X′ descent is increasingly encroached upon. With severe TR, no X′ descent is seen, and the jugular pulse wave is said to be "ventricularized."

results in a right-to-left "head bob" with each systole, best seen when observing the patient from the front.

d. Tall A and V waves may alternate in height (venous alternans) in the presence of severe true right ventricular failure plus tachycardia as may occur in an infant with severe pulmonary stenosis.

The Jugulars in Pericardial Tamponade and Constrictive Pericarditis

1. Why is the X′ descent in tamponade dominant?

   ANS.: Unlike constriction in which diastolic flow is not restricted until the end of early diastole, tamponade diastolic flow is restricted throughout diastole, including the period of early rapid expansion of the ventricle. Therefore, in tamponade, forward flow depends almost entirely on the descent of the base. It is not surprising that in the absence of diastolic forward flow the entire forward flow occurs during ventricular systole and a dominant X′ descent is always present. Cardiac output can be maintained only by tachycardia or more complete systolic emptying, or both.

   Note: In constrictive pericarditis, systole is often restricted as shown by the below-normal or low-normal cardiac output and stroke volume at rest (35).

2. How can a jugular contour help differentiate constrictive pericarditis, effusive constrictive pericarditis, and tamponade?

   ANS.: In tamponade there is an X′ descent but little or no Y because restriction occurs at the beginning of opening of the tricuspid valve (18). In constriction, restriction occurs only after the tricuspid valve has opened and the LV pressure has fallen to zero, thus making a good Y descent after a small or absent X′ descent. In effusive constrictive pericarditis the X′ is either dominant or equal to the Y descent, even in atrial fibrillation.

3. When should you suspect that a deep X′ descent is due to the presence of tamponade or effusive constrictive pericarditis?

   ANS.: If the venous pressure is high, a deep X′ is rarely seen unless there is tamponade or effusive constrictive pericarditis, especially if the patient is in atrial fibrillation.

   Note: a. In severe chronic MR the LV may bulge into the RV in diastole and prevent good filling of the RV. This Bernheim effect causes a reduced X′ descent and exaggerated V wave and Y descent. (See footnote 61, for explanation of Bernheim effect.)

    b. When constriction is caused by fibrosis and there is not much calcification in the pericardium, the jugular findings may show a good X' descent as well as an exaggerated Y, very much like effusive constrictive pericarditis.

    c. Constrictive pericarditis produces a square root sign in the jugulars, right atrium, and RV pressure tracings. This refers to an early diastolic dip and plateau that can be recognized in the jugular pulse as an abrupt, jerky rise following an exaggerated Y descent (Friedrich's sign) (3,17,21,34).[1]

    d. Right ventricular infarction and a restrictive cardiomyopathy (as with amyloid disease) also show this square root sign (3,17,21,34) (Figs. 24–26).

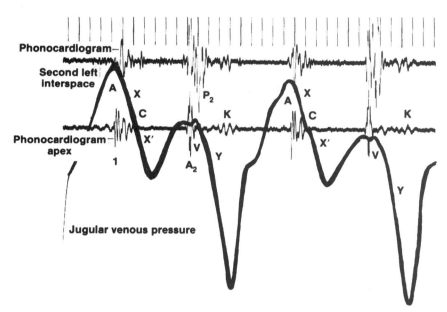

FIG. 24. Severe constrictive pericarditis. Shown is a jugular pulse tracing from a patient with a severe constrictive pericarditis. Note the double descent from a dominant Y descent and relatively small X' descent. K indicates a pericardial knock sound.

---

[1]The early diastolic dip caused by rapid expansion of the ventricle may be due to work performed on the fibrotic or calcified pericardium, so that the systolic deformation is like a loaded spring. The sudden release of the loaded spring in diastole causes an excess rate of "recoil." The encasement limits expansion, causing a steep rise after the dip (2).

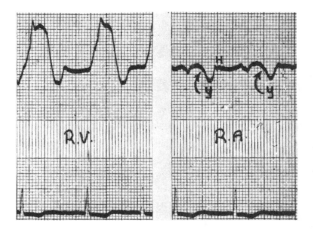

FIG. 25. Right ventricular (RV) and right atrial (RA) pressure from a patient with constrictive pericarditis and atrial fibrillation. Note the square root sign in the RV pressure curve reflected in the RA curves (i.e., a Y descent that terminates in a rapid rise to an H plateau). Note that despite atrial fibrillation, a small X′ descent is present.

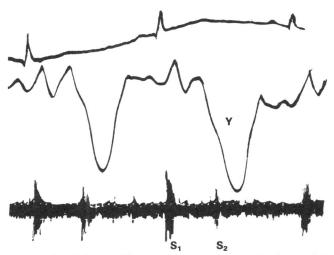

FIG. 26. This jugular tracing is from a 60-year-old woman 1 month after an inferior myocardial infarction that was diagnosed as extending to the RV. Note the "square root sign"; that is, the dominant Y descent rises steeply to a plateau-type H wave.

e. In constrictive pericarditis a pulsatile liver, reflecting the dominant jugular Y descent by liver movement away from the palpating hand, is a common finding (5).

Summary of Jugulars in Tamponade and Constrictive Pericarditis

1. In tamponade: A dominant X′ descent and almost absent Y.
2. In constriction: A dominant Y descent with a rebound wave after the Y trough and with a small X′.
3. In effusive constrictive or mild constrictive pericarditis: A dominant X′ with a fair Y almost equal to the X′.

THE JUGULAR PULSE IN ARRHYTHMIAS

1. How does atrial fibrillation affect the jugular pulse contour, besides the absence of an A wave?

    ANS.: There is a decreased X′ descent, usually with a dominant Y descent (Fig. 27).

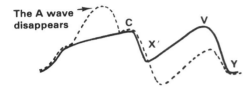

FIG. 27. The dominant descent in atrial fibrillation is almost always the Y descent; that is, it has the superficial appearance of the pulse wave of TR.

2. Why is there a diminished X′ descent in the presence of atrial fibrillation?

    ANS.: The absent atrial "kick" at the end of diastole causes a poor RV contraction, and an otherwise normal heart may decrease its stroke work by about 10%; but the heart with RV overload may decrease its stroke work by as much as 30% (Fig. 28).

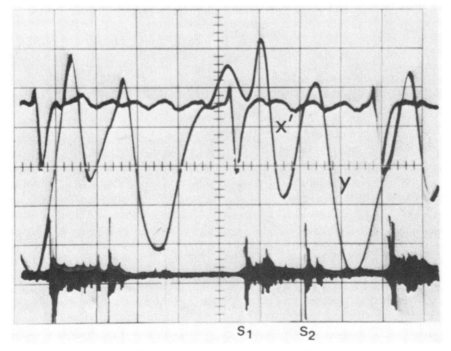

FIG. 28. The wave before the X′ cannot be an A wave because it is not due to atrial contraction. It is really a prolonged H wave. Note the good X′ descent, despite the dominant Y descent, in this patient with moderate rheumatic MR.

3. What other reasons are there for a poor X′ descent in atrial fibrillation if there is also a high venous pressure due to heart failure?

ANS.: a. A high venous pressure due to heart failure implies a poor RV contraction and therefore a poor descent of the base. The poor RV contraction also causes a smaller decrease in intrapericardial pressure, which in turn produces a smaller fall in right atrial pressure during systole.

   b. The right atrium in a patient in heart failure is under increased tension both from excess sympathetic stimulation and from the high pressure in the atrioventricle when the AV valve is open. Thus, the atrium is less compliant than normal and there is an earlier and steeper rise of V wave pressure as it receives its blood from the venae cavae during ventricular systole.

Note: a. Some TR tends to occur in the presence of atrial fibrillation and high venous pressure. This tends to obliterate the X′ descent still more.

   b. The wave that precedes the descent of the base or X′ descent in a patient in atrial fibrillation is the H wave. This supports the concept of naming descents rather than waves because physicians are not accustomed to describing H waves on jugular inspection.

4. How are jugular pulsations affected by atrial flutter?

ANS.: Multiple small A waves may result, one for each F wave, and this can often be recognized by eye since the average rate of flutter F waves is 300 per minute or about 5 per second. Atrial fibrillation F waves are too fast to be seen because they are 400 ± 50 per minute. The F waves of flutter become easier to see if the patient has a large right atrium due to congenital or rheumatic heart disease.

Note: a. The easiest way to recognize that the major descent is a Y descent in the presence of a rapid ventricular rate in atrial fibrillation is to use auscultation. This is because the rate may be too rapid to time with the radial pulse. At rapid rates, a Y descent falls on to the S_1. With rapid rates you may also make use of peaks as well as descents because while with an X′ descent the peak of the jugular movements occur with the S_1, with atrial fibrillation the peak is reached at the time of the S_2.

   b. With slow ventricular rates the dominant Y descent is easily recognized by noting that it occurs with a slight delay after the radial pulse.

5. How may ventricular tachycardia be recognized in the jugular pulse?

ANS.: A regular tachycardia with intermittent cannon A waves; that is, intermittent high jugular pulsations occurring whenever the atrium contracts against a closed tricuspid valve. This implies AV dissociation, which only occurs in about half the patients with VT.

REFERENCES

1. Baigrie RS, et al. The spectrum of right ventricular involvement in inferior wall myocardial infarction. *J Am Coll Cardiol* 1983;16:1396.
2. Burch GE, Giles TD. Theoretic consideration of the post-systolic "dip" of constrictive pericarditis. *Am Heart J* 1973;86:569.
3. Coma-Canella I, Lopez-Sendon J. Ventricular compliance in ischemic right ventricular dysfunction. *Am J Cardiol* 1980;45:555.
4. Constant J. The X prime descent in jugular contours: Nomenclature and recognition. *Am Heart J* 1974;88:372.
5. Coralli RJ, Crawley IS. Hepatic pulsations in constrictive pericarditis. *Am J Cardiol* 1986;58:370.
6. Davison R, Cannon R. Estimation of central venous pressure by examination of jugular veins. *Am Heart J* 1974; 87:279.
7. Dock W. Loud presystolic sounds over the jugular veins. *Am J Med* 1956;20:853.
8. Ducas J, et al. Validity of the hepatojugular reflux as a clinical test for congestive heart failure. *Am J Cardiol* 1983;52:1299.

9. Ewy GA. The abdominojugular test: Technique and hemodynamic correlates. *Ann Intern Med* 1988;109:456.
10. Fisher J, et al. Determinants and clinical significance of jugular venous valve competence. *Circulation* 1982; 65:188.
11. Fukuda N, et al. Phono-, mechano- and echocardiographic studies of patients with funnel chest. *J Cardiol* 1981; 11:161.
12. Gensini GG, et al. Persistent left superior vena cava. *Am J Cardiol* 1959;4:677.
13. Hamosh P, Cohn JN. Mechanism of the hepatojugular reflux test. *Am J Cardiol* 1970;25:100.
14. Hitzig WM. On the mechanism of inspiratory filling of the cervical veins and pulsus paradoxus. *J Mt Sinai Hosp* 1941;8:625.
15. Hoffman E, et al. Law of constant heart volume in humans. *J Am Coll Cardiol* 1987;9:38A.
16. Horwitz S, et al. Clinical diagnosis of persistent left superior vena cava. *Am Heart J* 1973;86:759.
17. Jensen DP, et al. Hemodynamic pattern resembling pericardial constriction after acute inferior infarction. *Am J Cardiol* 1978;42:858.
18. Kesteloot H, Denef B. Value of reference tracings in diagnosis and assessment of constrictive epi- and pericarditis. *Br Heart J* 1970;32:675.
19. Lange RL, et al. Diagnostic signs in compressive cardiac disorders. *Circulation* 1966;33:763.
20. Mackenzie J. *The Study of the Pulse.* London: Pentland, 1902.
21. Matsuhisa M, et al. Right ventricular infarction: Graphic studies of three cases. *J Cardiol* 1979;9:375.
22. Matsuhisa M, et al. Jugular phlebogram in congenital absence of the pericardium. *Am Heart J* 1986;112:1004.
23. Matsuhisa M, et al. Postoperative changes of jugular pulse tracing. *J Cardiol* 1986;6:403.
24. Matthews MD, Hampson J. Hepatojugular reflux. *Lancet* 1958;1:873.
25. McKay IFS, Walker RL. True venous pulse wave. *Nature* 1965;205:1220.
26. Nagel MR, et al. Left-to-right shunt at atrial level after rupture of papillary muscle. *Am Heart J* 1973;86:112.
27. Parikh DN, et al. Determinants and importance of atrial pressure morphology in atrial septal defect. *Br Heart J* 1984;51:473.
28. Pasteur W. Note on a new physical sign of tricuspid regurgitation. *Lancet* 1885;2:524.
29. Ranganathan N, Sivaciyan V. Abnormalities in jugular venous flow velocity in pulmonary hypertension. *Am J Cardiol* 1989;63:719.
30. Saunders DE Jr, et al. Relationship of sternal angle to right atrium in clinical measurement of jugular venous pressure. *J Am Coll Cardiol* 1988;11:89A.
31. Sharpey-Schafer EP. Venous tone. *Br Med J* 1961;2:1589.
32. Sivaciyan F, Ranganathan N. Transcutaneous Doppler jugular venous flow velocity recording. *Circulation* 1978; 57:930.
33. Sleight P. Unilateral elevation of the internal jugular pulse. *Br Heart J* 1962;24:726.
34. Swanton RH, et al. Systolic and diastolic ventricular function in cardiac amyloidosis. *Am J Cardiol* 1977;39:658.
35. Vogel JHK, et al. Left ventricular dysfunction in chronic constrictive pericarditis. *Chest* 1971;59:484.
36. Wood JE. The mechanism of the increased venous pressure with exercise in congestive heart failure. *J Clin Invest* 1962;41:2020.
37. Wood P. Chronic constrictive pericarditis. *Am J Cardiol* 1961;7:48.
38. Zelis R. Contribution of local factors to elevated venous tone of congestive heart failure. *J Clin Invest* 1974; 54:219.

5

Inspection, Palpation, and Auscultation of the Chest

EXAMINATION OF THE CHEST FOR VENTRICULAR ENLARGEMENT

Terminology Problems

1. What is the difference between cardiac enlargement and cardiac hypertrophy?

   ANS.: Cardiac enlargement refers to dilatation or increase in chamber volume with or without proportional hypertrophy; that is, not hypertrophy alone. Pure hypertrophy should *not* be called enlargement because the chamber volume may remain normal or even be encroached upon by the hypertrophied muscle (Fig. 1).

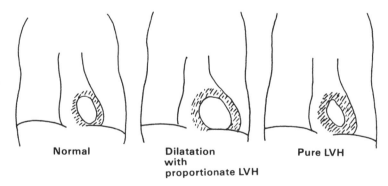

Normal   Dilatation with proportionate LVH   Pure LVH

FIG. 1. Pure LVH causes an encroachment inward on the cavity and has been called "concentric" hypertrophy. Dilatation with proportionate hypertrophy has been called "eccentric" hypertrophy.

2. What is usually meant by the term **apex beat**?

   ANS.: The term was originally meant to refer to the palpable apex of the left ventricle (LV). Unfortunately, in the sitting or supine position, the part of the heart that strikes the chest wall is not necessarily the apex, as seen on an x-ray or by direct examination of the heart. In patients with a large enough right ventricle (RV), an apex beat may be due to movement of the RV. Therefore, the apex beat really means the most lateral palpable ventricular movement or the most lateral cardiac impulse.

   Note: A recoil force produced by the ejection of blood into the aorta in an upward, rightward, and posterior direction thrusts the left ventricle against

94

the chest wall in an inferior leftward and anterior direction. However, the thrust against the chest wall is opposed by the systolic decrease in cardiac volume (Fig. 2).

3. What is meant by the term **point of maximum impulse** (PMI) and what are the term's drawbacks?

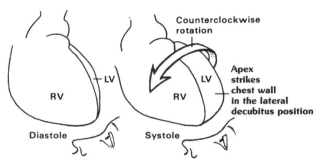

FIG. 2. This counterclockwise rotation occurs during isovulumic contraction; that is, before blood is ejected from the ventricles.

ANS.: The term *PMI* is often used as a synonym for an apex beat. However, it has also been used to mean point of maximum intensity; that is, the site of the loudest murmur. Second, as stated in the pamphlet prepared by Hurst and Schlant for the Committee on Medical Education for the American Heart Association, the term *PMI* should be avoided because the maximum precordial pulsations may be due to such abnormalities as a dilated pulmonary artery, a large RV, a ventricular aneurysm, or an aortic aneurysm. In describing what is thought to be the most lateral cardiac impulse nearest the true apex, the preferable term, even though not perfect, is apex beat (Fig. 3).

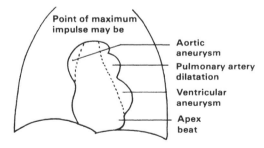

FIG. 3. The point of maximum impulse (PMI) should not be equated with the apical impulse.

Note: An ectopic left ventricular impulse caused by a ventricular aneurysm is most commonly above and medial to the expected location of an apex beat.

THE APEX BEAT

Chest Position to Find the Apex Beat

1. Why is the sitting position with the feet on the bed the best position to establish the site of the normal apex beat?

ANS.: It is the best compromise with the familiar normal apex site on a chest x-ray. In the sitting position the apex beat often becomes more palpable than it does standing, because with the legs on the bed the upward compression by the abdominal contents and diaphragm shifts the apex beat slightly to the left against the chest wall.
Note: The sitting position does not shift the apex beat laterally by any more than 1 cm when compared with the usual standing x-ray.

Palpability of the Apex Beat

1. About how often can you expect to feel an apex beat in normal sitting subjects?
   ANS.: Only in about one out of five adults over age 40 (11). However, in about 90% of children and teenagers, an apex beat is palpable.
   Note: a. An apex beat is much more likely to be palpable in the sitting than in the supine position because in the latter, the heart falls away from the anterior chest wall. In the left lateral decubitus position, however, the apex beat may be palpable in about four out of five older adults, and in most children and young adults. Elevation of the chest to about 30 degrees and various degrees of left lateral rotation may be required to palpate a subtle apex beat.
   b. Obesity does not necessarily make the normal LV impulse impalpable, probably because the heart is physiologically enlarged in obesity. However, if the chest wall is thick and the posteroanterior diameter is increased in a patient over age 50, the mere palpability of an apex impulse may be used as a sign of cardiomegaly.
2. What unusual approach may sometimes help you to feel a subtle apex beat or an unexpectedly posterior axillary line apex beat?
   ANS.: You should establish a routine of palpation from behind as well as from the front. A subtle apex beat may only be perceived when the hand palpates from a quiet immobile area like the back. The anterior chest is often disturbed by left parasternal movements and heart sound vibrations. Also, a frontal approach alone might mislead you into thinking that the movement you palpate on the anterior chest wall is the most lateral impulse when in fact it may be only an RV movement. The true LV apex beat may be missed because it may be near the posterior axillary line.
   Note: The apex beat may come out between the ribs during any phase of respiration.
3. Which part of which hand is best for feeling the faint localized movement of a subtle apex beat (Fig. 4)?
   ANS.: The fingertips or the area just proximal to them seems best for feeling a faint localized movement. Try each hand separately. Some examiners find that the fingers of one hand, usually the left in right-handed physicians, are more sensitive than the fingers of the other.
   Note: It is easy to mistake the vibrations of the first sound for a slight impulse, especially if it is not appreciated that heart sounds may be palpable.

The Normal Site of an Apex Beat

1. What is the disadvantage of using the midclavicular line as the site of the normal apex beat in the sitting position (with the feet on the bed)?
   ANS.: a. Some medical dictionaries equate the midclavicular line with the nipple line, to which it may bear no relation.

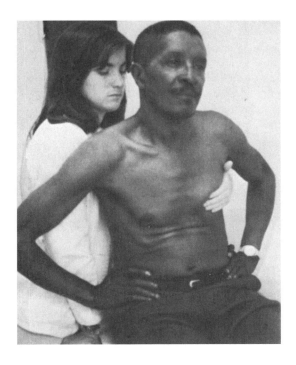

FIG. 4. A posterior in addition to an anterior approach may allow you to feel more subtle movements, especially if your left hand is more sensitive than your right.

    b. The lateral end of the clavicle is often difficult to locate accurately.

    c. There are faster and easier ways of showing whether an apex beat is displaced.

2. What are easier methods for finding the site of the normal apex beat in the sitting position?

    ANS.: a. A normal apex beat should not be more than 10 cm from the midsternal line in adults. In children use method b.

          b. Locate the mid-left thorax and measure the distance of the apex beat from that landmark. If the most lateral impulse is more than 2 cm to the left of the middle of the left hemithorax, cardiomegaly should be suspected. You can quickly find the mid-left thorax by using the method that artists employ to locate the center of any distant object. With your head in front of the left chest, place a horizontally held ruler or pen so that the left end is flush with the midsternal line. Now place your index finger on your ruler at a point that approximates the center of the left hemithorax. Test for accuracy by placing the right end of the ruler where you estimated the center of the left chest to be, and see if your index finger is now in line with the edge of the patient's chest. If it is not, shift your index finger until it is actually in the mid-left thorax; that is, until it is equidistant from the midsternum on the left and the edge of the chest on the right (Fig. 5).

          Note: a. The measurement of 10 cm from the midline is surprisingly useful because more than 10 cm has a good correlation with cardiomegaly even in a large chest. This may be due to the fact that when the chest is large enough for 11 cm to be normal, a ventricular impulse will not likely be palpable in such a chest. If it is palpable at all in a huge chest, cardiomegaly is probably present.

                  b. It is useless to estimate the site of the apex beat in the left lateral decubitus position because of variations in mediastinal mobility.

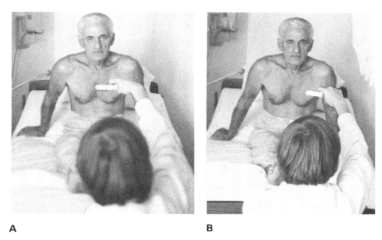

FIG. 5. A: The left edge of a tongue depressor is on the midsternal line while the forefinger marks off an estimated site of the mid-left thorax. **B:** The left edge of the tongue depressor is now on the estimated site of the mid-left thorax. If the left edge is really in the center of the left chest, the forefinger will be in a line with the edge of the left chest, as shown here.

     c. Stating the interspace in which the apex beat is present is of no value for two reasons.
       1. The ribs curve downward as they sweep forward from behind, so the interspace in the anterior axillary line is at a higher horizontal level than at the parasternal line.
       2. When the heart enlarges, it enlarges mostly in the X axis and very little in the Y axis.
     d. An apex beat that is displaced to the left does not necessarily indicate an increase in LV volume. This is because an apex beat may be displaced by marked left ventricular hypertrophy (LVH), as in a hypertrophic cardiomyopathy with a normal volume, as well as by a large left atrium (as in mitral stenosis), which can displace the LV laterally.

3. Why is chest percussion for cardiac size not employed by most cardiologists?

  ANS.: a. A palpable ventricular apical impulse indicates the heart size more quickly. When a ventricular impulse is not palpable because of a thick chest or overaeration due to pulmonary disease, percussion is most unreliable (i.e., when percussion is most needed, it is of least help).

     b. Dressler, who devoted 20 pages of his textbook on clinical cardiology to percussion, begins by stating that he finds it impossible to percuss cardiac borders (1). (His 20 pages are devoted to a system for defining "areas of cardiac dullness," which gave him information concerning specific chamber enlargements.)

     Note: A recent study that concluded percussion dullness in the fifth left interspace is better than palpation of the apex beat had several flaws (6).

       a. It did not palpate for the apex beat in the sitting position but only in the supine position. In this position most apex beats are not palpable unless the heart is enlarged.

       b. Patients with chronic obstructive pulmonary disease (COPD), increased chest diameter, low diaphragms, and those who did not take a deep breath for their x-rays were eliminated from the study.

    c. About 30% of patients were false-positives.

    d. The apex beat in the left lateral decubitus position was not used to look for signs of cardiomegaly.

CARDIAC DILATATION SIGNS IN THE LEFT LATERAL DECUBITUS POSITION

1. With the patient in the left lateral decubitus position, how can you tell that you are feeling a left or right ventricular apical impulse?

    ANS.: There are two methods.

        a. In the left lateral decubitus position an LV impulse often feels as if a ping-pong ball were protruding between the ribs in systole (sometimes called a left ventricular thrust). An RV impulse is usually more diffuse.

        b. Look for medial or lateral retraction. An LV impulse manifests medial retraction because the counterclockwise rotation of the heart during systole causes the medial aspect of the heart to withdraw from the chest wall and pull on any overlying chest wall structures, including the skin. The skin movement is best detected by observing the skin while palpating the apex beat. A mark on the skin made by a pen may aid in seeing slight medial retraction. A large RV often manifests lateral retraction (see p. 102 for explanation) (Fig. 6).

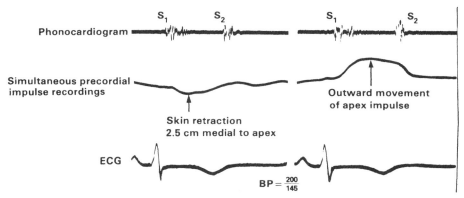

FIG. 6. Note the retraction medial to the apex that shows a sustained impulse due to the effect of LVH. Although these tracings were taken in the supine position, medial retraction is best seen in the left lateral decubitus position.

2. How can you tell that there is cardiac enlargement with the patient in the left lateral decubitus position?

    ANS.: Look for

        a. An enlarged area of apical impulse in the *Y* axis. An apical impulse should not be felt in more than one interspace (Fig. 7).

        b. An enlarged area of apical impulse in the *X* axis. An apical impulse should be no more than 3 cm from side to side (about 2 fingerbreadths) (2). This may not necessarily mean an increase in volume but may represent only hypertrophy (Fig. 8).

        c. An enlarged area of medial retraction. The normal area of medial retraction is not much larger than that of the normal apex beat.

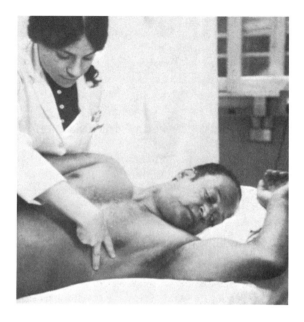

FIG. 7. The normal apex beat is not felt through two interspaces during the same phase of respiration.

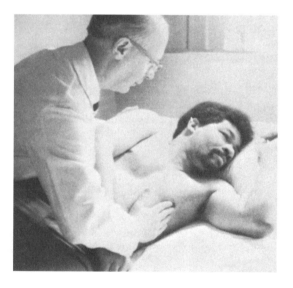

FIG. 8. A normal apical impulse is no larger than about 1.5 fingertip widths.

    d. The presence of a combination of both medial and lateral retraction. If the medial retraction is dominant, you are probably feeling a large LV. If the lateral retraction is dominant, a large RV is probably producing the apical impulse.

    e. A biventricular overload, as in a large ventricular septal defect (VSD), may be manifest on the chest wall as a biventricular rock; that is, both the left parasternal and apical areas may rise with systole with an area of retraction between them.

3. What cardiac diagnoses tend to be ruled out by the presence of a palpable LV impulse?

    ANS.: a. Any abnormality that causes a dilated RV without concomitant dilatation of the LV. For example, secundum-type atrial septal defects (ASDs) and primary pulmonary hypertension should not be readily diagnosed if an LV apex beat is found.

Note: a. In endocardial cushion defects there may be severe mitral regurgitation (MR) that enlarges the LV. Therefore, this type of ASD may be suggested by identifying an LV impulse.

   b. An LV impulse may occasionally be palpable in secundum ASDs even though the LV is often smaller than normal in patients with ASD. The reason is unknown, but this may be due to the exaggerated counter-clockwise rotation that occurs in ASDs.

b. The presence of a palpable LV apical impulse rules out any abnormality that causes pure right ventricular hypertrophy (RVH), such as pure pulmonary stenosis (PS). This is because a hypertrophied RV tends to rotate the heart clockwise (seen from below). This rotation places the LV more posteriorly, so that even if the RV is merely hypertrophied and not dilated, the LV is still usually not palpable.

Note: In severe PS with a marked right-to-left shunt through an intraatrial communication (ASD or patent foramen ovale), the LV may enlarge enough to become palpable in the left lateral decubitus position.

CAUSES OF A DISPLACED LEFT VENTRICULAR IMPULSE

1. Does left ventricular hypertrophy (LVH) displace the LV impulse to the left?

   ANS.: Not unless there is marked hypertrophic cardiomyopathy. Otherwise, there must be dilatation as well as LVH to displace an LV impulse. Pure LVH tends to encroach on the ventricular cavity by growing inward as much as outward. (Even if an LV free wall doubled its thickness from 1 to 2 cm, which would happen only with severe hypertrophy, and did not encroach on the volume, the border of the heart should not extend laterally more than 1 cm beyond normal.)

   Note: Dilatation without some hypertrophy of a ventricle is very rare. If a ventricle is dilated for a long enough period of time, it nearly always shows proportionate hypertrophy in obedience to Laplace's law, which states that pressure is proportional to tension and inversely proportional to radius or volume. This means that the larger the volume, the greater must be the wall tension to maintain pressure. The need for tension seems to stimulate hypertrophy, which in turn supplies the necessary tension. Laplace's law has been rewritten to bring hypertrophy into the equation

   $$T = \frac{(P \times R^4)}{2H}$$

   where T = tension, P = pressure, R = radius, and H = wall thickness.

   This shows that the greater the hypertrophy, the less the tension.

2. What kind of cardiac malposition besides dextrocardia will cause a ventricular impulse to be palpable on the right chest?

   ANS.: Dextroversion (see p. 102 for definition).

   Note: To confirm the presence of mirror-image dextrocardia by physical examination, percuss for a stomach bubble to reveal tympany on the right. To confirm dextroversion by physical examination, palpate for the aortic pulsations in the second right interspace. They may be present here because

of the anterior position of the aorta caused by the rotation of the LV anteriorly.

3. What can displace an LV impulse to the left in the absence of a large ventricle?
  ANS.: a. A marked pectus excavatum.
      b. Congenital complete absence of the pericardium.
      c. A large left atrium as in mitral stenosis can push the LV laterally.

Malpositions of the Heart (Abnormal Placement of Cardiac Chambers)

The three most common cardiac malpositions are situs inversus, dextroversion, and levoversion. **Situs solitus** (**solitus** means "usual") is the term used to denote a normal position of all chambers and vessels of the heart, and when used alone it implies that the viscera are also normally placed. It specifically means that the descending aorta, left atrium,
cardiac apex, and stomach are all on the left.

1. **Situs inversus:** The descending aorta, left atrium, apex, and stomach are all on the right.
  This is also known as mirror-image dextrocardia. *Dextrocardia* alone means that the
  heart and aorta are on the right, as in situs inversus, but the stomach is on the left; that is,
  there is a discordance between the heart and the gut.

2. **Dextroversion:** The aorta and stomach are situated as in situs solitus, but the heart is rotated so that the apex is on the right.

3. **Levoversion:** The aorta and stomach are in the same place as in dextrocardia, but the
  heart is rotated so that the apex is on the left. The term **levocardia** has been used to refer
  to situs solitus of the heart, but with the viscera inverted (stomach on the right).
  Dextrocardia and levocardia are almost always associated with other congenital abnormalities.
  Note: Kartagener syndrome is situs inversus with sinusitis and bronchiectasis.

RIGHT VENTRICULAR ENLARGEMENT

1. How can you best palpate for movement caused by a large RV?
  ANS.: a. Since the RV is an anterior structure, its enlargement may produce an increased
      left parasternal movement. Diffuse left parasternal movements are often best
      palpated with the proximal part (heel) of the palm. The shoulder becomes the
      fulcrum and this amplifies the hand movements that are at the end of the arm
      lever. Left parasternal pressure should be applied during held expiration (Fig. 9).
      b. Test for systolic downward movements of the RV in the epigastrium. If you
      place the pad of your right thumb pointing upward just below the xiphoid pro-
      cess, an impulse striking your thumb pad is usually due to a large RV. The
      downward impulse may be only palpable at the end of a deep, held inspiration
      with the chest at a 30- to 45-degree angle (Fig. 10).
      Note: a. Occasionally, the movement of a dilated pulmonary artery in the sec-
          ond left interspace imparts movement to the overlying skin even
          though it is impalpable. With the patient sitting and leaning forward,
          press firmly with one or two fingers over the second left interspace.
          Localized movements are best felt with the tips of the fingers. The de-
          gree of pulmonary artery dilatation that will cause a visible or palpa-
          ble movement is usually seen only with the dilated pulmonary artery
          caused by severe primary pulmonary hypertension or by volume over-
          loads, such as with ASD.

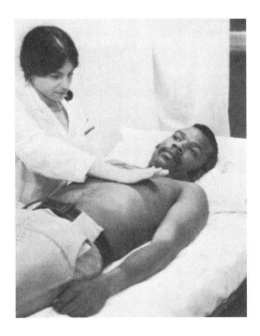

FIG. 9. In this patient with MS, the physician is palpating the movement of a large RV, which was producing a right ventricular rock; that is, a sustained left parasternal impulse and lateral retraction.

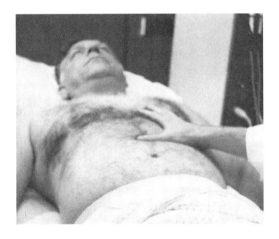

FIG. 10. If your fingernails are long enough to cause discomfort if you push up into the epigastrium, you can use the pad of your thumb to test for RV pulsations during a held deep inspiration.

You may also employ several fingers applied simultaneously and in parallel in the third, fourth, and fifth parasternal intercostal interspaces during held expiration. This can localize right ventricular systolic movements to the inflow portion (fourth and fifth intercostal interspaces) or to the outflow portion or infundibulum (third interspace).

When applied to a patient with tetralogy of Fallot, the right ventricular impulse may be confined to the fourth and fifth interspace and absent in the third interspace. This is because the infundibular stenosis relegates the elevated RV systolic pressure to the body or inflow portion of the chamber. An impulse in the third interspace as well as in the two lower interspaces suggests that the outflow tract also has a high pressure in it as in pulmonary valve stenosis or pulmonary hypertension.

b. Although the systolic left-to-right shunt in VSDs cannot enlarge the RV, VSDs with large left-to-right shunts can increase right ventricular end-diastolic volume up to 2.5 times normal because of significant shunting during isovolumic relaxation.

2. How can you diagnose the presence of a large RV in the left lateral decubitus position?
   ANS.: Look for dominant lateral retraction (Fig. 11).

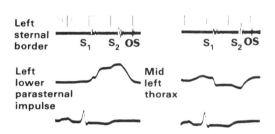

FIG. 11. A sustained left parasternal impulse with lateral retraction is a sign of a volume overload of the RV (and probably also of a pressure overload).

    Note: a. The lateral retraction seen with severe tricuspid regurgitation (TR) has been explained by two phenomena. First, there is an abnormally large inward movement of the apical region, which is formed by the dilated RV. Added to this is the simultaneous anterior thrust of the RV against the left parasternal area caused by the ballistic recoil response of the RV as it ejects its blood through the incompetent tricuspid valve.

    b. If the TR is severe, the anterior left parasternal movement together with the apical retraction creates a rocking motion that has been called a right ventricular rock. Sometimes the entire right precordium may expand during systole due to the expanding right atrium, while the entire left precordium, including the parasternal area, retracts, probably because the RV, like an overdistended balloon in diastole, empties during systole and may draw in the entire left parasternal area and even the entire left chest.

3. When will the most lateral ventricular impulse retract deeply in systole without the initial outward movement that is seen in RV overload?
   ANS.: In constrictive pericarditis. The systolic apical retraction is usually followed by a diastolic out-thrust. The outward impulse at the apex is diastolic. It is not systolic as is seen in the usual apex beat. Although retraction is maximal at the apex, it may extend medially to the left sternal border (Fig. 12).

4. What is the normal chest movement caused by the right ventricle at the left sternal border?
   ANS.: A small initial, almost impalpable outward movement, followed by a brief retraction of small amplitude finishing well before the second sound.

5. What movement is felt at the left parasternal area in patients with an atrial septal defect?
   ANS.: A dilated right ventricle with a volume overload but good function as in atrial septal defect will have a very-short-duration initial outward movement, followed by a prolonged deep-amplitude pansystolic retraction that ends at the S_2.

6. How does the left parasternal impulse caused by the RVH of pulmonary stenosis (PS) or pulmonary hypertension differ from normal?

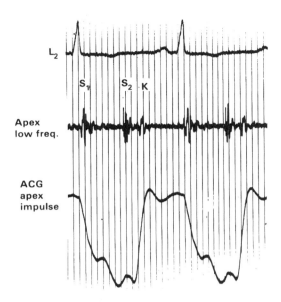

FIG. 12. Apex cardiogram and phonocardiogram of a 25-year-old man with constrictive pericarditis due to uremic pericarditis and hemopericardium. Note the early S_3 or pericardial knock (K), the systolic apical retraction, and the diastolic outward movement.

ANS.: It is a systolic outward movement with the peak in early or middle systole.
    a. The site of maximum RV impulse in patients with PS is often a few centimeters away from the parasternal area and may even be in the mid-left thorax.
    b. In valvular PS the parasternal impulse may be at the third left interspace, whereas in infundibular stenosis the impulse is confined to the fourth or fifth interspace.

7. What is the significance of feeling the impulse of a dilated pulmonary artery in the second left interspace in a patient with RVH?

ANS.: A palpable pulmonary artery movement is usually associated with a dilated RV, as in ASD or primary pulmonary hypertension.

8. What is the significance of a fixed anterior left chest bulge as seen from the front of the bed?

ANS.: You should suspect an ASD with pulmonary hypertension, because here the left chest bulge is presumably due to the occurrence in infancy of a large shunt with hyperkinetic pulmonary hypertension. The large hyperactive and hypertrophied RV under high pressure can push the left chest forward as the skeleton is developing. The RV never enlarges to the right on chest x-rays (e.g., the right border of the heart with no congenital malpositions is never due to the RV, no matter how large it becomes). Therefore, RV enlargement does not affect the right anterior chest but instead causes a left precordial bulge.

    Note: A large VSD with pulmonary hypertension due to increased flow in the lungs (hyperkinetic pulmonary hypertension) can cause a bulging sternum with an increased anteroposterior diameter of both sides of the chest.

LEFT-SIDED CAUSES OF LEFT PARASTERNAL MOVEMENT

1. When is mid-to-lower-left parasternal movement due to the LV?

ANS.: In young subjects with long, thin chests, the apex beat is medial. When the LV is

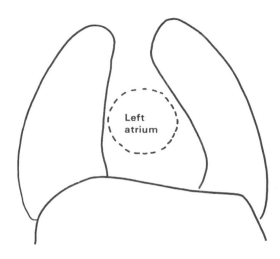

FIG. 13. The "left" atrium is really a posterosuperior atrium, since it is behind and above the right atrium. Although it is slightly to the left of the right atrium, the left atrium is a midline structure.

markedly enlarged and in the presence of a ventricular aneurysm, the left parasternal movement may be from an LV, in which case it is sustained; that is, with a late peak.

2. When is the left parasternal outward movement due to a large left atrium? Why?

   ANS.: In severe chronic MR. The left atrium is a midchest structure; that is, it is not really a left atrium but a posterior atrium (Figs. 13 and 14).

3. How can you tell whether or not an expanding left atrium due to severe chronic MR is the cause of a marked left parasternal movement?

   ANS.: Compare the LV apical movement with the left parasternal movement by placing a finger on each. A left atrial lift begins and ends slightly later than the LV thrust. The systolic impulse begins late, presumably because the LV must first contract

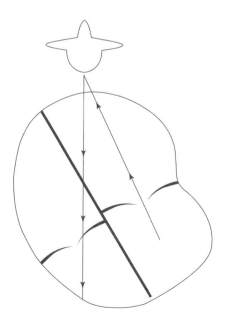

FIG. 14. Mitral regurgitation imparts a systolic thrust from the left ventricle to the left atrium and produces a ricochet-like effect off the spine, with a subsequent systolic anterior motion palpable at the left parasternal area.

and provide the regurgitant volume that expands the left atrium, which, in turn, pushes the RV forward. Primary RV movement begins and ends at the same time or even before the LV (Fig. 15).

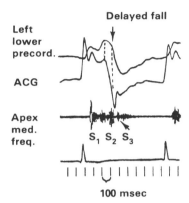

FIG. 15. The left lower parasternal area movement shows a delayed rise and fall in comparison with the apical impulse in this patient with severe chronic rheumatic MR.

4. How can the ventricular septum cause a forward displacement of the RV?
    ANS.: Dyskinetic motion of the ventricular septum during angina may displace the RV forward and result in a transient left parasternal impulse that disappears promptly with the relief of the angina. Postinfarction dyskinesis of the septum can cause a persistent anterior displacement of the RV. Thus, any paradoxical septal motion has the possibility of imparting a forward motion to the RV against the sternum.

X-RAY EVALUATION OF CARDIAC SIZE

1. How is determination of cardiac size by x-ray usually calculated?
    ANS.: By cardiothoracic (C/T) ratios. Fifty percent is considered by most radiologists to be the upper limit of normal. However, in one study on normal subjects, 2% of Caucasians, 4% of Asians, and 9% of African-Americans had C/T ratios of more than 50% (10).
2. How can we overcome the falsely normal C/T ratios in subjects who are short and underweight, or the falsely high C/T ratios in subjects who are overweight?
    ANS.: By use of the height and weight tables of Ungerleider and Clark (Table 1).
3. How can you measure cardiac volume to derive a more accurate cardiac size than any other x-ray method?
    ANS.: The cardiac volume uses the lateral chest film and body surface area. The length dimension (L) is measured in centimeters from the junction of the superior vena cava and right atrium to the cardiac apex. The broad diameter (B) is measured from the junction of the right atrium and diaphragm to the junction of the pulmonary

TABLE 1.

Theoretical transverse diameters of heart for various heights and weights

Height

5'0"	1"	2"	3"	4"	5"	6"	7"	8"	9"	10"	11"	6'0"	1"	2"	3"	4"	5"	6"
83	85	86	87	89	90	92												
85	86	88	89	91	92	93	95											
87	88	90	91	92	94	95	97											
88	90	92	93	94	96	97	99	100										
90	92	93	95	96	98	99	101	102										
92	93	95	96	98	99	101	103	104	106									
94	95	97	98	100	101	103	104	106	108									
95	97	99	100	102	103	105	106	108	110	111								
97	99	100	102	104	105	107	108	110	112	113								
99	101	102	104	106	107	109	110	112	114	115	117							
101	102	104	106	108	109	111	113	114	116	118	119	121						
103	104	106	108	109	111	113	115	116	118	120	121	123	125					
105	106	108	110	111	113	115	117	118	120	122	124	125	127	129				
106	108	110	112	113	115	117	119	121	123	124	126	128	129	131	133			
108	110	112	114	115	117	119	121	123	125	126	128	130	132	133	135	137		
110	112	114	116	117	119	121	123	125	127	129	130	132	134	136	138	140	141	
112	114	116	118	120	121	123	125	127	129	131	133	134	136	138	140	142	144	146
114	116	118	120	122	124	125	127	129	131	133	135	137	139	141	143	144	146	148
116	118	120	122	124	126	128	129	131	133	135	137	139	141	143	145	147	149	151
118	120	122	124	126	128	130	132	134	136	138	140	142	143	145	147	149	151	153
120	122	124	126	128	130	132	134	136	138	140	142	144	146	148	150	152	154	156
122	124	126	128	130	132	134	136	138	140	142	144	146	148	150	152	154	156	159
124	126	128	130	132	134	136	138	140	143	145	147	149	151	153	155	157	159	161
126	128	130	132	134	136	139	141	143	145	147	149	151	153	155	157	160	162	164
128	130	132	134	137	139	141	143	145	147	149	152	154	156	158	160	162	164	166
130	132	134	137	139	141	143	145	147	150	152	154	156	158	160	163	165	167	169
132	134	137	139	141	143	145	148	150	152	154	156	159	161	163	165	167	170	172
134	137	139	141	143	146	148	150	152	154	157	159	161	163	166	168	170	172	175
136	139	141	143	146	148	150	152	155	157	159	161	164	166	168	171	173	175	177
139	141	143	146	148	150	152	155	157	159	162	164	166	169	171	173	176	178	180
141	143	145	148	150	152	155	157	160	162	164	167	169	171	174	176	178	181	183
143	145	148	150	152	155	157	160	162	164	167	169	172	174	176	179	181	183	186
145	148	150	152	155	157	160	162	164	167	169	172	174	177	179	181	184	186	189
147	150	152	155	157	160	162	165	167	169	172	174	177	179	182	184	187	189	192
150	152	155	157	160	162	164	167	169	172	174	177	179	182	184	187	189	192	194
152	154	157	159	162	164	167	169	172	175	177	180	182	185	187	190	192	195	197
154	157	159	162	164	167	169	172	175	177	180	182	185	187	190	193	195	198	200
156	159	162	164	167	169	172	175	177	180	182	185	188	190	193	195	198	201	203
159	161	164	167	169	172	174	177	180	182	185	188	190	193	196	198	201	204	206
161	164	166	169	172	174	177	180	182	185	188	190	193	196	198	201	204	206	209
163	166	169	171	174	177	180	182	185	188	190	193	196	199	201	204	207	209	212
166	168	171	174	177	179	182	185	188	190	193	196	199	201	204	207	210	212	215
168	171	174	176	179	182	185	188	190	193	196	199	202	204	207	210	213	216	218
170	173	176	179	182	184	187	190	193	196	199	202	204	207	210	213	216	219	221
173	176	178	181	184	187	190	193	196	199	201	204	207	210	213	216	219	222	224
175	178	181	184	187	190	193	196	198	201	204	207	210	213	216	219	222	225	228
178	180	183	186	189	192	195	198	201	204	207	210	213	216	219	222	225	228	231
180	183	186	189	192	195	198	201	204	207	210	213	216	219	222	225	228	231	234
182	185	188	192	195	198	201	204	207	210	213	216	219	222	225	228	231	234	237
185	188	191	194	197	200	203	206	210	213	216	219	222	225	228	231	234	237	240
187	191	194	197	200	203	206	209	212	215	219	222	225	228	231	234	237	240	243
190	193	196	199	203	206	209	212	215	218	222	225	228	231	234	237	241	244	247
192	196	199	202	205	208	212	215	218	221	224	228	231	234	237	241	244	247	250
195	198	201	205	208	211	214	218	221	224	227	231	234	237	240	244	247	250	253
198	201	204	207	211	214	217	221	224	227	230	234	237	240	244	247	250	253	257
200	203	207	210	213	217	220	224	227	230	233	237	240	243	247	250	253	257	260
	206	210	213	216	220	223	227	230	233	236	240	243	247	250	254	257	260	264
			216	219	222	226	229	233	236	239	243	246	250	253	257	260	263	267
					225	229	232	236	239	243	246	249	253	256	260	263	267	270
							235	239	242	246	249	253	256	260	263	267	270	279
									245	249	252	256	259	263	266	270	274	277
											255	259	263	266	270	273	277	281
											259	262	266	270	273	277	280	284
													269	273	277	280	284	288
													273	276	280	284	287	291

Weight

Table for determining percent deviation from average

% Minus (−)						% Plus (+)				
25	20	15	10	5		5	10	15	20	25
75	80	85	90	95	**100**	105	110	115	120	125
76	81	86	91	96	**101**	106	111	116	121	126
77	82	87	92	97	**102**	107	112	117	122	128
77	82	88	93	98	**103**	108	113	118	124	129
78	83	88	94	99	**104**	109	114	120	125	130
79	84	89	95	100	**105**	110	116	121	126	131
80	85	90	95	101	**106**	111	117	122	127	133
80	86	91	96	102	**107**	112	118	123	128	134
81	86	92	97	103	**108**	113	119	124	130	135
82	87	93	98	104	**109**	114	120	125	131	136
83	88	94	99	105	**110**	116	121	127	132	138
83	89	94	100	105	**111**	117	122	128	133	139
84	90	95	101	106	**112**	118	123	129	134	140
85	90	96	102	107	**113**	119	124	130	136	141
86	91	97	103	108	**114**	120	125	131	137	143
86	92	98	104	109	**115**	121	127	132	138	144
87	93	99	104	110	**116**	122	128	133	139	145
88	94	99	105	111	**117**	123	129	135	140	146
89	94	100	106	112	**118**	124	130	136	142	148
89	95	101	107	113	**119**	125	131	137	143	149
90	96	102	108	114	**120**	126	132	138	144	150
91	97	103	109	115	**121**	127	133	139	145	151
92	98	104	110	116	**122**	128	134	140	146	153
92	98	105	111	117	**123**	129	135	141	148	154
93	99	105	112	118	**124**	130	136	143	149	155
94	100	106	113	119	**125**	131	138	144	150	156
95	101	107	113	120	**126**	132	139	145	151	158
95	102	108	114	121	**127**	133	140	146	152	159
96	102	109	115	122	**128**	134	141	147	154	160
97	103	110	116	123	**129**	135	142	148	155	161
98	104	111	117	124	**130**	137	143	150	156	163
98	105	111	118	124	**131**	138	144	151	157	164
99	106	112	119	125	**132**	139	145	152	158	165
100	106	113	120	126	**133**	140	146	153	160	166
101	107	114	121	127	**134**	141	147	154	161	168
101	108	115	122	128	**135**	142	149	155	162	169
102	109	116	122	129	**136**	143	150	156	163	170
103	110	116	123	130	**137**	144	151	158	164	171
104	110	117	124	131	**138**	145	152	159	166	173
104	111	118	125	132	**139**	146	153	160	167	174
105	112	119	126	133	**140**	147	154	161	168	175
106	113	120	127	134	**141**	148	155	162	169	176
107	114	121	128	135	**142**	149	156	163	170	178
107	114	122	129	136	**143**	150	157	164	172	179
108	115	122	130	137	**144**	151	158	166	173	180
109	116	123	131	138	**145**	152	160	167	174	181
110	117	124	131	139	**146**	153	161	168	175	183
110	118	125	132	140	**147**	154	162	169	176	184
111	118	126	133	141	**148**	155	163	170	178	185
112	119	127	134	142	**149**	156	164	171	179	186
113	120	128	135	143	**150**	158	165	173	180	188
113	121	128	136	143	**151**	159	166	174	181	189
114	122	129	137	144	**152**	160	167	175	182	190
115	122	130	138	145	**153**	161	168	176	184	191
116	123	131	139	146	**154**	162	169	177	185	193
116	124	132	140	147	**155**	163	171	178	186	194
117	125	133	140	148	**156**	164	172	179	187	195
118	126	133	141	149	**157**	165	173	181	188	196
119	126	134	142	150	**158**	166	174	182	190	198
119	127	135	143	151	**159**	167	175	183	191	199
120	128	136	144	152	**160**	168	176	184	192	200
121	129	137	145	153	**161**	169	177	185	193	201
122	130	138	146	154	**162**	170	178	186	194	203
122	130	139	147	155	**163**	171	179	187	196	204
123	131	139	148	156	**164**	172	180	189	197	205
Actual					**Predicted diameter (mm)**	Actual				

The heart is usually enlarged if the width is 10% greater than the average prediction shown in the boldface column on the right. Since this table was derived from thousands of male insurance applicants, subtract 8 mm for women (personal communication from Dr. H. E. Ungerleider). Instead of the table, one may use the formula (weight/height × 25) + 70 (for males), or + 62 (for females).

artery and left atrial appendage. The lateral dimension (*D*) is the greatest horizontal cardiac lateral diameter.

$$\text{Cardiac volume} = \frac{L \times B \times D}{\text{BSA}} \times 0.42$$

where BSA = body surface area and 0.42 is the correction factor for a 6-ft (1.8-m) distance of the heart from the film (Fig. 16).

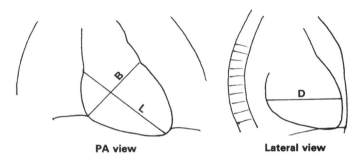

PA view   **Lateral view**

FIG. 16. PA and lateral views.

Note: The total cardiac volume is relatively fixed throughout the cardiac cycle because the atrial and ventricular volumes change reciprocally; that is, when the ventricles are filling in diastole, the atria are emptying. The lateral film takes left atrial volume changes into account.

EXAMINATION OF THE PRECORDIUM FOR VENTRICULAR HYPERTROPHY

Terminology Problems

1. What are the differences between the terms cardiac hypertrophy, dilatation, and enlargement?

   ANS.: The term **hypertrophy** refers to the thickening of the ventricular chamber. **Dilatation** refers to an increase in chamber volume. Although the term **enlargement** refers to hypertrophy and/or dilatation, it is best used as a synonym for dilatation.

2. What is meant by concentric versus eccentric hypertrophy?

   ANS.: **Concentric hypertrophy** refers to uniform hypertrophy of the ventricle and is usually used when there is pure hypertrophy without dilatation. The opposite of concentric used to be eccentric hypertrophy, which unfortunately, has many meanings. **Eccentric hypertrophy** suggests that the ventricle is eccentrically hypertrophied, but this is not at all its meaning. It has been applied to hearts with asymmetric septal hypertrophy, to dilated hearts that shifted the center eccentrically in the left, and to dilated hearts in which the hypertrophy was not proportional to the degree of dilatation. It should be apparent that the term *eccentric* hypertrophy should be avoided.

The Left Ventricular Impulse in Left Ventricular Hypertrophy

1. How can you establish by palpation that an LV apex beat is normal; that is, that there is no hypertrophy, dilatation, or loss of compliance?

   ANS.: In the supine and left lateral decubitus position the normal apex beat rises in systole and falls away rapidly to reach the S_2 at the bottom of the fall or even before the last one-third of systole. This is not a visual phenomenon, so compare only what you hear with what you *feel* (Fig. 17).

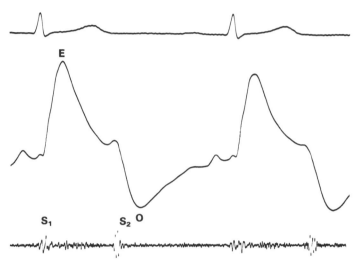

FIG. 17. This depicts a normal apex impulse (apex cardiogram, or ACG) recorded over the apex beat with the subject in the left lateral decubitus position. The fingers feel the E-O slope as a purely systolic retraction. The S_2-O portion of the slope is so short and rapid that the O nadir is perceived as ending at the S_2. The end-systolic hump of the ACG is not perceived by palpation as interrupting the E-O slope.

   Note: The O point is the nadir of the apex cardiogram (ACG) isovolumic relaxation phase. The letter *O* refers to opening of the mitral valve. However, the O point is actually slightly delayed with respect to mitral valve opening and is synchronous with the nadir of the LV pressure trace.

2. What is meant by a sustained apex beat?

   ANS.: It is one that remains outward throughout systole and begins to fall away only with the second heart sound. This is usually detected with the patient in the left lateral decubitus position (Fig. 18).

3. What is the significance of a sustained apex beat?

   ANS.: a. It may be due to a ventricular aneurysm involving the apex.

   b. It may be due to a complete absence of pericardium. (The apex beat in this case is displaced into the axilla.)

   c. In the presence of hypertrophic cardiomyopathy it may merely mean that there is severe LVH. In the absence of severe LVH, a sustained apex beat suggests a decrease in ejection fraction (13).

   Note: With mild to moderate aortic regurgitation (AR), the impulse may be overactive, but it falls to its lowest level before the S_2. When the AR is

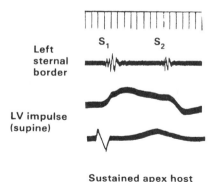

Left sternal border

LV impulse (supine)

Sustained apex host

FIG. 18. If you imagine a sound shortly after the S_2, the sustained apex beat will seem to fall onto it rather than onto the S_2.

moderately severe or severe, proportionate hypertrophy causes the apex beat to be sustained.

The A Wave or Palpable Atrial Hump

1. How does the cineangiogram show the effect of a contracting atrium on the ventricle?
   ANS.: When contrast material is injected into the LV, a cineangiogram can show that the LV suddenly expands at the end of diastole in response to atrial contraction.
2. When is this end-diastolic or presystolic expansion of the LV palpable?
   ANS.: It is normally not palpable. Only a very strong left atrial contraction can expand the LV with enough force to cause a palpable presystolic A wave or hump on the LV impulse.
      Note: a. If the A wave is too close to the outward movement of the ventricular contraction, it may be impalpable even if it is very high. This can be caused by a short PR interval (Fig. 19).

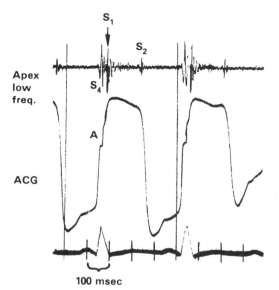

Apex low freq.

ACG

100 msec

FIG. 19. A short PR of about 80 msec due to a preexcitation abnormality has caused this high A wave (A) to be too close to the outward ventricular movement to be palpable.

b. In patients with normal systolic but impaired diastolic function, as in hypertension or hypertrophic cardiomyopathy, the A wave is not only high but sharp and so is more likely to be palpable and associated with an easily heard S_4 than is the rounded A wave in patients with a dominantly decreased systolic function (5).

3. What is the cause of a left atrial contraction strong enough to make a presystolic hump or A wave?

ANS.: Severe loss of LV compliance.

Note: The strong atrial contraction effect on the LV is often called the "atrial kick" or booster-pump effect because the stretch of the LV just before its contraction produces a Starling effect.

4. How does the left atrium "get the message" to contract harder when the LV is stiffer?

ANS.: In diastole, the mitral valve is open and the atrium and ventricle are in continuity; that is, they are, in effect, an "atrioventricle." When the ventricle is stiff, the atrioventricle is also stiff, and when blood pours into a stiff chamber, the pressure rises steeply. If the atrium is under high pressure at the end of diastole, then, due to the Starling effect, it contracts more strongly. Eventually, the atrium itself hypertrophies in response to its continued strong contractions and then contributes to the stiffness of the atrioventricle (Fig. 20).

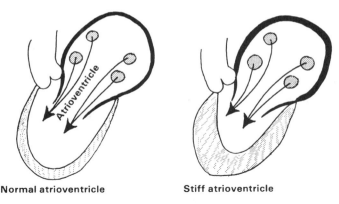

Normal atrioventricle   **Stiff atrioventricle**

FIG. 20. A stiff ventricle must be transmitting its loss of compliance to the atrium during diastole when the AV valves open.

Note: a. The most common cause of chronic increased stiffness of the LV is LVH secondary to hypertension. The next most common cause is LVH secondary to coronary disease (i.e., the confluent patchy areas of fibrosis or infarction plus the tendency to hypertrophy of the remaining healthy myocardium can cause a stiff LV).

b. A palpable A wave tells nothing about left ventricular function; that is, the ejection fraction may still be normal (13).

5. Which type of aortic stenosis (AS) is most likely to produce a palpable atrial presystolic hump (A wave) at the site of the LV impulse?

ANS.: Hypertrophic subaortic stenosis (HSS) or hypertrophic obstructive cardiomyopathy (HOCM), in which the septum is disproportionately hypertrophied in comparison with the free wall. Perhaps HOCM tends to produce a palpable atrial hump because, although the extremely thick septum causes a marked loss of compliance, the resulting strong atrial contraction can easily expand the rest of the LV, which is not nearly as thick as the septum that caused the strong atrial contraction in the first place. In valvular AS the entire LV is equally hypertrophied and therefore resists the expansion of a left atrial contraction.

> *Note*: A palpable atrial hump or A wave in the presence of valvular AS is strongly correlated with a gradient of at least 75 mm Hg in patients without angina or a history of infarction (3). In HOCM no such correlation can be made. A palpable A wave in the presence of valvular AS is unusual enough to point to suspicion of the addition of HOCM (7).

6. Why is it especially important to palpate for an A wave in AS?

   ANS.: The S_4 may be inaudible, or the S_4 may be mistaken for an S_1, and the murmur that follows may be thought to be midsystolic. You may be able to palpate an A wave but not hear an S_4 because the frequency of vibrations may be too low for audibility but not for palpation.

   > *Note*: a. The palpable A wave that is not associated with an auscultatory S_4 is usually a rounded A wave on an apical impulse picture (apex cardiogram), and this is usually found in patients who have cardiomyopathies that are not hypertrophic.
   >
   > b. An A wave tells you that there is no concomitant mitral stenosis (MS) because MS will not permit a large enough atrial hump to be palpable.

7. What does an atrial "kick" feel like to the palpating fingers?

   ANS.: When it is strong and far from the ventricular outward movement, it feels like a double outward movement. When it is slight or close to the ventricular outward movement, it feels like a notch or vibration on the apical upstroke (Fig. 21).

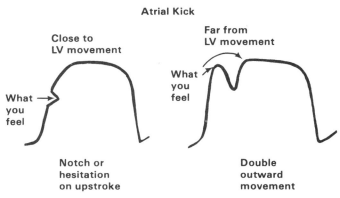

FIG. 21. If only a notch or slight hesitation is present on the upstroke, the tips of the fingers must be used to perceive it. If a large double movement is felt, it must be distinguished from a midsystolic dip.

> *Note*: These movements are best felt near the physician's fingertips with the patient in the left lateral decubitus position. Occasionally, a suspected faint atrial kick can be confirmed by observing a double movement of the patient's skin, your finger, or your stethoscope on the LV impulse. If the horizontal position does not yield a palpable A wave, raise the thorax about 30 degrees. Try a single fingertip while the chest is in full expiration. The

finger should be applied lightly because presystolic movement is low frequency and may be dampened by firm pressure.

AORTIC AND ARTERIAL PULSATIONS ON THE CHEST WALL

1. How do you look for an aortic **aneurysm** by palpating the chest wall?
   ANS.: Look for pulsations in the right or left sternoclavicular joint area.

   Note: a. An aortic aneurysm may occasionally be suspected if it depresses the left bronchus with each pulsation. Depression of a left bronchus in turn pulls down the trachea. If you stand behind the seated patient and apply steady upward pressure on the cricoid cartilage with the tip of one forefinger, you will readily detect the downward pull on the trachea with each pulsation. This phenomenon is known as the **tracheal tug**.

   b. A dilated right aortic arch may also cause a right sternoclavicular pulsation. In the presence of cyanosis, a right aortic arch suggests tetralogy, especially with pulmonary atresia, because only severe tetralogy (i.e., with severe PS or atresia) can cause a right aortic arch to be dilated enough to produce a palpable impulse. The more severe the PS, the larger the shunt into the aorta and the greater the diameter of the aorta. This pulsation should be sought specifically just below the right sternoclavicular junction.

   c. A large left coronary artery aneurysm can cause an abnormal systolic impulse at the left sternal border (15).

2. Where is coarctation most likely to produce pulsations on the chest wall? How are these brought out?
   ANS.: The posterior intercostal arteries (enlarged collaterals) may be both visible and palpable. You can best make their pulsations visible by asking the patient to bend forward, letting the arms dangle, thus stretching the skin of the back. Project a light from above to create a shadow below the posterior ribs (Fig. 22).

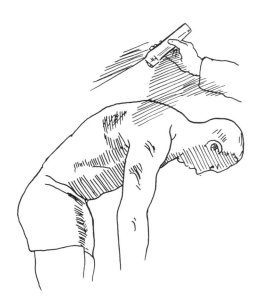

FIG. 22. In the proper light, the dilated subcostal collateral arteries can be seen to pulsate.

3. What should you suspect if a patient with coarctation has no posterior chest wall collateral vessel pulsations?

ANS.: Coarctation of the abdominal aorta.

Note: a. In the usual thoracic coarctation, there also may be no visible or palpable intercostal pulsations, no matter how severe the coarctation.

b. A large aneurysm of the descending aorta directly behind the heart can cause the entire left anterior chest wall to heave with systole.

THE NORMAL APEX CARDIOGRAM

1. What are the disadvantages of the term **apex cardiogram**?

ANS.: a. The noncardiologist is led to believe that an ACG is some sort of an electrocardiogram taken at the site of the LV impulse.

b. It usually refers to a method of recording any precordial pulsations and not just to movement of the apex beat.

2. In the normal ACG what causes the first outward movement that begins after the onset of the QRS?

ANS.: The beginning of LV systolic movement, the onset of which is the C point (Fig. 23).

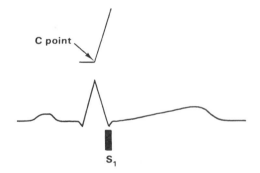

C point

S$_1$

FIG. 23. The beginning of contraction of the LV on the ACG is called the C point.

Note: The aortic valve opens near the peak of the initial outward movement (Fig. 24).

3. What does the normal ACG look like during ejection of blood through the aortic valve? Why?

ANS.: It looks like a sigmoid-shaped dropoff. The heart has struck the chest wall and is now retracting (Fig. 25).

Note: The nadir of the ACG isovolumic relaxation phase is called the O point. This refers to the opening of the mitral valve (Fig. 26).

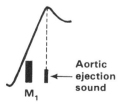

Aortic ejection sound

M$_1$

FIG. 24. The interval between M$_1$ and any sound simultaneous with the opening of the aortic valve is isovolumic contraction time.

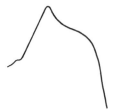

FIG. 25. The only reason that this curve does not look like the sustained outward motion of the LV pressure curve is because the kind of transducer used to record it has a shorter time constant than the ones used to record pressures at cardiac catheterization.

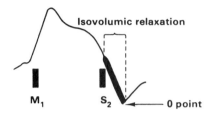

FIG. 26. If the mitral valve makes a snapping sound when it opens, as in mitral stenosis, the opening snap will occur near the O point of the ACG.

4. What happens to apical movement as the LV rapidly expands while it fills in early diastole?

ANS.: There is an outward movement, normally very rapid because it represents most of the phase of early rapid filling of the LV, when about 80% of the total diastolic blood volume enters the LV. This early diastolic wave has been called the rapid filling wave. The peak of the rapid filling wave is called the F point. (See Fig. 3 page 184.)

5. How does atrial contraction at the end of slow filling in diastole affect the ACG, and what is this wave called?

ANS.: By suddenly expanding the LV, it produces an outward movement called an A wave or an atrial hump (Fig. 27).

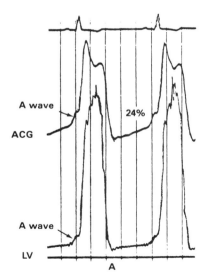
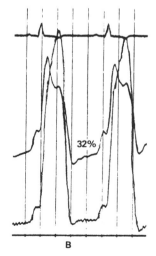

FIG. 27. A: Control LV pressure tracing and simultaneous ACG in a patient with an abnormally high A wave. B: After exercise there are parallel rises in LV end-diastolic and apex cardiographic A wave amplitude.

THE MIDSYSTOLIC DIP

1. With which abnormality do you often find a midsystolic dip in the presence of LVH?
   ANS.: Hypertrophic subaortic stenosis, or hypertrophic obstructive cardiomyopathy.
   Note: a. If an A wave is also present, a triple outward movement (almost pathognomonic of HOCM) is imparted to the fingers (Fig. 28).
   b. A prolapsed mitral valve may also produce a midsystolic dip.

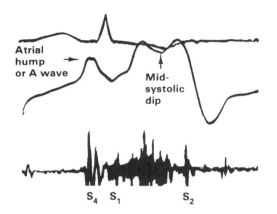

FIG. 28. This apex impulse tracing is from a 45-year-old man with HOCM. The atrial hump and the midsystolic dip give an impression of a triple outward movement.

2. When can an early diastolic hump, which is simultaneous with an S_3, be palpable?
   ANS.: This is most commonly felt in the presence of severe MR and a loud S_3 (Fig. 29).
   Note: A double diastolic outward movement is felt in some patients with sudden, severe AR. The second movement occurs after the mitral valve has closed in middiastole and further filling from the aorta occurs (14). See page 303, question 1, under "Sudden, Severe AR" for middiastolic mitral valve closure mechanism.

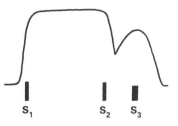

FIG. 29. A slight outward movement following the major out-and-back movement suggests a palpable early rapid filling of the LV and is most commonly felt together with an S_3 in severe MR.

AUSCULTATION OF THE CHEST FOR CRACKLES

Terminology Update

The term **rales** has had so many meanings and adjectives applied to it that it has given way to simply **fine** or **coarse** crackles (4). Continuous sounds due to bronchial obstruction or mucus are called **wheezes** or **rhonchi**.

Congestive Heart Failure Versus Bronchial Crackles

Compress the chest between one hand anteriorly and another posteriorly just before the end of expiration. If you listen with your ear close to the patient's mouth and the stethoscopic crackles are due to heart failure, nothing will be heard (12). If, however, they are due to bronchial disease, crackles will be heard. Different parts of the chest can be explored to localize the site of the bronchial abnormality.

Crackles due to heart failure will shift to the dependent side when the patient lies on the right or left side (8).

REFERENCES

1. Dressler W. *Clinical Aids in Cardiac Diagnosis.* New York: Grune & Stratton, 1970.
2. Eilen SD, et al. Accuracy of precordial palpation for detecting increased left ventricular volume. *Ann Intern Med* 1983;99:628.
3. Epstein EJ, et al. The "A" wave of the apex cardiogram in aortic valve disease and cardiomyopathy. *Br Heart J* 1968;30:591.
4. Forgacs P. *Lung Sounds.* New York: Macmillan, 1978.
5. Fuseno H, et al. The apex cardiographic A-wave peak-time in assessing left ventricular dysfunction. *J Cardiol* 1984;14:143.
6. Heckerling PS, et al. Accuracy of precordial percussion. *Am J Med* 1991;91:328.
7. Johnson AD, et al. Combined hypertrophic subaortic stenosis and calcific aortic valvular stenosis. *Am J Cardiol* 1975;35:706.
8. Lawson JD. The shifting rales of left ventricular failure. *Am J Med Sci* 1960;241:459.
9. Miyagi S. Auscultation of the lungs. *Nihon-Iji-Shimpo* 1992;550:140.
10. Nickol K, Wade AJ. Radiographic heart size and cardiothoracic ratio in three ethnic groups. *Br J Radiol* 1982;55:399.
11. Niehauss FW, Wright WD. Facts and fallacies about the normal apex beat. *Am Heart J* 1945;30:604.
12. Power L. Manual compression of the chest as an aid to demonstrating adventitious respiratory sounds. *Lancet* 1958;1:458.
13. Ranganathan N, et al. The apical impulse in coronary heart disease. *Clin Cardiol* 1985;8:20.
14. Wigle ED, Labrosse CJ. Sudden severe aortic regurgitation. *Circulation* 1965;32:708.
15. Zitnik RS, Giuliani ER. Clinical recognition of atrial myxoma. *Am Heart J* 1970;80:689.

6

The Stethoscope

THE BELL CHESTPIECE

1. What is the relation between the tautness (stiffness) of a membrane that collects sound from the chest wall and the ability of the membrane to transmit high or low frequencies?

   ANS.: The stiffer the membrane, the higher its natural frequency of oscillation and the more efficient it is at higher frequencies.

   Note: a. The terms **frequency** and **pitch** are usually used interchangeably. However, **frequency** refers to the number of oscillations per second made by a sound-producing structure, whereas **pitch** refers to what you hear when those vibrations act on your hearing apparatus.

   b. The skin can be turned into a taut diaphragm by the bell chestpiece if enough pressure is applied to the skin to produce pain.

2. Which chestpiece diameter picks up the most sound, a very small one or a very large one?

   ANS.: A very large one. The ability of a chestpiece to collect sound is proportional to its diameter.

   Note: A large chestpiece diameter also picks up low frequencies better.

3. How much pressure should be applied with a bell chestpiece?

   ANS.: Just enough to prevent room-noise leak. Any more pressure tightens the skin and tends to damp out the low frequencies.

   Note: An exception to this occurs when you are listening for an S_4. Firm pressure with the bell often brings out an S_4.

4. What is the relationship between the internal volume of a stethoscope (air space enclosed by the chestpiece and tubing) and the loudness of the transmitted sound?

   ANS.: There is an inverse relationship; that is, the smaller the internal volume, the greater the loudness of the sound, provided the diameter is large.

   Note: a. A shallow bell gives the smallest internal volume and can be coupled with a large diameter.

   b. It is believed by some cardiologists, with no explanation or testing other than their own ears, that a third chestpiece consisting of a large-diameter corrugated diaphragm applied with light pressure (only the weight of the three-headed stethoscope) is sometimes best for hearing low frequencies. They still advise having a bell handy, however, because it is needed for auscultation in small places such as the supraclavicular fossa or between the ribs on a bony chest and because the bell is occasionally superior for certain low frequencies.

5. What kind of murmurs and sounds are best heard with the bell?

ANS.: Murmurs: Dominantly low-frequency diastolic murmurs through mitral and tricuspid valves. Sounds: The S_3 and S_4.

Note: Adults can hear frequencies of up to 14,000 cycles per second (cps). However, since cardiac sound does not extend much above 1,000 cps, loss of ability to hear frequencies above 3,000 cps, which is the usual type of hearing loss in older physicians, should not interfere with the hearing of any cardiac sounds or murmurs (1).

THE SMOOTH DIAPHRAGM

1. What is meant by "masking" of sounds?

ANS.: Masking of sounds refers to the inability to hear a sound well because of interference by another loud sound just before or just after it (2). Loud low frequencies mask high ones easily.

2. What is the purpose of the smooth, stiff diaphragm?

ANS.: To damp out low frequencies and unmask high frequencies. If the resonance frequency of the diaphragm happens to be the same as that of the murmur, it may actually amplify the murmur.

Note: a. Amplification of sound may also be due to the summation of reflected or standing waves in the tubing. Different tubing lengths, therefore, may amplify different frequencies.

b. Although a bell brings out low frequencies considerably better than a diaphragm, high-frequency sounds and murmurs are actually heard just as well with the bell as with the diaphragm (5,8).

3. Why not use the bell chestpiece as a diaphragm by merely applying pressure, thus eliminating the need for two chestpieces?

ANS.: The stretched skin is an inefficient diaphragm for filtering out low frequencies. The skin does not become stiff enough to be a good filter.

Note: a. X-ray film has been shown to be about as good as no diaphragm at all for filtering out low frequencies.

b. A greater degree of pressure variation with the diaphragm has been attained through prestressing a nylon diaphragm by bowing it slightly forward. A small raised area in the center of the diaphragm can further increase the tension by exerting pressure against the skin (6).

4. Which murmurs and sounds are usually heard well only with the stiff, smooth diaphragm?

ANS.: Murmurs: Soft high-frequency aortic and pulmonary blowing diastolic murmurs and soft mitral regurgitation murmurs. Sounds: Splitting of first or second heart sounds and nonejection clicks.

Note: a. It is very difficult to hear splitting of heart sounds with a bell because there are so many low-frequency "reverberations" surrounding each component that the ear cannot separate them if the splitting is close. The ear can separate two short, high-frequency sounds placed close to each other more easily than it can separate two prolonged low- or medium-frequency sounds.

b. Because high-frequency sounds do not radiate as widely as do low frequencies, the diaphragm may help you to localize murmurs to their site of origin (1).

THE TUBING

1. Which frequencies are attenuated by too long a tubing?

   ANS.: High frequencies. The low frequencies are relatively unaffected by tube length (7).

   > *Note*: a. The shortest length that can maximize high frequencies and still not be too short for comfort is 12 inches (30 cm). However, 15 inches (37.5 cm) is a good compromise between the ideal of 12 inches and the usual length of 20 to 22 inches (50 to 55 cm) that are commercially available.
   >
   > b. Reflected waves in the tubing may amplify sounds. Therefore, different tubing lengths may amplify different frequencies.

2. How can the thickness of the tubing affect auscultation?

   ANS.: The thicker the tube, the better is the elimination of room noise. A vinyl tube has been found to be better than rubber for this purpose.

   > *Note*: Very narrow tubes carry low frequencies best, and wide tubing carries high frequencies best. An internal diameter of 3 mm was once recommended as the ideal compromise for carrying both frequencies. However, it has recently been found that 4.6 mm is even better.

3. Which is more efficient, a single or a double tube?

   ANS.: The single-tube stethoscope appears at first glance to be more efficient because it eliminates the necessity for binding parallel tubes together to prevent collision sounds and it is more flexible and portable. However, tests have shown that the double tube is *more efficient for high frequencies* because it allows less interference from reflected waves (1,2). However, a single tube attenuates only frequencies of over 400 cps, which suggests that only the softest- and highest-pitched murmurs will be missed by using a single tube (8).

AIR LEAKS AND EARTIPS

1. How important are air leaks at either the changeover valve or chestpiece?

   ANS.: The greatest impairment of the efficiency of a stethoscope is the air leak (4). Room noise due to air leaks tends to mask high frequencies more than low ones.

   > *Note*: You can test for air leaks at the chestpiece or changeover valve by blowing into one tube while occluding the opposite eartip and tubing. Your fingers will feel the air escaping. Also, if, when you withdraw the chestpiece quickly from the precordium, a change in pressure is produced that is painful to the ear, there are no significant air leaks.

2. Why may small eartips become partially obstructed when being inserted into the ear?

   ANS.: The usual stethoscope headpieces are designed to point the eartips slightly anteriorly. If the eartips are too small, their aperture may impinge partially or completely against the cartilaginous meatus, which points backward (3) (Fig. 1).

SUMMARY OF GOOD STETHOSCOPE CHARACTERISTICS

1. A shallow bell with a large diameter for low frequencies.
2. A smooth, stiff, thin diaphragm for high frequencies.
3. A pediatric-sized bell and diaphragm accessories.
4. An internally smooth vinyl tubing, not over 12 inches (30 cm) long and three-sixteenths of an inch (4.6 mm) in internal diameter.

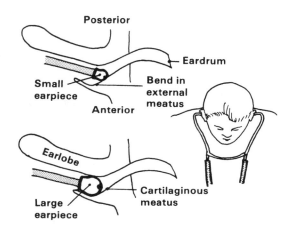

FIG. 1. Headpieces are designed to point the eartips slightly anteriorly. Small eartips can therefore be partly occluded against the backward-directed meatus.

5. Double-tubing with some method of binding the tubes together.
6. The largest eartips possible, preferably of slightly soft, rubbery material.
7. Metal headpieces that can be rotated so that the eartips can be pointed in the most comfortable direction.

REFERENCES

1. Ertel PY, et al. Stethoscope acoustics. *Circulation* 1966;34:889.
2. Ertel PY, et al. Stethoscope acoustics. Transmission and filtration patterns. *Circulation* 1966;34:899.
3. Groom D, Chapman W. Anatomic variations of the auditory canal pertaining to the fit of the stethoscope earpieces. *Circulation* 1959;19:606.
4. Groom D. Comparative efficiency of stethoscopes. *Am Heart J* 1967;68:220.
5. Hampton CS, Chaloner A. Which stethoscope? *Br Med J* 1967;4:388.
6. Howell WL, Aldridge CF. The effect of stethoscope-applied pressure in auscultation. *Circulation* 1965;32:430.
7. Johnston FD. An acoustical study of the stethoscope. *Arch Intern Med* 1940;65:328.
8. Kindig JR, et al. Acoustical performance of the stethoscope. *Am Heart J* 1982;104:269.

7

Diagraming and Grading Heart Sounds and Murmurs (The Auscultogram)

A graphic method for illustrating auscultatory findings is offered here not only as a means of keeping records as conveniently and efficiently as possible, but also as an aid to learning auscultation. One such "auscultogram" (see figures) can equal a 639-word description of the auscultatory findings. The graph can tell the story at a glance once the symbols are understood (1) (Figs. 1 and 2).

Filling in an auscultogram serves a self-teaching function in auscultation because one is forced to dissect out and listen separately to each component of the cycle, a method that is the hallmark of a good auscultator. Although listening to the total effect of all the sounds and murmurs as a single unit is also important, beginners tend to listen this way to the exclusion of the dissection method.

The auscultogram uses widely spaced wavy lines for low frequencies and closely spaced straight lines for high frequencies because this resembles the way they look on a phonocardiogram. We show medium or mixed frequencies by means of low-frequency wavy lines with diagonal lines drawn through them. An explanatory example of the frequency symbols should be included on each auscultogram.

The loudness of sounds and murmurs is indicated by their height on a vertical column divided into six parts to represent six grades of loudness. Drawing versus numbering them is analogous to the difference between looking at a complicated column of numbers and looking at a simple bar graph.

Grading amplitude on a scale of 6 is acceptable if we can separate grades 3 and 4. In 1933, when Freeman and Levine introduced the grading of murmurs up to 6, only grades 1, 2, and 6 were described in detail (2). Grade 6 was a murmur heard with the stethoscope off the chest, and grade 1 could be missed on first applying the stethoscope. Grade 2 was an easily heard, faint murmur. By 1959, Levine had proposed that grade 5 was a murmur that could be heard when the edge of the chestpiece (preferably the diaphragm) was applied to the precordium (3). However, he left the distinction between grades 3 and 4 to be made by the listener. This problem has been solved by using palpability as a means of separating these grades; that is, if the murmur is accompanied by a thrill, it is grade 4 or more.

Note: a. A grade 1 murmur is best defined as one that requires "tuning in." **Tuning in** is a term used to describe a psychological state in which you must first have an expectation (i.e., you must know what you are listening for); you then eliminate room noise by an act of concentration. It has been facetiously stated that a grade 1 murmur is one that "a medical student cannot hear." This has some truth since a medical student

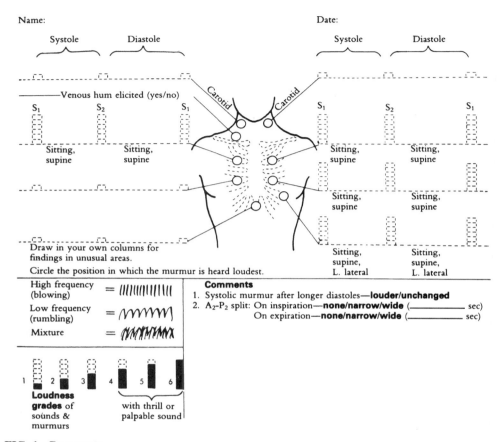

Name: Date:

FIG. 1. Comments
1. **Systolic murmur after longer diastoles—louder/unchanged**
2. **A₂–P₂ split: On inspiration—none/narrow/wide; on expiration—none/narrow/wide**

does not have the experience of knowing what to listen for. You cannot tune in to nothing.

   b. It is not necessary to add *palpable* to the word *thrill* because all thrills are palpable.

Using palpability to separate grade 3 from grade 4 murmurs has many advantages:

1. It facilitates the teaching of grading because grades 3 and 4 are the only stumbling blocks.
2. It teaches the relationship between a thrill and a murmur, making the physician realize that a long thrill is never felt in the absence of a loud murmur. (Widely split components of loud heart sounds or a slight bisferiens pulse may feel like *short* thrills.)
3. It lends itself to the grading of heart sounds.
   Note: Thrills and sounds are best perceived with the distal palm. One hand may be more sensitive than the other, so test each hand on a patient with a faint thrill or palpable sound to find your better hand (Fig. 3).
       The auscultogram can serve as a means of training the cardiology student to acquire any habits of auscultation that a teaching service desires. For example, providing a place on the graph for noting the width and movements of the second sound split with respiration

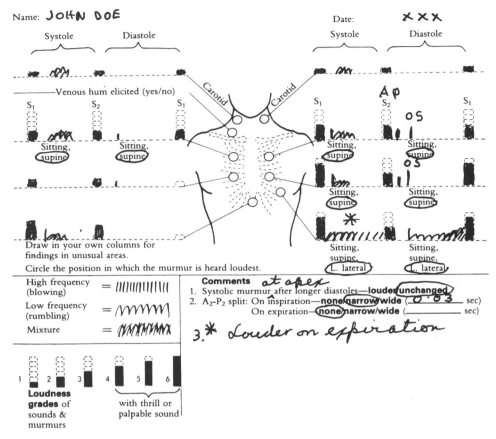

Name: JOHN DOE

Date: X X X

FIG. 2. Comments
1. **Systolic murmur at apex after longer diastoles—louder/unchanged**
2. **A_2–P_2 split: On inspiration—none/narrow/wide (0.03 sec); on expiration—none/narrow/wide**
3. **Louder on expiration**

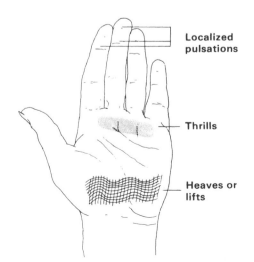

Localized pulsations

Thrills

Heaves or lifts

FIG. 3. Although small, localized movements are best perceived by the distal finger pads, thrills are best felt with the distal palm.

serves as a constant reminder to listen for such movements. Because we wish to teach auscultators the value of listening in the neck for heart sounds and murmurs, we include the neck on our diagram. We also provide a place for noting the effects of intermittent long diastoles. (See p. 210 for the reason for this.)

The writing and listening should be done simultaneously; the art of auscultation should not be a memory test. It is best for a right-handed physician to carry out his examination from the patient's left side because this position allows one to hold the stethoscope with the left hand while writing with the right (Fig. 4).

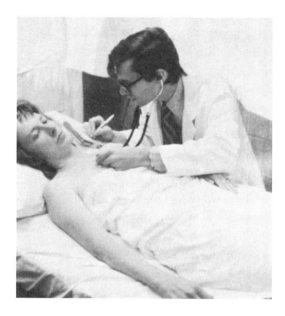

FIG. 4. Simultaneous writing and listening are keys to this method of ear training and accuracy of recording.

It is convenient to print auscultogram pads that are small enough to fit on about half a hospital chart page. A sticky backing makes for easy attachment.

REFERENCES

1. Constant J, Lippschutz EJ. Diagramming and grading heart sounds and murmurs. *Am Heart J* 1965;70:326.
2. Freeman AR, Levine SA. The clinical significance of the systolic murmur. *Ann Intern Med* 1933;6:1371.
3. Levine SA, Harvey WP. *Clinical Auscultation of the Heart.* Philadelphia: Saunders, 1959.

8

The First Heart Sound (S₁)

PHYSIOLOGY OF FIRST SOUND COMPONENTS

1. What events are responsible for the two major components of the first heart sound (S_1)?

   ANS.: We should not consider the mere coaptation of valve cusps to be the cause of heart sounds. The sounds are produced by the vibrations of the cusps and ventricles as the upward movement of the cusps' bellies is suddenly checked when they reach their full extent of movement (39). The high-frequency component of the S_1 occurs about 20 msec after echocardiographic valve closure (apposition) and after the crossover of pressure pulses in the left ventricle and left atrium (12,25). Mitral valve closure is a continuous movement; the leaflets make contact near their leading free edge, after which the area of contact spreads toward the basal attachments as both leaflets are propelled toward the left atrium until restrained by the chordae to produce the mitral component of the first heart sound (M_1). This sudden tension of the elastic coapted cusps causes them to stretch and recoil in a rapid vibratory movement that produces the M_1. When the mitral valve is removed experimentally, the M_1 is absent.

   Note: If a low-frequency phonocardiogram is analyzed, there are four discrete vibrations of the S_1. If, however, only medium or high frequencies are used, or if the paper speed is not very fast, there are usually only two or three distinct vibrations. Splitting of the S_1 is audible only in about 85% of patients.

2. Which of the four phonocardiographic distinct vibrations are audible?

   ANS.: The S_1 commonly has two distinct components. The following explanation for each component is a synthesis of many theories.

   The first audible (and major) component of S_1 (simultaneous with the second phonocardiographic component) is called the M_1 because it is caused by events associated with mitral closure. The origin of the second audible (third phonocardiographic) component depends on the width of the split. When the split is narrow, the origin is probably tricuspid closure, and the sound is called the T_1. When the split is wide, the second audible (fourth phonocardiographic) component may be caused by the opening of a stiff aortic or pulmonary valve, as occurs with systemic or pulmonary hypertension or aortic or pulmonary valve stenosis. The second component of a wide split is called an ejection sound, but if the semilunar valves are stiff enough, the sound may be so short and sharp that it has the quality of a click. It may then be called an "ejection click." (See Fig. 1.).

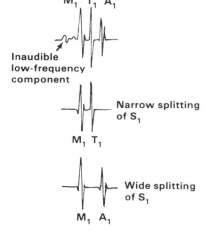

FIG. 1. Narrow splitting of S_1 (less than the usual isovolumic contraction time of about 50 msec [0.05 sec]) may be due to M_1, T_1 components. Wide splitting (50 msec or longer) is probably due to the M_1, A_1[146] components, unless there is a right ventricular volume-to-pressure overload.

Note: a. Although the initial low-amplitude inaudible vibration of S_1 (also called the "M" sound) is occasionally due to atrial contraction, it sometimes occurs in atrial fibrillation, in atrioventricular (AV) dissociation, and when the ventricles are paced (2,24). Therefore, it may emanate from the ventricular wall as it becomes taut (Fig. 2).

b. An aortic root sound theory has been proposed to explain the second component (A_1) of a widely split S_1 in subjects with no valvular abnor-

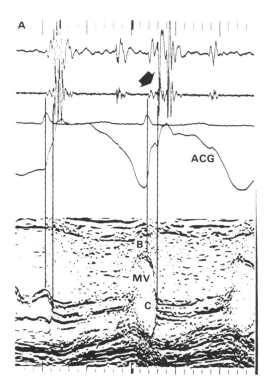

FIG. 2. The initial low-frequency component of the S_1 (*arrow*) recorded in this patient with atrial fibrillation occurs during the preisovolumic contraction period of the left ventricle as seen on the apex cardiogram (ACG) and before mitral valve echocardiogram.

malities; that is, A_1 is caused by a change in the rate of pressure rise in the left ventricle (LV) that suddenly tenses the aortic root structures just as the aortic valve begins to open (26). However, all aortic ejection sounds correlated with echocardiograms have been timed to be simultaneous with the peak of opening of either the aortic or tricuspid valves (14,20) (Fig. 3).

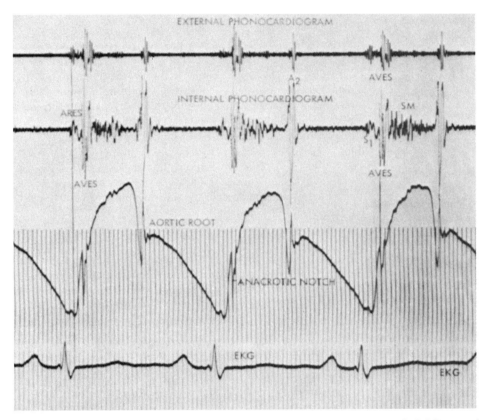

FIG. 3. This aortic root tracing from a 16-year-old boy with minimal congenital AS was taken with a catheter-tip electromanometer to avoid any delays due to tubing. An aortic root ejection sound (ARES) is present, coincident with the onset of pressure rise in the aortic root. There is no M_1 in this area. An aortic valve ejection sound (AVES) is also present, occurring 40 msec (0.04 sec) later and simultaneously with the anacrotic notch. (Reproduced with permission from A. V. Whitaker et al. Sound pressure correlates of the aortic ejection sound. *Circulation* 39:475. © 1969 American Heart Association.)

    c. The arguments against attributing the easily heard second component of a widely split first sound to tricuspid valve closure are as follows.
      1. When the right ventricle (RV) is completely bypassed or destroyed, so that it cannot contract, the S_1 may still be split.
      2. If the heart is explored with a microphone placed directly on the myocardium, all components of the S_1 become softer over the RV, and

there is no amplification of any component of the first heart sound (16).

3. In subjects with left bundle branch block (LBBB), the S_1 often shows the same degree of splitting and the same number of components despite the marked delay in the onset of the M_1 in LBBB (23). Whenever wide splitting is heard in right bundle branch block (RBBB), the second component can often be shown to be due to an ejection sound and not a T_1 (42). In one series, 40% of patients with RBBB showed no clearly detectable split of S_1 (by auscultation), and in another 44%, the usual narrow physiologic splitting was observed (35).

4. In a study of 16 normal subjects by echocardiography, the first major component of the S_1 coincided with mitral closure in all subjects, and it coincided also with tricuspid valve closure in the majority. The second major component of the S_1 coincided with aortic valve opening in all subjects and with tricuspid valve closure in one-third (29).

5. The RV has been found by radionuclide angiography to contract an average of about 7 msec after the LV. The mitral and tricuspid sounds therefore would occur too close together to be distinguished only with difficulty if at all by expert auscultators (41).

3. When is it likely that tricuspid closure *does* contribute to the S_1 in the presence of a normal tricuspid valve?

ANS.: Whenever the RV has a volume or pressure overload (e.g., in atrial septal defect [ASD] or in pulmonary hypertension). This is supported by the following findings.

a. In subjects with an ASD, the second major component of the S_1 coincides with the peak of the right atrial C wave.

b. In 75% of children with an ASD, the second component of a split S_1 at the apex occupied by the RV is louder than the M_1 (15,34). This relationship of component loudness is unusual in normal children.

c. In one study of subjects with an ASD, only those with a complete RBBB were found to have a widely split S_1 (13). (Although this suggests that the second component was a T_1, it may have been a pulmonary ejection sound.)

Note: a. In at least one report, it has been shown that the second loud component of the split S_1 in ASD is not always due to T_1, because it was found by intracardiac phonocardiography that the second component was absent in the RV in half the patients tested, that it often occurred after the rise in pulmonary artery pressure, and that it showed a constant time relationship with the onset of rise of aortic pressure (28).

b. In mitral stenosis (MS) a tricuspid component may precede the delayed M_1. Intracardiac phonocardiography has shown that a right-sided S_1 component precedes a left-sided S_1 component in about a fourth of patients with MS.

c. If the second component of the split S_1 increases on inspiration, you may then be justified in calling it a T_1. If it is more than 40 msec from the M_1 (in the absence of RBBB), it is probably an aortic ejection sound.

d. In the Ebstein anomaly not only is the second component tricuspid, but it may be markedly delayed and accentuated.

THE M₁ PLUS AORTIC EJECTION SOUND AS THE CAUSE OF A SPLIT S₁

1. How long after the M₁ does the aortic ejection sound (A₁) occur in normal subjects?
   ANS.: The usual A₁ occurs at the end of isovolumic contraction (i.e., about 40 to 60 msec [0.04 to 0.06 sec] after the M₁). A moderately wide 40-msec split takes as long as it does to say "pa-da" as quickly as possible. The 60-msec split can be imitated by saying "pa-ta" as quickly as possible.
   Note: a. It may be easier to hear a split of the S₁ in older subjects because isovolumic contraction times tend to lengthen with age. (The differentiation of an M₁ ejection sound interval from an S₄S₁ is described on p. 203.)
   b. About two-thirds of acute myocardial infarction patients have very widely split first sounds (more than 60 msec) in the first 3 days, especially if heart failure is present.
2. Which valvular abnormalities are the usual causes of an aortic ejection sound (or click)?
   ANS.: a. A bicuspid aortic valve.
   b. A stiff aortic valve, such as that occurring in **aortic stenosis** (AS) or hypertension.
   Note: Hypertension may stretch the aortic root, causing the cusps to become taut and therefore to open with an easily audible sound (Fig. 4).

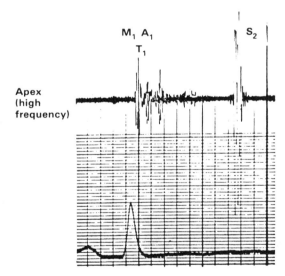

FIG. 4. This phonocardiogram is from a 40-year-old woman with mild hypertension. The third component is probably an aortic ejection sound. This sounded simply like a widely split S₁, probably because the T₁ was too close to the M₁ to be audible.

3. What features suggest that the aortic ejection sound or click, as in AS, is due to an opening snap of the aortic valve and not merely to forceful ejection into the aorta?
   ANS.: a. It disappears with severe calcification of the aortic valve; conversely, the louder the sound, the more mobile the valve can be shown to be.
   b. It is not a feature of supravalvular AS or of obstruction below the valve (e.g., hypertrophic subaortic stenosis [HSS, or HOCM] or discrete subvalvular stenosis [a fibrous ring just below the aortic valve]) (22).
4. Why is the aortic ejection sound of diagnostic help in the presence of AS?

ANS.: a. It helps to locate the site of the AS because only valvular AS characteristically has an audible ejection sound.

b. The absence of an ejection sound warns you of two possibilities: either there is no valvular stenosis, or there is valvular stenosis with heavy calcification with a gradient of more than 50 mm Hg (11). Calcification is likely if the A_2 is soft or absent.

Note: a. In some patients with HSS or HOCM an aortic ejection sound (as well as a dilated ascending aorta) is occasionally present (44). This is not surprising considering the increased rate of flow into the aorta in early systole. This is also the cause of the ejection sounds heard in aortic regurgitation (AR) and thyrotoxicosis.

b. The loudness of the ejection sound is correlated with the degree of leaflet mobility and their distance of excursion.

5. Where is the aortic ejection sound best heard?

ANS.: The ejection sound is best heard wherever aortic events are best heard (i.e., anywhere in a "sash area" from the second right interspace to the apex). (See Fig. 221.) The ejection click of AS, however, is most often heard best at the apex because the AS murmur may be loud enough at the second right interspace and left sternal border to obscure the click.

6. What features may suggest that an aortic ejection sound is due to a nonstenotic bicuspid aortic valve?

ANS.: a. If it is loud, especially if it is louder than the M_1 and associated with a louder A_2 than normal.

b. If it is associated with AR. (AR, usually of only mild or moderate degree, is commonly associated with a bicuspid aortic valve.)

Note: A bicuspid aortic valve may calcify in patients over 50 years old and lead to aortic stenosis of any degree, or it may remain nonstenotic permanently (21).

THE PULMONARY EJECTION SOUND

Ejection Sounds in Pulmonary Stenosis

1. What is responsible for the ejection sound heard in valvular pulmonary stenosis (PS)? What proof can be offered?

ANS.: It is an opening sound of the pulmonary valve. The evidence is as follows.

a. The ejection sound is not present in pure infundibular stenosis.

b. It is not present if the valve is severely dysplastic.

c. It occurs at the peak of opening of the pulmonary valve on echophono-cardiography (Fig. 5).

2. Why does the pulmonary ejection sound tend to disappear on inspiration in valvular PS?

ANS.: The sudden upward movement of a dome-shaped pulmonary valve produces the sound. If the valve is already in the domed or near-domed position when the RV contracts, there will be no sound or only a soft sound. On inspiration, the increased blood drawn into the right atrium causes it to contract more strongly, and the stronger atrial contraction at the end of diastole raises the pressure in the RV just before the ventricle contracts. This rise in end-diastolic pressure in the RV may be higher than the pulmonary artery pressure. This is easy to understand if you realize that pulmonary artery diastolic pressure in PS may not be much more than 7

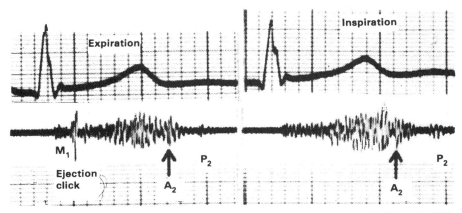

FIG. 5. High-frequency tracing from the third left interspace of a patient with PS and a RV pressure of 100 mm Hg. The ejection click that disappears on inspiration shows that the site of obstruction is at the valve. The A_2-P_2 interval increases slightly from 100 to 120 msec (0.10 to 0.12 sec) on inspiration.

mm Hg, and RV end-diastolic pressure in PS can easily exceed 7 mm Hg. Thus, the pulmonary valve will be raised into the domed position at the end of diastole if the end-diastolic pressure in the RV rises to as little as 8 mm Hg with a strong atrial contraction (Fig. 6).

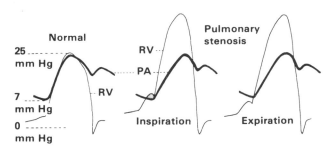

FIG. 6. These RV and pulmonary artery pressure tracings show how inspiration can raise the end-diastolic RV pressure above pulmonary artery pressure because of a strong right atrial contraction plus a thick RV.

On expiration, the end-diastolic pressure in the RV falls, and the pulmonary valve is in the *down* position at the beginning of RV systole. Ventricular contractions can now balloon the pulmonary valve upward into a dome, causing a click (Fig. 7).

Note: a. A click or sound can occur *before the QRS* at the end of diastole if the RV end-diastolic pressure is higher than the pulmonary artery diastolic pressure due to atrial systole. (It can even occur in early diastole at the peak of early rapid ventricular filling if the RV pressure exceeds pulmonary artery pressure at that time.)

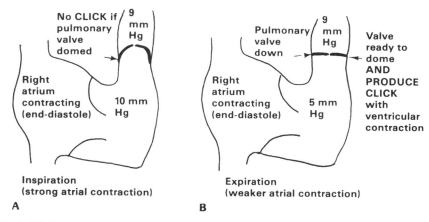

FIG. 7. A: Right atrial contraction is assisted by inspiration in raising RV pressure higher than pulmonary artery pressure. This causes the pulmonary valve to dome up before the RV contracts. B: The effect of a reduction in RV diastolic pressure caused by expiration results in a downward position of the pulmonary valve when the RV begins to contract.

   b. The aortic ejection click does not change significantly with respiration because the end-diastolic pressure in the LV in AS, even when very high (the normal end-diastolic pressure is not much higher than 10 mm Hg), can never exceed the usual diastolic pressure in the aorta (which is rarely lower than 50 mm Hg).

3. Why may the pulmonary ejection sound or click of PS show respiratory variation only in the sitting position?

   ANS.: If the PS is moderately severe, the supine pressure in the RV may be high enough at the end of diastole to keep the valve in the domed position even on expiration, and respiration will have no effect on the click. In the sitting position, however, the decrease in venous return may cause a lower RV pressure at the end of diastole and may allow the pulmonary valve to fall to the downward position on expiration.

   Note: In very mild PS, there may be a pulmonary ejection click on both inspiration and expiration, with only a little attenuation on inspiration.

4. Where is the pulmonary ejection sound best heard?

   ANS.: Wherever pulmonary sounds and murmurs are best heard (i.e., anywhere along the left sternal border). The pulmonary ejection click may be heard well toward the mid-left thorax if the RV is enlarged.

5. Why is there a good correlation between ejection clicks and poststenotic dilatation beyond a valvular stenosis (i.e., dilatation of the pulmonary artery just beyond the valve)?

   ANS.: Most patients with ejection clicks have systolic murmurs due to turbulent blood flow through the stenosed valve. The turbulence causing the murmur may disrupt the elastin structure of the artery just beyond the valve (5,6). One theory of poststenotic dilatation is based on the principle that turbulent blood flow increases the forces that tend to drag the lining of a vessel downstream. The distorted endothelial cells then initiate changes in the subjacent layers that can modify the lumen (32).

Low-frequency vibrations, even if inaudible, can cause dilatation of a young artery (5).

Note: a. The absence of poststenotic dilatation beyond a purely infundibular PS has not been explained. Perhaps the turbulence that produces the murmur here is dissipated before it can reach the pulmonary artery walls with enough force to destroy the molecular structure.

b. Poststenotic dilatation is so common in the presence of an ejection click that it was originally believed all ejection clicks were caused by distention of the dilated segment.

6. What is the likely cause of an ejection sound heard in patients with tetralogy of Fallot?

ANS.: If there is severe enough tetralogy (tetralogy that is almost pulmonary atresia, also known as pseudotruncus arteriosus), there is usually an aortic ejection sound due to the dilated and volume-overloaded aorta receiving the blood volume from the two ventricles. In mild (acyanotic) tetralogy, it is probably a pulmonary ejection sound due to pulmonary valve stenosis (17).

Note: a. About one-third of patients with tetralogy have pure valvular stenosis. (Embryologically, this is not true tetralogy.) The others have either pure infundibular or mixed infundibular and valvular stenosis. If it is purely valvular and not severe (acyanotic type), there may be an audible pulmonary second sound (P_2) in addition to an ejection sound.

b. The rare pulmonary ejection sound with mild tetralogy does not usually decrease with inspiration because the ventricular septal defect (VSD) does not allow the stronger right atrial contraction to increase the RV diastolic pressure; that is, the right atrium may contract very strongly with inspiration, but instead of doming the pulmonary valve, its energy may be dissipated through the VSD.

7. Which early sounds or clicks are neither aortic nor pulmonary?

ANS.: a. The nonejection click of the mitral valve prolapse syndrome (see p. 254) may come so early that it imitates an aortic or pulmonary ejection click.

b. VSDs often close spontaneously either by development of a membranous septal aneurysm (a pouch with a small opening at the end) or by adherence of tricuspid valve tissue to the edges of the defect (4). The click may be due to the aneurysm as it is abruptly distended under high pressure from the LV, or it may be a tricuspid valve click (27). The VSD clicks are loudest on expiration, localized to the left lower sternal border, and are usually present with the pansystolic crescendo murmur of the pinhole VSD. Their Q-click intervals are in the range of 100 to 130 msec, similar to that of late pulmonary or aortic ejection clicks.

c. A persistent truncus arteriosus quadracuspid valve almost always produces an ejection sound, often louder than any of the heart sounds, and is not influenced by respiration (43).

8. What happens to RV isovolumic contraction time and the Q-click interval with increasing PS? Why?

ANS.: They become shorter because as PS becomes more and more severe

a. The rate of RV pressure rise becomes faster.

b. The pulmonary diastolic pressure becomes lower.

Note: a. If the stenosis is severe, the ejection sound may merge with the M_1. A clue to its presence, however, may be detected by respiratory variation in S_1 loudness.

b. The earliness of an aortic ejection click does not correlate with the degree of AS.

Ejection Sounds in Pulmonary Hypertension

1. Why is an ejection sound heard in pulmonary hypertension?
   ANS.: The high pressure in the pulmonary artery may cause a dilated pulmonary artery root, which stretches and tightens the valve ring and cusps, which produce the valve click. Echophonocardiography has shown that the click occurs at the peak of opening of the pulmonary valve (20).
2. How does an ejection sound heard in pulmonary hypertension differ from one heard in PS?
   ANS.: In pulmonary hypertension the ejection sound is often heard better lower down on the chest and is rarely changed by respiration (Fig. 8).

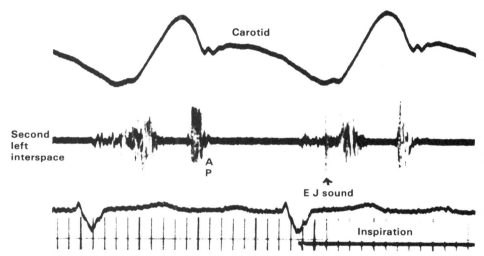

FIG. 8. This high-frequency phonocardiogram and simultaneous carotid tracing is from a patient with severe pulmonary hypertension secondary to a VSD (Eisenmenger syndrome). Note that the pulmonary ejection sound does not diminish inspiration.

Note: a. Primary pulmonary hypertension often produces a vibratory S_1, which is thought to be due to a loud T_1 (40).
   b. The ejection sound of pulmonary hypertension is often followed by a short murmur that ends in midsystole.

Ejection Sounds in Idiopathic Dilatation of the Pulmonary Artery

1. How can you explain the ejection sounds in idiopathic dilatation of the pulmonary artery?
   ANS.: Idiopathic dilatation of the pulmonary artery implies an abnormal artery with marked loss of elasticity. A jerky expansion of this lax pulmonary artery may cause a sound or a click.
      Note: a. Sudden expansion of a distal pulmonary artery was the only reasonable explanation for the ejection click heard in a patient with an absent pulmonary valve and dilated pulmonary artery in whom intracardiac phonocardiograms showed that the ejection murmur preceded the click by 50 msec (1).

b. The ejection sounds of idiopathic dilatation of the pulmonary artery tend to be far from the M_1, suggesting that a distal event, such as dilation of a lax pulmonary artery, may be the cause of the click (2).

2. What lesion produces rapid ejection into a dilated pulmonary artery without an ejection sound or click?

ANS.: An ASD produces rapid flow through the pulmonary artery, but there is often no audible ejection sound unless pulmonary hypertension is present or the pulmonary artery is markedly dilated.

Note: With most ASDs, a split first sound is usually present, with the second component louder than the first component at the apex, which is usually usurped by the RV in patients with ASDs. This reversal of normal loudness of the S_1 components has been proposed as a helpful clue to the presence of an ASD (15). Although the second component has been timed on echocardiograms with closure of the tricuspid valve (T_1), it is still possible that it is sometimes a pulmonary ejection sound (P_1).

LOUDNESS OF THE M_1 COMPONENT OF S_1

1. What factors other than chest wall shape and thickness control the loudness of the M_1?

ANS.: a. The rate of rise of ventricular pressure. The faster the rise at the time the LV pressure exceeds left atrial pressure, the louder the M_1 (10).

b. The duration of LV contraction before it exceeds left atrial pressure. Because the LV accelerates in the early phase of its contraction, the longer the LV must contract before it can close the mitral valve, the louder the M_1 (36).

c. The stiffness of the mitral valve bellies. An immobile valve can produce little sound.

Note: With large pericardial effusions, the heart is suspended by the great vessels and swings in a pendular arc whose period is twice the heart rate. Therefore, the heart is closer to the stethoscope during every other cycle and may produce an auscultatory (as well as electrical) alternans of the loudness of S_1.

Ventricular Pressure Rise and M_1 Loudness

1. What is the physiologist's way of expressing the rate of rise of pressure?

ANS.: delta *P*/delta *t* = change of pressure/change of time. This is usually shortened to *dP/dt*. The greater the *dP/dt* (i.e., the faster the rate of LV pressure rise), the louder the M_1 (10).

Note: a. An increased *dP/dt* of the LV means increased contractility. Increased contractility is due either to the Starling effect of a large volume or to positive inotropic agents such as catecholamines, digitalis, or thyroxine. Sympathetic stimulation is probably the cause of the loud M_1 in sinus tachycardia and in exercise. A decrease in the *dP/dt* of the LV resulting in a soft M_1 may be due to drugs that decrease contractility.

b. For some unknown reason, in one study, the M_1 was more likely to be softer in posterior than in anterior myocardial infarction (30).

c. The M_1 is said to be soft in acute myocardial infarction because the acutely infarcted area tends to balloon outward paradoxically with systole so that part of the energy developed by the LV is absorbed. This ar-

gument is weakened by the finding that in most patients with ventricular aneurysms the S_1 is no softer than in patients with a previous infarction and no aneurysm (18). Also, in some patients with anteroseptal
aneurysms, the S_1 actually may be loud. This has been explained by the
fact that a sudden tensing of the tissue of a ventricular aneurysm (suspended between two rubber stoppers in a tank of water) can produce as
loud a sound as tensing of mitral valve leaflets, especially in the low-frequency range (9).

d. In acute myocardial infarction the softness of the S_1 correlates with a
prolonged isovolumic contraction time. As patients recover from the infarction, the S_1 becomes louder and the isovolumic contraction time becomes shorter.

e. The first sound is also made softer by drugs, such as beta blockers, that
decrease contractility, and also by advancing age. The S_1 is softer in old-
age groups because of the decreasing contractility, longer PR interval,
and increase in anteroposterior diameter of the chest that often occurs.
These soft first sounds are often described as muffled because they have
lost most of their high frequencies.

PR Interval and M_1 Loudness

1. Why does a short PR interval cause a loud M_1 and a long PR a soft M_1?
   ANS.: The P controls the timing of atrial contraction, which raises left atrial (LA) pressure and opens the mitral valve further at the end of diastole. If the PR interval is
   short, ventricular contraction occurs so quickly after the atrium has contracted that
   the LA has not had time to relax (short X descent). Therefore, atrial pressure is still
   at a high level when the pressure in the LV exceeds it enough to close the mitral
   valve (36). This means that the ventricle has a long time to contract before it overcomes the relatively high LA pressure. Therefore, the LV has time to accelerate to
   the more rapid dP/dt part of its pressure curve by the time it closes the mitral valve.
   If the PR is long, the delayed LV contraction gives the LA pressure a chance to
   drop to low levels (deep X descent) by the time the LV begins to contract. Thus,
   LV pressure exceeds LA pressure at the very early slow part of its acceleration
   curve (Fig. 9).

   Note: a. It has usually been taught that the reason for the loud M_1 with a short PR
   interval is that the mitral leaflets are wide open at the time of the LV
   contraction onset; atrial relaxation, which can close mitral valves by a
   kind of suction effect, has not had much time to act (14). The analogy of
   a wide-open door making more noise when it closes than a slightly open
   door is often used but is not valid unless the door is made to accelerate
   as it closes.

   b. The paradox of a long PR interval and a loud S_1 is seen in mitral stenosis (MS). This is due to the high left atrial pressure present in MS and,
   therefore, the long time the LV has to accelerate before it closes the mitral valve. In the Ebstein anomaly with a long PR, although the M_1 may
   be soft, the second component of the S_1 may be loud and clicking because it is caused by a closure of a large deformed tricuspid anterior
   leaflet. Because this leaflet has been likened to a large sail flapping in
   the breeze, this loud T_1 has been called a "sail sound." This sound often

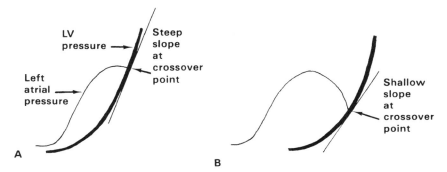

FIG. 9. **A:** If the PR interval is short, the LV contracts before the left atrium has had a chance to relax and drop its pressure. Therefore, the LV pressure will not exceed left atrial pressure until it has contracted for a long enough time to accelerate to a stage of rapid pressure rise by the time the mitral leaflets are closed. This produces an abrupt deceleration of forward flow and a loud sound. **B:** If the PR interval is long, the LV contracts later than in A, so that the left atrium has time to drop to a low pressure when the LV pressure exceeds it. The pressure crossover point is on the slow part of the LV acceleration curve, and the valves are closed at a relatively slow rate, producing a soft sound.

increases with inspiration and is usually associated with a very late tricuspid opening snap.

S₁ Loudness in Arrhythmias and Bundle Branch Block

1. Which situations can be diagnosed by hearing the effect of a changing PR interval on the S₁?

    ANS.: Any AV dissociation, as in complete AV block or some ventricular tachycardias (Fig. 10). (If the ventricular tachycardia has retrograde ventriculoatrial conduction into the atria, there is no AV dissociation.)

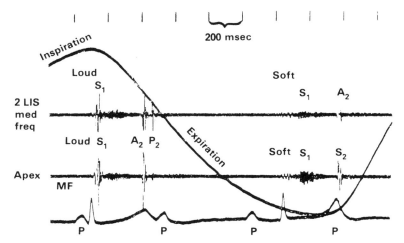

FIG. 10. This medium-frequency (MF) phonocardiogram is from a patient with complete AV block; that is, the P waves and QRS complexes are independent, thus causing the PR intervals to vary. Note the loud S₁ after the short PR (first one) and the soft one after the long PR.

Note: Type 1 second-degree AV block (Wenckebach periods) also has gradually longer PR intervals until complete AV block occurs and a beat is dropped. The gradually longer PR interval has been said to cause a softer and softer first sound until a pause occurs. However, if the longest PR is very long (e.g., about 260 msec), the valves may open again owing to continued pulmonary venous return, and so produce a slight increase in loudness. Often, though, the PR changes are so small that no perceptible first sound changes occur.

2. In atrial fibrillation, how will the different lengths of diastole and the absence of atrial contraction control the loudness of the M_1?

ANS.: With no P waves, only changes in LV contractility can affect the loudness of the M_1. A series of short cycles can cause an increase in contractility due to a **postextrasystolic potentiation effect** (see p. 211) and produce a loud M_1 for the next normal cycle. At the end of a short diastole, a decrease in LV stretch makes a soft M_1 (see Note b for the exception). Long diastoles make a loud M_1 (Starling effect).

Note: a. Although the preceding RR interval, in general, controls the loudness of the S_1, the pre-preceding (penultimate) RR interval controls it also, by a postextrasystolic potentiation effect; that is, the shorter the cycle length before the preceding RR interval, the greater the contractility and S_1 loudness. This is the major reason that at the bedside it is difficult to relate the observed intensity of the S_1 to cycle length.

b. In atrial fibrillation the loudest M_1 occurs when the diastole is so short the M_1 coincides with or occurs just after an S_3 (33). This suggests that when a ventricle contracts just after it has been expanding rapidly, it takes longer than usual to reverse the forward flow, so there is more time for acceleration by the time the mitral valve is closed.

3. How does LBBB affect the loudness of the M_1?

ANS.: It tends to cause a soft M_1 because

a. The *dP/dt* of early contraction is often decreased in LBBB, probably because initial conduction is almost entirely septal; therefore, the main LV mass may not participate in preisovolumic contraction (i.e., in the pre-M_1 contraction phase) (7,8).

b. The onset of left ventricular contraction may be delayed so that the effect is the same as that of a long PR interval (19).

Valvular Heart Disease and M_1 Loudness

1. When is the M_1 in AS soft?

ANS.: When the systolic gradient exceeds 50 mm Hg, LV contractility has been shown to decrease, especially in patients over age 40 (37).

2. How does a gradient across the mitral valve at the end of diastole in mitral stenosis affect the loudness of the M_1? Why?

ANS.: It makes the M_1 loud because the high pressure in the left atrium that makes the gradient at the end of diastole requires the ventricle to reach a higher pressure before it can close the valve. The LV, therefore, has more time to accelerate before it closes the valve.

Note: Some patients with constrictive pericarditis have a loud S_1 if there is localized AV groove calcification, causing an "external mitral stenosis" effect (36).

3. How does a relatively stiff mitral valve, as in mitral stenosis, affect the quality of the M_1? Why?

    ANS.: It makes the M_1 short and snapping (i.e., it causes a "closing snap") (3). The resistance to movement of the fibrotic and tethered edges causes the still flexible bodies or bellies of the anterior leaflet to billow upward like a snapping sail.

        Note: a. The posterior leaflet usually has relatively little "belly" to billow unless it has redundant tissue, as in the mitral valve prolapse syndrome. Therefore, the anterior leaflet is mainly responsible for the M_1 snapping effect.

           b. When porcine mitral valves become fibrosed, the high frequencies become dominant (38).

           c. When the belly of the anterior leaflet is very stiff and immobile due to either calcium or severe fibrosis, there is no snapping M_1.

4. In MS, how does the M_1 loudness vary if atrial fibrillation is present?

    ANS.: At least three types of M_1 loudness variations are seen.

    Type 1. If the MS is mild and although there is softening with short diastoles as with a normal valve, there is less tendency for the M_1 to become louder after long diastoles (31).

    Type 2. If the valves are severely stenosed and calcified (i.e., no opening snap is present), the M_1 depends entirely on end-diastolic volume and on the preceding and pre-preceding RR intervals (Starling and **postextrasystolic potentiation effect**). Thus, the S_1 becomes louder in proportion to the length of the previous diastole (31).

    Type 3. If the valves are moderately stenosed, the S_1 loudness varies inversely with the duration of the previous diastole (i.e., the shorter the previous RR interval, the louder the M_1 because of dependence on the end-diastolic left atrial-to-LV gradient) (31).

The M_1 in Mitral Regurgitation

1. How does the duration of the forward diastolic gradient across a mitral valve due to torrential flow across the mitral valve, as in mitral regurgitation (MR), differ from that of MS?

    ANS.: The torrential flow may cause a gradient only in early and middiastole, whereas a stenotic valve, even with less-than-normal flow, causes a gradient across the mitral valve throughout diastole. (See p. 283 for illustration of mitral valve gradient.)

2. Is the M_1 loud or soft if MR is present?

    ANS.: About half the patients with pure MR have a soft M_1. If the LV is not damaged, the M_1 may be loud.

        Note: About 70% of patients with papillary muscle dysfunction murmurs have a loud S_1.

REFERENCES

1. Ahuja SP, Coles JC. Further observations on the genesis of early systolic clicks. *Am J Cardiol* 1966;17:291.
2. Armstrong TG, Gotsman MS. Initial low frequency vibrations of the first heart sound. *Br Heart J* 1973;35:691.
3. Barrington WW, et al. Mitral stenosis: Left atrial dimensional changes and mitral "dome" ascent and descent. *Circulation* (Abst) 1983;68:308.
4. Beerman LB, et al. Ventricular septal defect associated with aneurysm of the membranous septum. *J Am Coll Cardiol* 1985;5:116.
5. Boughner DR, Roach MR. Effect of low frequency vibration on the arterial wall. *Circ Res* 1971;20:136.
6. Bruns DL, et al. Experimental observations on post-stenotic dilatation. *J Thorac Cardiovasc Surg* 1959;38:662.
7. Burgraff GW, Craige E. The first heart sound in complete heart block. *Circulation* 1974;50:17.
8. D'Cunha GF, et al. The first heart sound in intermittent left bundle branch block. *Am J Cardiol* 1971;27:447.
9. Dock W. The genesis of diastolic heart sounds. *Am J Med* 1971;50:178.

10. Gould L, et al. The genesis of the first heart sound with varying P-R intervals. *Dis Chest* 1967;52:817.
11. Hunt D, et al. Quantitative evaluation of cineaortography in the assessment of aortic regurgitation. *Am J Cardiol* 1973;31:696.
12. Laniado S, et al. Temporal relation of the first heart sound to closure of the mitral valve. *Circulation* 1973; 47:1006.
13. Leatham A. Heart murmurs, mechanism, intensity, and pitch. *Lancet* 1958;2:757. (Classic article.)
14. Leech G, et al. Mechanism of influence of the PR interval on loudness of the first heart sound. *Br Heart J* 1980; 43:138.
15. Lopez JF, et al. The apical first heart sound as an aid in the diagnosis of atrial septal defect. *Circulation* 1962; 26:1296.
16. Luisada AA, et al. Normal first heart sounds with nonfunctional tricuspid valve. *Circulation* 1967;35:119.
17. Martin CE, et al. Genesis, frequency, and diagnostic significance of the ejection sound in tetralogy of Fallot. *Br Heart J* 1973;35:402.
18. McGinn FX, et al. The phonocardiogram and apexcardiogram in patients with ventricular aneurysm. *Am J Cardiol* 1968;21:467.
19. Mikawa T, et al. Mitral component of the first heart sound in complete left bundle branch block: The mechanism of the decreased intensity. *J Cardiol* 1986;16:963.
20. Mills PG, et al. Echocardiographic and hemodynamic relationships of ejection sounds. *Circulation* 1977;56:430.
21. Mills PG, et al. The natural history of a non-stenotic bicuspid aortic valve. *Br Heart J* 1978;40:951.
22. Oakley CM, Hallidie-Smith KA. Assessment of site and severity in congenital aortic stenosis. *Br Heart J* 1967; 29:367.
23. Oravetz J, et al. Dynamic analysis of heart sounds in right and left bundle branch blocks. *Circulation* 1967; 36:275.
24. Ozawa Y, et al. Experimental studies on the genesis of low-frequency vibrations (M-sound) of the first heart sounds using a miniature accelerometer. *J Cardiol* 1983;13:137.
25. Parisi AF, Milton BG. Relation of mitral valve closure to the first heart sound in man. *Am J Cardiol* 1973; 32:779.
26. Piemme TE, et al. Relationship of heart sounds to acceleration of blood flow. *Circ Res* 1966;18:303.
27. Pieroni DR, et al. Auscultatory recognition of aneurysm of the membranous septum. *Circulation* 1971;44:733.
28. Plass R, et al. Intracardiac sounds and murmurs in atrial septal defect. *Am J Cardiol* 1971;28:173.
29. Prakash R. Genesis of heart sounds. *JAMA* 1978;240:2732.
30. Price WH, Brown AE. Alterations in intensity of heart sounds after myocardial infarction. *Br Heart J* 1968; 30:835.
31. Ravin A, Bershoff E. The intensity of the first heart sound in auricular fibrillation with mitral stenosis. *Am Heart J* 1951;41:539.
32. Rodbard S, et al. An analysis of mechanisms of post-stenotic dilatation. *Angiology* 1967;18:349.
33. Rytand DA. The variable loudness of the first heart sound in auricular fibrillation. *Am Heart J* 1949;37:187.
34. Sanchez J, et al. Diagnostic value of the first heart sound in children with atrial septal defect. *Am Heart J* 1969; 78:467.
35. Segall HN, Sharp A. Heart sounds in bundle branch block. *Jpn Heart J* 1967;8:468.
36. Shah PM, Kramer DH, Gramiak R. Influence of timing of atrial systole on mitral valve closure on the first heart sound in man. *Am J Cardiol* 1970;26:231.
37. Simon H, et al. The contractile state of the hypertrophied left ventricular myocardium in aortic stenosis. *Am Heart J* 1970;79:587.
38. Stein PD, et al. Frequency of the first heart sound in the assessment of stiffening of mitral bioprosthetic valves. *Circulation* 1981;63:200.
39. Stein PD, Sabbah HN. Origin of the second heart sound. *Am J Cardiol* 1978;41:108.
40. Tanaka K, et al. Diagnostic significance of phonocardiography and apex cardiography in patients with primary pulmonary hypertension. *CV Sound Bull* 1975;5:385.
41. Underwood SR, et al. Patterns of ventricular contraction in patients with conduction abnormality studied by radionuclide angiocardiography. *Br Heart J* 1974;51:568.
42. Van Bogaert A. A new concept on the mechanism of the first heart sound. *Am J Cardiol* 1966;18:253.
43. Victorica BE, et al. Persistent truncus arteriosus in infancy. *Am Heart J* 1969;77:13.
44. Weintraub AM, et al. Poststenotic dilatation of the aorta with muscular subaortic stenosis. *Am Heart J* 1964; 68:741.

9

The Second Heart Sound (S_2)

1. What produces the normal second heart sound (S_2)?
    ANS.: Events associated with closure of the aortic and pulmonary valves (Fig. 1).

    Note: Valve "closure" itself probably produces no noise. Echocardiography shows that sounds occur slightly after the coaptation of the leaflets. Shortly after apposition the sealed cusps are made tense and then vibrate due to the rapid force of aortic or pulmonary artery recoil.

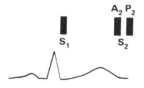

FIG. 1. A_2 is the aortic valve closure component of S_2. P_2 is the pulmonary valve closure component of the S_2. Note that the S_2 occurs near the end of the T wave of the ECG; that is, the T wave is a systolic event.

2. How can you use the QS_2 interval to diagnose excess cardiac sympathetic stimulation?
    ANS.: Normally, the QS_2 is longer than the QT by 26 ± 13 msec. Sympathetic stimulation shortens the QS_2 so that it encroaches on the QT interval and may even make the QS_2 shorter than the QT (6,14). This can occur in pheochromocytoma (36) and thyrotoxicosis (58) and is called the Hegglin syndrome (21).

    Note: When the QS_2 is prolonged to 40 msec or more beyond the QT, it is called the anti-Hegglin syndrome. This syndrome has been reported to occur in Takayasu arteritis and in anulo-aortic ectasia (34).

EXPLANATION OF NORMAL SPLITTING SEQUENCE OF S_2

1. At what pressure does the A_2 occur; that is, does it occur at aortic systolic or some intermediate pressure?
    ANS.: The aortic valve closes when the force of ventricular ejection decreases and when the peripheral resistance plus the elastic recoil of the expanded aorta overcomes the decreasing pressure in the LV. This occurs at just below aortic systolic pressure (e.g., if the systolic pressure in the aorta is 120 mm Hg, the A_2 probably occurs at a pressure of about 110 mm Hg) (Fig. 2).

    Note: The pulmonary artery pressure tracing also has a dicrotic notch or incisura where the P_2 occurs. The normal pulmonary artery pressure is about 25/10 mm Hg.

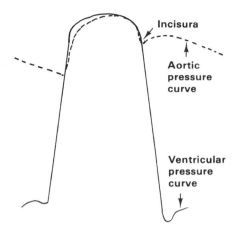

FIG. 2. Note that when the LV pressure rise exceeds aortic pressure, the aortic valve opens and produces a single chamber effect or an "aortoventricle." The point at which ejection is finished and the aortic and LV pressure curves separate is called the incisura and is simultaneous with the aortic second sound, or A₂.

2. How is the actual aortic valve closure related in time to the incisura and the A_2?

    ANS.: The actual closure or coaptation (apposition) of the aortic and pulmonary valves has been shown by echophonocardiography to occur usually slightly before (0 to 20 msec) their respective incisurae and sounds (3). This occurs because blood flow has inertia that continues the forward flow even after the LV pressure has dropped below aortic pressure and the valve has closed. Forward flow continues for a short time after the onset of the sound (42).

        Note: The duration of forward flow that takes place even after aortic pressure exceeds LV pressure is controlled by the impedance or resistance to forward flow, namely, the size of the vascular bed (capacitance), the resistance of the vascular bed, the compliance or distensibility of the vascular bed into which the blood is ejected, and the inertia of the mass of blood flowing into the vascular bed. Thus, if impedance is low, forward flow continues for a long time after the pressure crossover point and A_2 (or P_2) occurs very late. The leaflet coaptation-to-A_2 interval has been called the "hangout" interval (49) (Fig. 3).

3. If the aortic valve closes at a pressure of about 100 mm Hg and the pulmonary valve closes at about 20 mm Hg, why will aortic closure occur first?

    ANS.: The second heart sounds occur simultaneously with the incisurae of the pulmonary artery and aorta. The timing of the incisurae, in turn, has been shown to be related to the impedance to flow. For example, the less the arteriolar resistance and elastic recoil and the greater the capacity of the pulmonary arteries, the longer will forward flow continue and the later will the incisura occur on the pressure curve of the pulmonary artery. The pulmonary vascular resistance is about a tenth that of the systemic resistance. The elastic recoil power of the normal pulmonary artery is probably less than that of the aorta, and capacitance of the pulmonary vascular bed is greater than that of the aorta. Therefore, forward flow continues longer in the pulmonary circuit than in the aortic circuit after their respective pressure crossovers. This causes the pulmonary pressure and closure sound (P_2) to occur later than the aortic incisura and A_2.

        Note: a. Although the conduction system feeds the left ventricle (LV) before the right ventricle (RV) and contraction begins slightly earlier in the LV

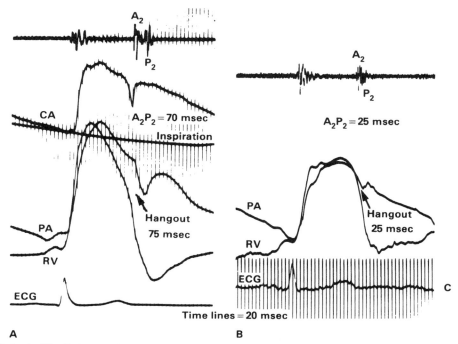

FIG. 3. A: The RV and PA pressure curves during inspiration from a normal 20-year-old male. **B:** The same pressure curves also during inspiration, from a normal 61-year-old male. The distance separating the pulmonary incisura from the RV pressure curve is called the "hangout interval" and is seen to be nearly equal to the A$_2$P$_2$ interval in each patient. This interval is the time necessary to overcome the inertia of forward flow.

than in the RV, this contributes very little to the relative timing of the respective closure sounds.

b. In truncus arteriosus the single truncal valve theoretically should be incapable of causing a split S$_2$. However, when the cusps are abnormal or when there are more than three, the S$_2$ is likely to be split and may even increase in width on inspiration. The cause of this split is unknown. It seems to be the "true reduplicated second sound" that all split sounds were formerly called, before it was recognized that they came separately from the aortic and pulmonary valves. The split may be a double movement of the valves due to a different impedance of the pulmonary and aortic circuits or possibly due to asynchronous closure of multiple unequal cusps.

c. Split P$_2$'s have been recorded in some normal subjects; the cause of this is also unknown.

PHYSIOLOGY OF THE NORMALLY MOVING SPLIT

1. It is well known that the normal split of S$_2$ widens on inspiration and narrows on expiration. Is this movement due to the movement of the A$_2$ or to the movement of the P$_2$?

ANS.: Both. The P$_2$ moves out, away from the A$_2$, and the A$_2$ moves inward, away from the P$_2$.

Note: In all age groups, but especially over age 40, there are normal subjects in whom the A_2 does not move at all. When it does move, it can contribute up to 30% of the total movement (Fig. 4).

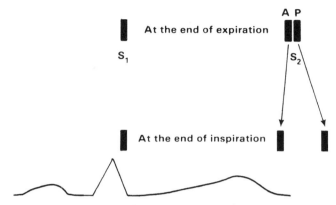

FIG. 4. The P_2 outward movement contributes more to the inspiratory widening of the S_2 than does the inward movement of the A_2.

2. Why does the P_2 occur later with inspiration?
   ANS.: There are at least two explanations.

   a. The RV becomes larger with inspiration because inspiration lowers the intrathoracic pressure. The lungs act as bellows; that is, when they expand the lungs function like a suction apparatus that sucks blood from the venae cavae into the right atrium and ventricle. This increased RV volume on inspiration delays pulmonary closure because when a ventricle increases its volume and has only one outlet for systole, it takes longer to eject that extra volume.

   b. On inspiration the pulmonary impedance falls because the capacitance of the pulmonary vasculature is increased. This contributes to the delay in pulmonary valve closure.

   c. The A_2 occurs earlier with inspiration because the LV becomes smaller with inspiration. By enlarging the chest volume, inspiration enlarges the vascular capacity of the lungs to such an extent that they cannot compensate by drawing enough blood from the RV. (The lungs do not fill from the RV in proportion to their increase in blood space potential during inspiration.) This excessive increase in lung capacity withholds some blood from the LV.

   Note: Maximum widening of the split A_2P_2 occurs at the peak of inspiration. Maximum narrowing occurs almost equally between mid- and end-expiration (38).

3. Does the normally moving split phenomenon (i.e., widening on inspiration and narrowing on expiration) refer to (a) held expiration and inspiration or moving respiration and to (b) deep respiration or normal respiration?
   ANS.: a. It refers to moving respiration.
   b. It refers to normal depth of respiration.

   Note: a. Held expiration results in a steady state in which the split remains fixed somewhere between the width on inspiration and expiration, with the A_2 coming first as usual.

b. A split S$_2$ at end-expiration is so rare after age 50 that it should be considered abnormal.

c. Over age 50 the S$_2$ usually remains single on both phases of respiration. A persistently single S$_2$ in a young person should make you think of all the causes of a soft or absent P$_2$ such as tetralogy of Fallot, pulmonary atresia, or transposition of the great vessels.

LOUDNESS OF COMPONENTS OF THE S$_2$

The Physics of Loudness

1. Is the greatest amplitude or loudness of the components of the S$_2$ in the low-, medium-, or high-frequency range?
   ANS.: In the low- and medium-frequency range.

2. Since the bell is best for bringing out low and medium frequencies, why is it usually better to listen to the splitting of the S$_2$ with the diaphragm?
   ANS.: The diaphragm separates the two components of the split better. Soft, high-frequency components may be masked by louder and longer low and medium frequencies if the split is narrow. Because the diaphragm damps out the louder low and medium frequencies, which reverberate around the high ones, volume is sacrificed for clarity in separating the components. Therefore, if one of the components of the S$_2$ is very soft, the bell may actually bring it out better (Fig. 5).

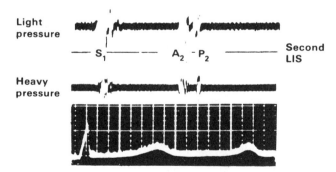

FIG. 5. With light pressure, the low and medium frequencies dominate and cause the split sounds (about 50 msec [0.05 sec] apart) to run together. Heavy pressure, by turning the skin into a diaphragm, attenuates the reverberations of the low and medium frequencies and helps to separate the components of the split.

3. What makes an A$_2$ or P$_2$ loud when there is more volume going through the valve?
   ANS.: If the aortic or pulmonary artery root is distended by an increased volume, the aorta or pulmonary artery beyond the valve has a greater recoil velocity, which closes the valve with more energy.

Sites of A$_2$ and P$_2$ Loudness

1. What is meant by the expression "A$_2$ is louder than P$_2$" or vice versa?
   ANS.: Before 1958, the A$_2$ meant the entire S$_2$ in the second right interspace (traditional "aortic area"), and the P$_2$ meant the entire S$_2$ in the second left interspace (tradi-

tional "pulmonary area"). Today they refer only to individual components of the split S_2.

2. Which *component* of the S_2 is best heard at the second left interspace (formerly called the "pulmonary area") in normal subjects? What is the clinical significance of this?

   ANS.: The A_2 is louder than the P_2 in the second left interspace in 70% of normal subjects under age 20. Over age 20, the A_2 is always louder than the P_2 in the second left interspace (45). (Even with severe pulmonary hypertension, as in Eisenmenger reactions, the A_2 is often louder than the P_2 in the second left interspace.) The P_2 is often best heard in the third or fourth left interspace, another reason why the second left interspace should not be considered the "true pulmonary area." Because this term is misleading, we encourage use of the term **second left interspace** instead (Fig. 6).

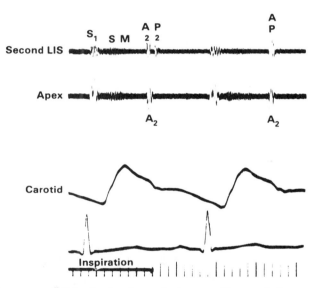

FIG. 6. This simultaneous carotid pulse tracing and phonocardiogram is from a normal 16-year-old with a normal split of S_2 on inspiration. Note that (a) only the A_2 would be audible at the apex, and (b) the A_2 has a greater amplitude than the P_2 at the second left interspace (LIS).

   Note: a. The second left interspace may be called the "classic" or "traditional" pulmonary area.

   b. Normally, the rate of change of the aortic-LV gradient at the time of aortic valve closure is greater than the pulmonary artery-RV gradient at the time of pulmonary valve closure. This helps to explain why the A_2 is louder than the P_2 in the second left interspace. In addition, the aortic valve is closest to the second and third left interspace, further reason for not naming the second right interspace the "aortic area" (Fig. 7).

3. Where is the P_2 normally heard on the chest wall?

   ANS.: In adults the P_2 is normally heard along the left sternal border, often only a few centimeters to the left of the sternum. In infants and young children, and in young

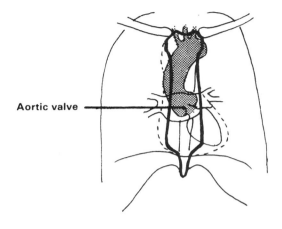

FIG. 7. The root of the aorta with its aortic valve is behind the middle of the sternum.

adults with a thin chest wall and a narrow anteroposterior chest diameter, it may also be heard at the apex.

Note: a. This implies that if the P_2 (split S_2) is also heard to the right of the sternum or at the apex in a thick-chested adult, the P_2 is probably louder than normal. When the P_2 is heard unexpectedly at the apex, you often find that the RV is enlarged and the apex beat is not due to the LV but entirely to the RV. Thus, in atrial septal defects (ASDs), it is expected that the large RV will make the P_2 audible at the apex, even though there may be no pulmonary hypertension.

   b. The A_2 is normally heard anywhere on the chest.

4. Where is the splitting of the S_2 most often heard on the chest wall?

   ANS.: At the second or third left interspace parasternally.

   Note: a. In obese patients, the split S_2 often is best heard at the *first* left interspace (39).

   b. The split second sound may be best heard to the right of the sternum in dextrocardia, persistent truncus arteriosus, or in transposition of the great vessels, whether they are congenitally corrected or not (Fig. 8).[1]

   c. In cyanotic tetralogy of Fallot, the S_2 is usually single and consists entirely of A_2 because the A_2 is attenuated by

   1. A deformed pulmonary valve when there is valvular stenosis (this occurs in only about one-third of tetralogies).

   2. The anterior placement of an enlarged aorta relative to a posteriorly placed small pulmonary artery.

   3. The low pulmonary artery pressure resulting from the diversion of RV blood through the high subaortic ventricular septal defect (VSD) directly into the aorta.

---

[1]In transposition of the great vessels, the aortic root is anterior to the pulmonary artery root so that the RV sends its venous blood to the aorta, and the LV ejects its oxygenated blood to the lungs. The patient dies unless adequate shunting occurs through an atrial septal defect (ASD, best), VSD, or persistent ductus arteriosus (PDA). If the ventricles are also reversed (congenitally corrected), shunts are not necessary for survival because an anatomic RV feeds the aorta and an anatomic LV feeds the pulmonary circuit with venous blood.

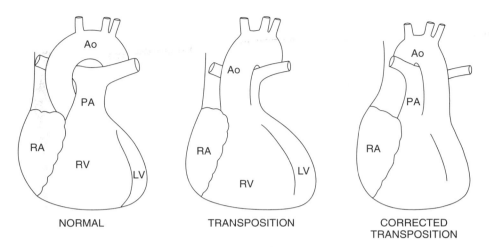

NORMAL   TRANSPOSITION   CORRECTED
                                               TRANSPOSITION

FIG. 8. In corrected transposition an anatomic left ventricle feeds the pulmonary artery and an anatomic right ventricle ejects into the aorta and must achieve systemic pressures. Note that the convexity of the left upper border of a chest x-ray could easily be mistaken for a pulmonary artery.

Causes of a Loud A_2 or P_2

1. What conditions tend to make the aortic component of the second sound louder than normal?

   ANS.: a. Conditions that raise aortic systolic pressure (e.g., systemic hypertension). Systemic hypertension occasionally produces a drumlike or "tambour" S_2.

   Note: A tambour is a small drum that is covered only on one side. The tambour S_2 is often heard in hypertensive patients and has been said to occur in some patients with only a dilated aortic root that stretches the valve cusps. In hypertensive subjects it may disappear with acute lowering of the blood pressure, as with amyl nitrite, but may persist even when the blood pressure is lowered chronically by treatment.

   b. Conditions that produce a hyperkinetic systemic circulation (e.g., youth, thyrotoxicosis, and aortic regurgitation).

   Note: The loudness of the aortic closure depends on the recoil of the aorta and the rate of systolic contraction of the LV. Therefore, it is related to ventricular performance. It follows, then, that a hypertensive patient in heart failure may not have a loud A_2.

   c. Any condition that brings the aorta close to the chest wall as when the aortic root is dilated, when the aorta is in front of the pulmonary trunk as in transposition of the great arteries, or when the aorta is behind an atretic pulmonary trunk.

2. What conditions other than a thin chest wall and pulmonary hypertension tend to make the P_2 louder than normal?

   ANS.: Conditions that produce increased blood flow into the pulmonary artery, as in an ASD or VSD.

   Note: a. The increased pulmonary flow due to an ASD does not necessarily make the P_2 louder than the A_2 unless the pulmonary artery pressure is at least 50 mm Hg (32). If pulmonary stenosis (PS) is present with the ASD, the

P_2 will probably be much softer than the A_2 and the split will be wide (60 msec or more) (31).

    b. In mitral stenosis (MS) the absolute loudness of the P_2 is a good sign of pulmonary hypertension only if it is loud. A P_2 that is louder than the A_2 in the second left interspace, however, is also a good sign of pulmonary hypertension but it does not tell you the degree of pulmonary hypertension.

    c. The P_2 is as loud as or louder than the A_2 in pulmonary hypertension even though pulmonary artery pressure may not be quite as high as aortic pressure because

        1. The pulmonary valve is more distensible and has a larger surface area than the aortic valve.

        2. The pulmonary valve is anterior to the aortic valve.

        3. In massive pulmonary embolism the P_2 may not be accentuated because of the decrease in ejection caused by the increase in afterload.

3. Why does the A_2 tend to be loud in hyperkinetic states such as thyrotoxicosis and aortic regurgitation (AR)?

    ANS.: The intensity of the A_2 is increased if the aortic valve closes when the aorta is energetically recoiling from the violent stretch caused by the increased volume flung into it during systole. The loudness of the A_2 is proportionate to the energy present when closure of the aortic valves decelerates the forward flow through the valve.

        Note: a. With severe AR the A_2 may be soft, presumably because of the absence of adequate valve substance to cause a sudden deceleration of forward flow. Also, when AR is severe, the peripheral resistance may be so low that the aortic recoil energy may be dissipated peripherally.

        b. One study using an intracardiac phonocatheter placed across the aortic valve found a softer than normal A_2 with all degrees of AR (44). This finding contradicts clinical experience with the stethoscope and must be considered to be due to a technical artifact that occurs when a phonocatheter is placed above a regurgitant valve.

4. How does inspiration affect the loudness of each component of the S_2?

    ANS.: The P_2 commonly becomes louder because extra blood in the pulmonary artery on inspiration causes more energetic elastic recoil. The A_2, on the other hand, becomes softer because inspiration decreases the volume ejected into the aorta and places the aorta farther from the stethoscope.

        Note: All sounds tend to become softer on inspiration if you listen over the upper chest, where excess lung space is interposed between the stethoscope and the heart on inspiration.

Causes of a Soft A_2 or P_2

1. What can make either the A_2 or the P_2 softer than normal, besides the effect of respiration and abnormal chest shapes and thickness?

    ANS.: a. Conditions that lower systolic pressure, as in severe pulmonary stenosis, which is associated with low pulmonary artery pressure, especially if there is a right-to-left shunt through an ASD or a VSD.

        b. Conditions that decrease the recoil power of the aortic or pulmonary roots such as

        1. Poor myocardial contractility.

2. Idiopathic pulmonary artery dilatation or poststenotic dilatation of the pulmonary artery or aorta, both of which are associated with damage to the elastic tissue of the arterial root area. Aortic distensibility is decreased in the poststenotic segment even more if coronary disease is present, probably because the vasa vasorum of the ascending aorta are derived from the coronary arteries (52).

c. Conditions that stiffen the semilunar valves (e.g., calcification, sclerosis, or fusion of the cusps, as in aortic stenosis [AS] or pulmonary stenosis [PS]).

Note: a. In PS the pulmonary valve is thick and leathery, and viewed from the pulmonary artery the stenotic valve resembles a uterine cervix. It is often adherent at its base to the surrounding pulmonary artery. This not only makes the P_2 soft but also adds to its lateness because the RV pressure must drop considerably below the pulmonary artery pressure before it can move the relatively immobile valve.

b. A massive pulmonary embolus that touches the pulmonary valve makes the P_2 soft even in the presence of pulmonary hypertension.

c. Conditions that place the pulmonary artery farther from the stethoscope (e.g., transposition of the great vessels [see p. 150], congenitally corrected or not) soften the P_2 even in the presence of pulmonary hypertension.

d. If the PS is purely subinfundibular due to hypertrophic cardiomyopathy (very rare), the P_2 may be of normal loudness, although delayed. In congenital infundibular PS the P_2 may be inaudible.

e. When the aortic or pulmonary valves are calcified or fibrosed, low frequencies tend to be attenuated; that is, the dominant frequencies are higher than they are when the valves are normal (53). Similarly, with porcine xenograft aortic prosthesis the low frequencies are lost over the years, probably due to degenerative changes (53).

Relative Loudness, Pitch, and Duration of the S_1 and S_2

1. The S_1 and S_2 usually make groups of two because diastole is longer than systole. When are there no groups of two?

ANS.: a. When diastole becomes relatively shorter than systole, as with marked tachycardias. This is called embryocardia because this is what is heard when listening to fetal heart sounds after the fifth month of pregnancy. A more appropriate term would be **fetocardia**.

Note: Embryocardia may occur even after birth because the heart rate in the first year of life may be as high as 190, and in the second year up to 160. Even in the fourth year it can normally be 130. At the time of puberty, it may normally be as high as 100.

b. In adults, systole may become long relative to diastole for unknown reasons. This is called "ticktack rhythm" and is comparable to the ticking of a clock.

Note: A long QT by itself cannot prolong systole because the QS_2 can be concomitantly shortened by excess sympathetic stimulation of coronary disease with or without an old infarction (6,14). Therefore, ticktack rhythm without a tachycardia to shorten diastole implies an absence of significant coronary disease.

c. Severe AR can produce a ticktack rhythm even without a tachycardia because the increased volume ejected in systole can prolong systole relative to diastole. It is common in severe AR to mistake systole for diastole.

2. How may the relative loudness of the S$_1$ and S$_2$ help distinguish one from the other?

   ANS.: In a completely normal subject the S$_2$ is louder than the S$_1$ at the second right or left interspace (i.e., at the base of the heart), possibly because this is where the aortic and pulmonary valve structures are closest to the chest wall. At the apex, the S$_1$ is usually louder than the S$_2$.

   Note: If the S$_1$ is louder than the S$_2$ at the base it suggests that an extra-loud S$_1$ is present, as in MS, or that there is an extra-soft S$_2$.

3. How can you tell at the bedside which heart sound is the S$_2$ when relative loudness is of no help?

   ANS.: a. The S$_2$ is higher in pitch and is sharper and shorter than the S$_1$ because it is usually single on expiration. The S$_1$ is relatively muffled and rough because of its three components. This is implied by the term **lub-dup**, often used to mimic the sounds of the S$_1$S$_2$.

   b. Palpate the carotid while listening with the stethoscope. The S$_1$ is heard just before the carotid impulse is felt. The carotid has the same relationship to the S$_1$ as the peak of an early systolic murmur; that is, if we use the letter *C* to represent the carotid impulse, then the rhythm goes "1-C-2, 1-C-2." This is due to the slight delay between the beginning of ventricular contraction, which produces the S$_1$, and the arrival of the carotid impulse in the neck (Fig. 9).

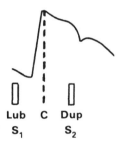

Lub   C   Dup
S$_1$ S$_2$

FIG. 9. The tap of the carotid pulse on your fingers is felt *after* and *not with* the first heart sound.

   c. Place the stethoscope or a finger over the apex beat and note the outward impulse that occurs during systole. It should bulge outward with or just after the S$_1$. The stethoscope itself rises during systole, and this tells you which sound is the S$_1$. The S$_1$ appears to "produce" the rise in apical impulse.

   d. If you hear inspiratory splitting of one sound at the left sternal border and therefore know which sound is the S$_2$, "inch" toward the apex. Inching means keeping the rhythm intact by moving the stethoscope rhythmically a few inches at a time exactly in time with the heart sounds.

THE WIDELY SPLIT S$_2$

1. What do physiologists often call heart sounds in contrast to heart murmurs?

   ANS.: Transients. This merely implies noises of short duration.

   Note: The smallest time interval between transients that the ear is capable of distinguishing as two separate sounds is 20 msec. This narrow interval allows a distinction of two separate sounds only if they are very short and high in frequency as, for example, the sounds of a camera shutter or a snare drum. For practical purposes, a split of 20 msec sounds merely like an impure or dirty sound rather than a sharp and clean one. This means that the narrowest split of heart sounds that the ear can clearly separate is about 30 msec.

2. What is meant by a wide split of the S_2?

   ANS.: There are two ways of defining a wide split.

   a. A sound that splits widely on inspiration (i.e., to at least 60 msec [0.06 sec]), even if it is single on expiration.

   b. A persistent split of S_2 on expiration that widens still more on inspiration.

   Note: The concept of wide and narrow splitting is best understood if you practice the vocal imitation of splitting widths as follows. A normal narrow split on inspiration is 30 to 40 msec (0.03 to 0.04 sec). Imitate this by rolling the tongue as in a Spanish *dr* or *tr*. For a slightly wider split of 50 to 60 msec (0.05 to 0.06 sec), say "pa-da" quickly. For a wide split of 70 to 80 msec (0.07 to 0.08 sec), say "pa-ta" quickly. Articulate both the *p* and the *t* sharply. A very wide split is 90 to 100 msec (0.09 to 0.10 sec). For this, say "pa-pa" as quickly as possible.

3. What conditions can cause wide splitting of the S_2 as a result of a delay in pulmonary valve closure?

   ANS.: Delays of P_2 are caused by

   a. Conditions that cause electrical delay of activation of the RV (e.g., right bundle branch block [RBBB]).

   Note: The delay in P_2 with RBBB is due not only to delayed onset of right ventricular contraction but also to a slower rate of rise of right ventricular pressure (24). Type A atrioventricular preexcitation also causes a wide split (usually 50 to 70 msec) because the accessory bundle in type A enters the LV first and therefore acts like a RBBB.

   b. Conditions that cause an increased volume in the RV in comparison with the LV (e.g., at least a moderately sized ASD or a moderate amount of pulmonary regurgitation [PR]).

   Note: For some unknown reason, even in severe congenital PR, the S_2 may occasionally be narrowly split.

   c. Conditions that cause a gradient across the pulmonary valve due to valvular or infundibular PS.

   d. Conditions that cause either acute or chronic RV failure, as in massive pulmonary embolism, or in the late stages of chronic pulmonary embolism or primary pulmonary hypertension (11).

   e. Conditions that decrease elastic recoil and increase capacitance of the pulmonary artery (e.g., idiopathic dilatation of the pulmonary artery) (43,48).

   Note: The reason for the lack of wide splitting in some patients with idiopathic dilatation of the pulmonary artery may be a relatively smaller loss of elastic tissue. The exceptionally broad P_2 heard in some patients with idiopathic dilatation is unexplained.

   f. Bilateral pulmonary artery branch stenosis (13,23).

   g. Congenital absence of the pericardium.

4. What has been shown to cause the delay of P_2 in patients with a VSD besides the volume overload of the RV?

   ANS.: The QP_2 interval is lengthened because in VSDs there is a delay in the onset of RV contraction. The interval from Q to the onset of the RV contraction (electromechanical interval) may be prolonged by as much as 60 msec more than the normal 40 to 60 msec.

> *Note*: a. The P$_2$ occurs late in ASDs because the pulmonary incisura is late due to the difficulty in halting the high velocity of flow into the low-impedance pulmonary vascular bed, which is partly due to dilatation of the main pulmonary artery (increased capacitance).
>
>   b. In more than 70% of postoperative ASD patients the wide splitting of the S$_2$ persists. This suggests that the theory claiming a dilated pulmonary artery causes delay of the incisura might be correct, because the pulmonary artery remains dilated after corrective surgery. This theory is further supported by the absence of a significant relationship between the width of the split and the size of the shunt (9).

5. When can a wide split occur due to early closure of the A$_2$?

   a. In patients with pulsus paradoxus wide splitting may be present at the onset of inspiration due to marked shortening of systole. It then becomes single within a few beats. In tamponade the early occurrence of the A$_2$ is due to markedly disproportionate decrease in the size of the LV in comparison with the RV on inspiration (20). (The Q-P$_2$ does not change with inspiration in tamponade.) The Q-A$_2$, on the other hand, shortens due to marked decrease in LV volume.

   b. In the presence of a left atrial tumor, usually a myxoma, there is underfilling of the LV (27).

   > *Note*: a. It has been assumed in the past that a widely split S$_2$ occurring in severe mitral regurgitation (MR) is due to an early A$_2$ secondary to shortening of the ejection time because of the presence of two outlets for systole. This is unreasonable because
   >   1. There may be two outlets, but there is also more volume to be ejected.
   >   2. The S$_2$ is not widely split in mild to moderate MR.
   >   3. Left ventricular ejection times are normal in MR unless the output is decreased at rest.
   >   4. MR can delay the onset of LV contraction (28).
   >
   >   b. It is important to know that MR can produce a widely split S$_2$ because a wide split tells you the MR is at least moderately severe and that you must not assume that a widely split S$_2$ with MR is due to an A$_2$-opening snap. (Differentiating between an A$_2$P$_2$ and an A$_2$-opening snap is discussed on pp. 176–177.)

6. In tamponade, why does the LV decrease in size so markedly in comparison with the RV during inspiration?

   ANS.: a. The increase in RV volume during inspiration stretches the entire pericardium, which also covers the atria. The rise in intrapericardial pressure restricts the expansion of the left atrium so that it cannot dilate with the blood it receives from the pulmonary veins. During inspiration the left atrial pressure may actually rise higher than the pulmonary venous pressure, and blood may flow backward into the pulmonary veins.

   b. An exaggerated shift of the ventricular septum toward the LV during inspiration also decreases LV volume in tamponade.

7. What is the widest normal split heard during held expiration?

   ANS.: On held expiration or at the end of normal expiration, the widest normal split is about 30 msec; this is rare over age 40.

Note: a. Over age 50, the S_2 closes on expiration in 95% of normal subjects in the recumbent position (1). Exceptionally wide splitting (80 msec on inspiration) is found in some normal children (16); the reason for this is unknown.

b. When both ventricles are volume-overloaded as when a **Sinus of Valsalva** ruptures into the right atrium or RV, the split S_2 widens except with a VSD-to-right atrial shunt.

THE A_2P_2 IN PULMONARY STENOSIS

1. Why will a stenotic RV outflow tract or valve cause a delay of the P_2?

   ANS.: In PS, RV pressure is much higher than pulmonary artery pressure. It therefore takes an extra-long time for the RV pressure to drop to the closing pressure of the pulmonary artery valve. (See Fig. 15, p. 163.) Also, a stiff pulmonic valve requires a greater fall in RV pressure below the pulmonary artery pressure before it can move the rigid valve into the closed position. Furthermore, if there is poststenotic dilatation, the increased pulmonary capacitance plus the poor elastic recoil increases the delay in P_2.

   Note: There is less delay in RV emptying in supravalvular PS than in valvular PS because in the former there is a high pressure between the valve and the supravalvular obstruction. In supravalvular PS or in unilateral pulmonary artery stenosis, the A_2P_2 split is usually normal or narrow (13,41).

2. Does the PS seen in severe tetralogy of Fallot produce a wide split of the S_2?

   ANS.: In actual practice, the P_2 is audible in only about one-third of cyanotic adults with tetralogy of Fallot (22). Intracardiac phonocardiography with the microphone in the pulmonary artery, however, has always shown the delayed P_2 (17). Also, after shunt operations that increase pulmonary flow, the P_2 has been seen to be very delayed.

   Note: A long systolic murmur that continues into or through the A_2 along the left sternal border can obscure the widely split S_2. This occurs with the murmur of VSD or with severe PS (Fig. 10).

Left sternal border

A_2 P_2

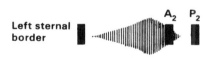

Apical area

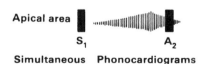

S_1 A_2

Simultaneous   Phonocardiograms

FIG. 10. At the apex, the easily recorded A_2 may be heard despite the murmur, which is much softer in that area.

3. How can the A_2P_2 interval tell you the probable RV pressure in PS?

   ANS.: In general, the more severe the obstruction and the higher the RV pressure, the longer the A_2P_2 interval.

   Note: a. If the A_2P_2 interval is 40 msec or less, the RV pressure ranges from normal to about 45 mm Hg. If 50 msec, the RV pressure ranges from normal to about 55 mm Hg. If 60 msec, the RV pressure is no longer likely to be normal but ranges from 60 to 120 mm Hg. If 100 msec, the range is from 70 to 160 mm Hg (19). If there is marked poststenotic dilatation of the pulmonary artery, the increase in capacitance of the pulmonary artery may delay pulmonary valve closure so that the RV pressure is thought to be higher than it really is. Therefore, the lower end of the range of RV pressure is more likely to be the correct one if pulmonary artery dilatation is marked (49). This is also true if the infundibulum is hypertrophied (usually secondary to valvular PS), because contraction of the infundibulum may occur considerably later than that of the body of the RV even with only moderate gradients.

   b. The wide split of S$_2$ in PS is relatively fixed, either with mild PS and marked dilatation of the pulmonary artery or with severe PS and marked RV hypertrophy (RVH) (50).

THE FIXED SPLIT OF THE S$_2$

1. What is meant by a fixed or relatively fixed split of the S$_2$?
   ANS.: If the split changes less than 20 msec (0.02 sec) with quiet respiration, it is called a fixed or relatively fixed split.
2. What can cause a fixed or relatively fixed split of the S$_2$?
   ANS.: a. ASDs.
      b. Heart failure, because the heart in failure is relatively insensitive to changes in filling pressure (40). For example, a rise in LV end-diastolic pressure of a few millimeters of mercury in the normal ventricle can almost double cardiac output; in the failing ventricle the output rises only slightly or not at all.
      c. Moderate to large VSDs (5). An obviously moving split in a patient with a VSD usually implies a small shunt (with a pulmonary-systemic flow of less than 2:1) and a pulmonary artery systolic pressure of less than 50 mm Hg (25).
      d. Pulmonary stenosis in some patients (50).
      e. Pulmonary embolism, massive pulmonary embolism, or the late sequelae of chronic pulmonary embolism, when the pulmonary artery pressure is at least two-thirds of the systemic pressure (11).
      f. Idiopathic dilatation of the pulmonary artery. In six of eight patients with idiopathic dilatation of the pulmonary artery in one series, the split was relatively fixed (26).
         Note: A relatively fixed split is a variation of normal in about 15% of children and young men, especially in the supine position (10). The reason is unknown. If the split is fixed when the patient is supine, it will not be fixed in the sitting position, and occasionally vice versa.
      g. Constrictive pericarditis, for the same reason as for the fixed split in heart failure (i.e., an inability to respond to a change in diastolic volume).

The Fixed Split of the S$_2$ in ASD

1. Why is the S$_2$ split in ASD relatively fixed?
   ANS.: In ASD the LV does not become smaller on inspiration and may even become

larger. This occurs because on inspiration vena caval blood is drawn into the right atrium, where the pressure then rises, thereby decreasing the left-to-right shunt through the ASD. This nonshunted left atrial blood passes through the mitral valve into the LV and thus tends to keep LV volume constant during inspiration (Fig. 11).

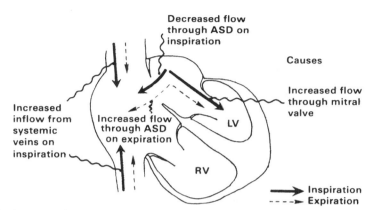

FIG. 11. The increased inflow into the right atrium on inspiration (*vertical solid arrows*) causes a decreased flow through the ASD and thus increased flow through the mitral valve.

Note: a. If the left-to-right shunt is *markedly* decreased on inspiration due to a poorly compliant RV, the LV volume may even *increase* with the large inflow of blood from the left atrium during inspiration, and the A_2 may move in the same direction as the P_2.

b. There is physiologic proof that the shunt from the left to the right atrium in ASD is decreased by inspiration. Oxygen saturation in the pulmonary artery has been shown to be less during inspiration in subjects with ASD (4). It has been found that a 50% decrease in left-to-right shunt can occur with inspiration.

c. The volume of the left-to-right shunt is decreased on inspiration, thus minimizing the increase in volume of the RV during inspiration.

2. Does the P_2 move normally with respiration in the presence of an ASD?

ANS.: With normal respiration, the P_2 moves only slightly or not at all. The QP_2 interval moves less than 20 msec in ASDs during quiet inspiration (4). (In normal subjects the QP_2 is almost always lengthened on quiet inspiration by at least 20 msec and in most cases by about 40 msec.) With deep inspiration, however, the P_2 in patients with ASDs can move almost normally because deep inspiration can increase the flow into the RV as shown by the following evidence.

a. A tricuspid diastolic flow murmur due to torrential flow through the valve is often heard only on deep inspiration.

b. The P_2 may become louder on deep inspiration on both external and intracardiac phonocardiograms (18) (Figs. 12 and 13).

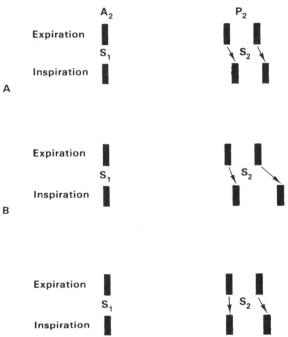

FIG. 12. If, as in A, the A_2 moves forward on inspiration exactly the same amount as the P_2, the split will be absolutely fixed on respiration. This is uncommon. Usually, even when the A_2 moves forward with inspiration, it does not move as much as does the P_2 as in B and C.

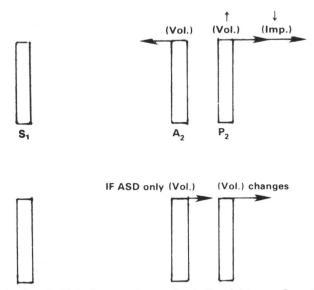

FIG. 13. On inspiration the P_2 is shown to be moving to the right away from the S_1 by two mechanisms, the increased volume in the RV and the decreased impedance of the pulmonary circuit. The A_2 is shown moving to the left (toward the S_1) by only one mechanism, the decreased volume in the LV. In ASDs the P_2 moves with inspiration due only to its increased volume, because there is no significant impedance effect when the lung vessels are overfilled because of the shunt flow. The A_2 either may not move at all with inspiration or may actually move in the same direction as the P_2.

NARROW SPLIT OF THE S$_2$ IN ASD

1. How common is a narrow split of the S$_2$ with ASDs?

    ANS.: Although ASDs are noted for their wide splits, the majority of adults with ASDs do not have a split of more than 60 msec. Some normal young subjects have wider inspiratory splits than this.

    Note: a. In subjects with an ASD, a narrow split of the S$_2$ is unrelated to the size of the shunt. The duration of RV ejection is not necessarily proportional to the stroke volume of the RV because the larger the stroke volume, the faster the RV contracts.

    b. A narrow split on inspiration that remains split on expiration, especially during sitting or standing, is an excellent sign of a relatively fixed split, because if a split is narrow on inspiration, it should *close* on expiration, especially in the sitting or standing position. It is not surprising that in ASD patients even a narrow split of the S$_2$ remains open in the sitting or standing position, because it has been shown that in uncomplicated left-to-right shunts the shunt flow increases in the upright position (8). In ASD patients there is often more variation of the split S$_2$ with respiration in the sitting position; the longer the subject sits, the more variation there may be.

    c. Tachycardias also narrow the split in patients with ASDs.

    d. Marked dilatation of the pulmonary artery, which is common with ASDs, perhaps as an associated anomaly, can increase the capacitance of the pulmonary vascular tree and so delay closure of the P$_2$. With a narrow split in patients with an ASD, one should suspect that the pulmonary artery is only minimally dilated.

2. How can a long pause after a premature ventricular contraction or in atrial fibrillation suggest the presence of a fixed split in a patient with an ASD?

    ANS.: After a long pause, the split widens markedly (56). This widening may be due to an increase in the left-to-right shunt during long diastoles. (In the normal heart the split S$_2$ is also widened after long diastoles but not as much as in the presence of an ASD.) The left-to-right shunt in diastole is controlled largely by the relative resistance to expansion of the RV and the LV. It may be that the difference in distensibility between the RV and the LV is exaggerated by a long diastole.

DIFFERENTIAL DIAGNOSIS OF THE FIXED SPLIT

1. Why is the split S$_2$ of some patients with PS relatively fixed?

    ANS.: There are at least two possibilities.

    a. Because the split is usually fixed when there is marked poststenotic dilatation of the pulmonary artery, poor elastic recoil may somehow be responsible. The dilated segment has been shown to be more distensible than normal (43).

    b. The markedly hypertrophied RV often has much fibrosis and may not be able to respond well to the increased blood volume brought to it by inspiration.

    Note: Suspect the presence of PS in addition to an ASD when the split on expiration is 60 mm Hg or more and the P$_2$ is softer than the A$_2$.

2. What may mimic a wide fixed split of the S$_2$?

    ANS.: a. A paradoxical split in complete left bundle branch block (LBBB), especially with heart failure. (The paradoxical split is explained on p. 165.)

   b. The A$_2$ followed by an opening snap. (The six ways of distinguishing an A$_2$P$_2$ from an A$_2$-opening snap are detailed on p. 176.)
   c. A very wide split in which normal movements of the A$_2$P$_2$ are difficult to perceive by auscultation. It is much easier to perceive movement of two sounds when they are close together than when they are far apart. The solution to this dilemma is to make the two sounds approach one another by causing less blood to return to the heart, as with sitting or standing (Fig. 14).

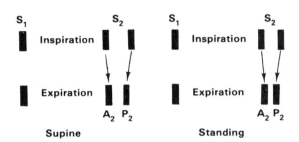

FIG. 14. It would be difficult to perceive movement of the split in the supine position shown in the S$_2$ on the left, and you might call it a relatively fixed split until the patient sits or stands up.

   Note: The split S$_2$ in the normal subject tends to narrow on sitting or standing because when both ventricles receive less blood (due to pooling in the abdomen and the legs), the RV responds by ejecting its blood relatively faster than the LV (35). The RV responds more to changes in filling pressure than does the LV (46).

3. How can placing a patient in the sitting position help distinguish the supine expiratory splitting of the S$_2$ in a normal young patient from the relatively fixed split of a patient with an ASD?
   ANS.: The normal patient usually shows increased respiratory variation on sitting or standing, and the split closes on expiration (33). On sitting or standing, the ASD patient maintains the split on expiration, even though respiratory variation may also increase in these positions.

4. What happens to the splitting of the S$_2$ after the release of a Valsalva? How can you use this maneuver to detect the presence of an ASD?
   ANS.: The Valsalva maneuver dams up venous blood behind the RV. On release of this dammed-up blood, there is extra filling of the RV for a few beats, in contrast to the LV, and the split widens.
      A few seconds after the release of the strain, the split S$_2$ becomes very narrow or single because the dammed-up blood now reaches the LV after a few beats, pushing a comparatively greater volume into the LV than into the RV for a few beats.
      In patients with ASDs, however, the atria act almost as a single chamber, so that any rise in right atrial pressure is also reflected in a rise in left atrial pressure. Thus, on release of the Valsalva, any increased venous blood that rushes into the RV also causes more blood to enter the LV, and there is only slight immediate widening and no delayed narrowing of the S$_2$ (4).
      This test is useful after surgery on an ASD, because the wide and relatively fixed split may persist for at least a year. The post-Valsalva effect does, however, indicate the true situation.

Note: Overcoming difficulties in a patient's understanding of how to perform a Valsalva maneuver is explained on p. 64.

5. Which abnormalities other than an ASD may produce a relatively fixed split of the S_2 as well as a *wide* split?

ANS.: a. RBBB plus heart failure. The RBBB makes the split wide, and the heart failure fixes it.

   b. Right ventricular failure secondary to pulmonary hypertension. The wide split is probably due to a prolonged isovolumic contraction time in the failing RV.

   c. Some moderately large VSDs have wide and relatively fixed splits. The widening here is partly due to a delayed P_2 (5).

   d. Some patients with partial **anomalous pulmonary venous drainage** into the right atrium have relatively fixed, wide splits.

   Note: Although this anomaly may cause the same physical, ECG, and x-ray signs of an ASD, the effect of respiration on the split of the S_2 often enables you to distinguish the two lesions. If the splitting is normal, the differentiation is easy. Some subjects with partial anomalous pulmonary venous drainage, however, have relatively fixed splits due to a prolongation of the QP_2 interval on expiration (29).

6. How can you distinguish the wide, fixed split and loud P_2 of RV failure due to pulmonary hypertension from that of ASD with pulmonary hypertension?

ANS: Exercise widens the split further only in RV failure because it delays the P_2. This probably occurs because a rise in pulmonary artery pressure with exercise increases the isovolumic contraction time of the failing RV and leaves the isovolumic contraction of the normal LV relatively unchanged.

THE NARROWLY SPLIT S$_2$

1. List the usual causes, other than aortic stenosis (AS), of a narrowly split S_2 due to a delayed A_2.

ANS.: a. Conditions that cause electrical delay of LV conduction: LBBB and some types of Wolff-Parkinson-White (WPW) preexcitation that imitate LBBB by causing premature depolarization of the RV.

   b. Conditions that increase the volume of the LV without an extra outlet (MR or a VSD has an extra outlet), for example, PDA and AR.

   Note: a. Hypertension can prolong the QA_2 more than the QP_2 probably by delaying the onset of LV contraction (electromechanical interval) and by slightly prolonging the ejection time. If myocardial damage is superimposed on the hypertension, the isovolumic contraction time is prolonged as well, and a paradoxical or reversed split (P_2A_2) may result.

   b. Aging not only prolongs the LV ejection time, thus delaying the A_2, but also causes a shortening of the QP_2 interval, thus bringing the P_2 earlier. In the elderly, the A_2 often does not move at all.

2. What causes the narrow or reversed split S_2 in AS?

ANS.: AS causes a significant gradient across the outflow of the LV so that there is a delay in LV pressure dropping below aortic pressure (Fig. 15).

   Note: a. The delay in the A_2 in AS is not due to prolonged LV contraction. The time from the Q wave to the end of the LV systole (i.e., from the Q to the beginning of the fall in LV pressure [end of LV systole] on the LV pressure curve) is *shorter* than the time from the Q wave to the end of the RV systole in all degrees of AS.

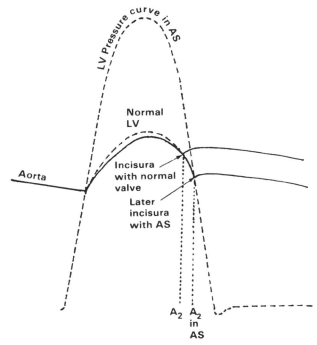

FIG. 15. In AS the LV pressure rises high above aortic pressure during systole. It then takes so long to drop down to aortic diastolic pressure and close the valve that the incisura is low and late on the aortic pressure curve. The A₂ is also late because it is simultaneous with the incisura.

        b. Marked poststenotic dilatation may further delay the A_2 by decreasing the impedance beyond the valve (43).

3. List the causes of a narrowly split S_2 due to an early P_2.

    ANS.: a. Conditions that increase impedance of the pulmonary vasculature (e.g., early stages of pulmonary hypertension). (In the late stages the split widens due to RV failure.)

        b. As a person grows older, the P_2 occurs slightly earlier (i.e., the QP_2 interval shortens due to the increase in impedance in the pulmonary circuit with aging) (12). The isovolumic contraction time of the LV also becomes slightly longer, tending to delay the A_2 (51).

        c. Shortening the RV systole due to underfilling of the RV secondary to a right atrial tumor, usually an atrial myxoma (27).

         Note: About 30% of normal subjects under age 50 and 60% of those over age 50 will have a single S_2 on quiet respiration (1).

4. How can you tell that an S_2 is split on inspiration even if you do not hear two distinct components?

    ANS.: If the S_2 is clean and sharp on expiration and becomes impure or rough on inspiration, then it probably has opened up slightly on inspiration (to about 20 msec [0.02 sec]).

        Note: Too deep an inspiration interposes too much lung between the stethoscope and the heart, causing one or both of the S_2 components to disappear. Too shallow an inspiration may not open the S_2 at all.

5. How can you control the respiration of a patient so that there are enough cardiac cycles on inspiration and expiration for you to distinguish normal from abnormal splitting?

ANS.: Ask the patient to follow your arm, raising it for inspiration and lowering it for expiration; you may "conduct" the patient's respiration so that there are at least two or three cycles during each phase of respiration. Be certain that the patient does not breathe too deeply.

THE SPLIT S$_2$ IN PULMONARY HYPERTENSION

1. What are the three general types of pulmonary hypertension?

ANS.: a. Hyperkinetic pulmonary hypertension; that is, that due to excess volume flow, as in large left-to-right shunts. The pulmonary arterioles can dilate to accommodate up to three times the normal cardiac output before the excess flow causes the pulmonary artery pressure to rise, due also to some vasoconstriction.

b. Obstructive pulmonary hypertension; that is, that due to fixed lumen obliteration, as with pulmonary emboli, or that due to narrowing, as with the endothelial and medial hypertrophy seen in some ASDs, PDAs, and VSDs with bidirectional shunting (Eisenmenger reaction).

c. Primary pulmonary hypertension.

2. In which of the preceding causes of pulmonary hypertension do you expect (a) normal or narrow splitting, (b) wide splitting, or (c) no splitting?

ANS.: a. Normal or narrow splitting is expected in the early stages of primary pulmonary hypertension in some subjects and with the pulmonary hypertension of most subjects with PDA or MS (55). The increased impedance due to the high resistance and tense pulmonary artery ordinarily causes an early P$_2$, making the S$_2$ single. However, the dilated pulmonary artery, so often found in patients with pulmonary hypertension, decreases the impedance to pulmonary flow and may cause separation of the S$_2$ to normal degrees on inspiration.

Note: The level of pulmonary hypertension does not correlate with the width of splitting in MS or MR (55).

b. Wide splitting is expected in ASDs, in massive pulmonary embolism, and in some patients with severe primary pulmonary hypertension, with a prolonged RV isovolumic contraction time.

c. No splitting is expected in VSDs with an Eisenmenger reaction, but in VSDs with hyperkinetic pulmonary hypertension the S$_2$ may be either single or split normally (55).

Note: Although a single S$_2$ in VSD does not indicate whether or not the pulmonary hypertension is too fixed to be operable, a split S$_2$ usually implies that an operation is feasible.

3. How much obstruction is necessary before an acute pulmonary embolism can produce wide, relatively fixed splitting of the S$_2$?

ANS.: Almost the entire pulmonary tree on both sides must be obstructed. If pulmonary hypertension is already present due to previous disease, however, a further embolus to one branch may cause wide, fixed splitting.

Note: a. Moderate exercise can bring out the wide splitting in borderline cases and exaggerate it still more in advanced obstruction. In severe obstruction, the split may be almost 80 msec. Because it is relatively fixed, it may be mistaken for an opening snap. This wide split often narrows with lysis of the embolus over 3 to 6 days.

   b. The cause of the wide split in acute pulmonary embolism is due to a shortened QA$_2$ and a normal QP$_2$.
4. What is an ASD, VSD, or PDA with bidirectional shunting called?
   ANS.: An Eisenmenger situation, syndrome, or reaction. The pulmonary hypertension may be so severe that only right-to-left shunting occurs.
      Note: When a VSD is the cause of the pulmonary hypertension, it is often called an Eisenmenger complex because this is the original lesion described by Eisenmenger in 1897.
5. How does the S$_2$ differ among the three different levels of Eisenmenger syndromes (i.e., VSD, ASD, and PDA)?
   ANS.: In VSD the S$_2$ is single, in ASD it is split and fixed (often widely split), in PDA it is normally or narrowly split, and when split, it moves normally (55).
      Note: a. Early in the course of development of an ASD Eisenmenger reaction, the high resistance beyond the pulmonary valve may narrow the split S$_2$. As the RV begins to fail, its isovolumic contraction time is prolonged, and the split becomes wide again.
         b. The S$_2$ of a VSD with an Eisenmenger reaction becomes single on both phases of respiration because only a large VSD can produce an Eisenmenger reaction, and such a large communication between the ventricles tends to make them function as a single chamber.
         c. The A$_2$/P$_2$ loudness ratio at the second left interspace can suggest the presence of hyperkinetic pulmonary hypertension in a subject with a VSD. In a VSD with normal pulmonary artery pressure, the A$_2$ is generally louder than the P$_2$. Therefore, if the P$_2$ is louder, pulmonary hypertension is probably present.
         d. Primary pulmonary hypertension tends to have a vibratory S$_1$, which is thought to be due to loud tricuspid valve closure (56).

THE REVERSED OR PARADOXICALLY SPLIT S$_2$

Physiology and Etiologies

1. What is meant by a reversed or paradoxical split of the S$_2$?
   ANS.: This is the split in which the order of components is P$_2$A$_2$ instead of the normal A$_2$P$_2$.
      Note: A reversed split caused by too early a P$_2$ is very rare. A reversed split is nearly always caused by a delayed A$_2$.
2. What can delay the A$_2$ enough to cause paradoxical splitting?
   ANS.: a. Conduction defects that delay depolarization of the LV, such as complete LBBB and some types of WPW preexcitation that imitate LBBB. The type of WPW preexcitation that acts like LBBB is one in which the initial conduction passes to the RV muscle first. This is known as type B, in which the QRS in V$_1$ points predominantly posteriorly (i.e., it is predominantly negative).
      b. A marked systolic gradient across the aortic valve, causing a delay in the fall of LV pressure to below aortic pressure, as in severe AS (see p. 163).
         Note: Poststenotic dilatation can contribute to the delay in A$_2$ by producing a loss of elastic recoil as well as by increasing the capacitance of the aorta.
      c. Marked volume loads on the LV with only one outlet for systole (e.g., a large PDA or AR).

       d. Rarely, acute ventricular dysfunction, as in acute myocardial infarction, acute myocarditis, or during angina pectoris.

       e. Hypertension plus myocardial damage, especially if the increase in blood pressure is transiently higher than average for that patient.

3. What causes the widest reversed split?

   ANS.: Complete LBBB (i.e., with a QRS of 120 msec [0.12 sec] or longer). This is also the most common cause of reversed splits and the only one that is easily recognized by the noncardiologist (Fig. 16).

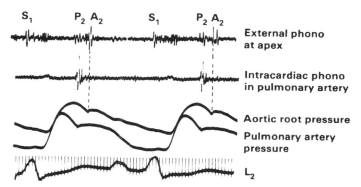

FIG. 16. These simultaneous intraarterial and phonocardiogram tracings are from a 59-year-old man in heart failure due to an idiopathic cardiomyopathy. Because of LBBB, the incisura of the pulmonary artery and its simultaneous P_2 comes before the aortic incisura and its simultaneous A_2. (His pulmonary artery systolic pressure was 35 mm Hg; his LV pressure, 120 mm Hg; and his cardiac index, 2.4). These are catheter-tip electromanometer tracings, so there are no tubing delays.

4. What produces the delayed A_2 in LBBB?

   ANS.: The delay is usually due to prolongation of isovolumic contraction time (7). This has been shown in subjects with intermittent LBBB. Prolongation of the electromechanical interval (i.e., Q to onset of ventricular contraction) is prolonged in some patients but not in others (47).

5. What is the significance of a reversed split in AS?

   ANS.: It implies that the gradient is at least 60 mm Hg or more. This is more reliable in congenital than in rheumatic stenosis because in the latter, myocardial damage may add extra delays to the A_2 by delaying the onset of the aortic valve opening (i.e., the isovolumic contraction time may be prolonged).

      Note: In hypertrophic subaortic stenosis (HSS, or HOCM) there may be day-to-day variation in S_2 splitting, so that splitting may change from normal to single to reversed. The highest incidence of audible reversed split in AS apparently occurs in severe HSS or HOCM, probably because there is no calcification of the valve to cause the A_2 to disappear (57).

6. When do reversed splits occur in patients with ischemic heart disease in the absence of LBBB?

   ANS.: It is rare to observe reversed splitting in chronic coronary disease. It does, however, occur in the following situations:

       a. During acute angina or after exercise in the presence of significant coronary obstruction (15).

    b. During the first three days of acute myocardial infarction in about 15% of patients (54).

    c. In patients over 70 years old with coronary disease and usually enough heart damage to produce an S$_3$ (2).

    d. In hypertensive patients with myocardial damage, or during acute hypertensive crisis.

        Note: a. The reversed split is so narrow in coronary disease problems that the only sign of reversal may be a pure S$_2$ on inspiration and an impure sound on expiration.

           b. The delay of the S$_2$ in patients with coronary disease is usually due to a prolonged isovolumic contraction time.

7. What is the significance of expiratory splitting of the S$_2$?

    ANS.: Expiratory splitting indicates either a wide split, a fixed split, or a paradoxical split.

        Note: In normal subjects over age 50, expiratory splitting of the S$_2$ is rare. Therefore, when expiratory splitting is found in this age group, it may be abnormal and should be accounted for.

8. What can be confused with paradoxical splitting of the S$_2$?

    ANS.: a. An S$_2$-opening snap. (This is discussed in detail on p. 177.)

        b. A widely split A$_2$P$_2$ in atrial fibrillation. After short diastoles there is narrow splitting. Inspiration, however, because of its autonomic effect on the AV node, may cause a faster rate. Therefore, the split may narrow on inspiration because of the shorter RR intervals. The widening on expiration and narrowing on inspiration sounds like a reversed split (30).

        c. An electronic pacemaker in the RV in a patient with complete AV block may not produce a reversed split when a P wave precedes the QRS. This reversal does not occur because the booster pump action of the atrial kick affects the RV ejection time more than the LV ejection time, thereby prolonging the RV ejection time more than that of the LV (46).

9. How can you use S$_2$ splitting to tell a PAC from a PVC?

    ANS.: If a premature ventricular beat manifests narrow or no splitting of S$_2$, it is probably supraventricular. If splitting occurs, it could be either a PAC or a PVC.

Eliciting and Recognizing Reversed Splits

1. What should make you suspect paradoxical or reversed splitting?

    ANS.: A split that widens on expiration and narrows on inspiration suggests that the P$_2$ comes first (Fig. 17).

2. How can you confirm by auscultation that a wide split is reversed when the respiratory movements are so erratic that the respiratory change cannot be recognized?

    ANS.: a. At the apex the A$_2$ is either the only sound heard, or it is the loudest component of the S$_2$ if both are heard there. Therefore, you should gradually move your stethoscope from the left sternal border toward the apex as you listen to the split second sound. The S$_2$ component that either disappears or becomes softer at the apex is the P$_2$. If it is the second component that disappears or becomes softer, then you know that the order of components is A$_2$P$_2$. If, on the other hand, you hear the first component becoming softer or disappearing in relation to the second component, then the order is P$_2$A$_2$. Since the A$_2$ is usually the only component of S$_2$ heard at the second right interspace, the same maneuver can be used by gradually shifting your chestpiece toward the second right interspace.

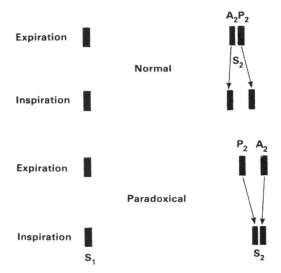

FIG. 17. If the split narrows on inspiration, the P_2 must come first, and the split S_2 is reversed.

b. The component that increases in loudness with inspiration is the P_2 (Fig. 18).

c. Have the patient perform a Valsalva maneuver for about 10 sec. During the strain, while blood is being withheld from both ventricles, the P_2 comes relatively early, and the reversed split widens. In normal subjects, the S_2 split usually becomes narrower during a Valsalva strain.

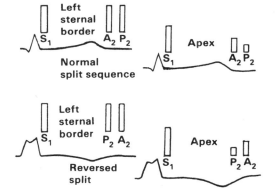

FIG. 18. If the split is fixed at the left sternal border, it may be difficult to tell whether it has a normal or paradoxical sequence. Toward the apex, the component that becomes relatively softer must be the P_2.

Immediately on release of the Valsalva maneuver, more blood comes back to the right side, and the P_2 occurs later. If the split S_2 narrows, the order is P_2A_2. In normal subjects, the sudden return of blood into the RV causes an immediate widening of the S_2 split.

A few beats after the release of the Valsalva, the reversed split widens again markedly. In normal subjects, on the contrary, the split narrows as the excess pulmonary blood reaches the LV after traversing the lungs.

3. What is meant by nonparadoxical reversed splitting?

ANS.: The order is P_2A_2 but the S_2 splits more widely on inspiration than on expiration.

It can occur in the presence of LBBB in a patient with a cardiomyopathy or acute myocardial infarction. It is apparently due to an excessively early P_2 on inspiration and can be diagnosed only by simultaneous phonocardiograms or pulse tracings, but it can be suspected if a patient with a known LBBB has an apparently normal movement with a widely split S_2.

Note: Some patients with severe chronic obstructive pulmonary disease (COPD) (hyperinflated lungs and low diaphragm) have a paradoxical decrease in flow into the thorax on inspiration, resulting in narrowing of the A_2P_2 interval on inspiration but without a reversal of components (37).

REFERENCES

1. Adolph RJ, Fowler NO. The second heart sound. *Mod Concepts Cardiovasc Dis* 1970;39:91.
2. Agnew T, et al. Delayed closure of the aortic valve in ischemic heart disease. *Br Heart J* 1967;29:775.
3. Anastassiades PC, et al. The aortic valve closure: Echocardiographic, phonocardiographic and hemodynamic assessment. *Am Heart J* 1976;91:228.
4. Aygen MM, Braunwald E. The splitting of the second heart sound in normal subjects and in congenital heart disease. *Circulation* 1962;25:328.
5. Blazek WV, Bliss HA. The second sound in uncomplicated ventricular septal defect. *Med Clin North Am* 1966; 50:111.
6. Boudoulas H, et al. Prolonged electrical systole and QT > QS₂ secondary to coronary artery disease. *Am J Cardiol* 1985;55:915.
7. Bourassa MG, et al. Hemodynamic studies during intermittent left bundle branch block. *Am J Cardiol* 1962; 10:792.
8. Bruce RA, John GG. Effect of upright posture and exercise on pulmonary hemodynamics in patients with central cardiovascular shunts. *Circulation* 1957;16:776.
9. Castle RF. Variables affecting the splitting of the second heart sound in atrial septal defect. *Am Heart J* 1967; 73:468.
10. Castle RF, et al. Variables affecting the splitting of the second heart sound in normal children. *Pediatrics* 1969; 43:183.
11. Cobbs BW, Jr. The second heart sound in pulmonary embolism and pulmonary hypertension. *Am Heart J* 1966; 71:843.
12. Curtiss EI, et al. New concepts in physiologic splitting of the second heart sound. *Am Heart Assoc Monograph* 46, 1975.
13. D'Cruz IA, et al. Stenotic lesions of the pulmonary arteries. *Am J Cardiol* 1964;13:441.
14. DeCaprio L, et al. QT/QS₂ ratio as an index of autonomic tone changes. *Am J Cardiol* 1984;53:818.
15. Dickerson RB, Nelson WP. Paradoxical splitting of the second heart sound. *Am Heart J* 1964;67:410.
16. Ehlers KH, et al. Wide splitting of the second heart sound without demonstrable heart disease. *Am J Cardiol* 1969;23:690.
17. Feruglio GA, Gunton RW. Intracardiac phonocardiography in ventricular septal defect. *Circulation* 1960;21:49.
18. Feruglio GA, Sreenivasan A. Intracardiac phonocardiogram in thirty cases of atrial septal defects. *Circulation* 1959;22:1087.
19. Gamboa R, et al. Accuracy of the phonocardiogram in aortic and pulmonary stenosis. *Circulation* 1964;30:35.
20. Golinko RJ, et al. The mechanism of pulsus paradoxus during tamponade. *J Clin Invest* 1963;42:249.
21. Hegglin R, Holzmann M. Abnorme Verzeitigkeit Des 2. Herztones bei Verlängerter QT-Distanz im EKG. *Klin Wochenschr* 1937;33:1146.
22. Higgins CB, Mulder DG. Tetralogy of Fallot in the adult. *Am J Cardiol* 1972;29:837.
23. Honey M. Delayed closure of the pulmonary valve. *Lancet* 1966;5:318.
24. Johnston RR, et al. Effect of intermittent right bundle branch block on right ventricular contractility. *Am J Cardiol* 1966;1:813.
25. Kardalinos A. The second heart sound. *Am Heart J* 1962;64:610.
26. Karnegis JN, Wang Y. The phonocardiogram in idiopathic dilatation of the pulmonary artery. *Am J Cardiol* 1964;14:75.
27. Kaufmann G, et al. Heart sounds in atrial tumors. *Am J Cardiol* 1951;8:350.
28. Kinoshita M, et al. Phonocardiographic findings of mitral insufficiency due to ruptures of the chordae tendineae. *CV Sound Bull* 1964;5:263.
29. Kraus Y, et al. Splitting of the second heart sound in partial anomalous pulmonary venous connection. In *Proceedings of Fourth Asian-Pacific Congress of Cardiology.* New York: Academic Press, 1969, p. 147.
30. Leacham RD, et al. Narrowed splitting of the second heart sound on inspiration in patients with giant left atrium. *Chest* 1971;60:151.
31. Leatham A, Gray I. Auscultatory and phonocardiographic signs of atrial septal defect. *Br Heart J* 1956;18:193.

32. Macieira-Coelho E, Guimaraes C. Phonocardiography in atrial septal defects. *Cardiologia* 1964;44:78.
33. MacKenzie JC, et al. Postural variation in second sound splitting. *Chest* 1973;63:56.
34. Matsuhisa M, et al. Anti-Hegglin syndrome in Takayasu's arteritis. *J Cardiol* 1984;14:169.
35. Moss WG, Johnson V. Differential effects of stretch upon the stroke volumes of the ventricles. *Am J Physiol* 1943;139:52.
36. Nakamura T, Sawayama T. A case of pheochromocytoma with marked Hegglin syndrome. *JECCS* 1988;4:72.
37. Nakhjavan FK, et al. Influence of respiration on venous return in pulmonary emphysema. *Circulation* 1966;33:8.
38. Nandi PS, Pigott VM, Spodick DH. Sequential cardiac responses during the respiratory cycle: Patterns of change in systolic intervals. *Chest* 1973;63:380.
39. Nelson WP, North RL. Splitting of the second heart sound in adults 40 years and older. *Am J Med Sci* 1967; 56:805.
40. Perloff JK, Harvey WP. Mechanisms of fixed splitting of the second heart sound. *Circulation* 1958;18:998.
41. Perloff JK, Lebauer EJ. Auscultatory and phonocardiographic manifestations of pulmonary artery stenosis. *Br Heart J* 1969;31:314.
42. Piemme TE, et al. Relationship of heart sounds to acceleration of blood flow. *Circ Res* 1966;18:303.
43. Roach MR. Changes in arterial distensibility as a cause of poststenotic dilatation. *Am J Cardiol* 1963;12:802.
44. Sabbah HN, et al. Aortic closure sound in pure aortic insufficiency. *Circulation* 1977;56:859.
45. Sainani GS, Luisada AA. "Mapping" the precordium. *Am J Cardiol* 1967;19:788.
46. Sakai H, et al. Influence of the atrial contraction on systolic time intervals. *J Cardiol* 1979;9:363.
47. Sakamoto T, et al. QRS dependence of the split interval of the second heart sound in bundle branch block. *Jpn Heart J* 1967;8:459.
48. Schrire V, Vogelpoel L. The role of the dilated pulmonary artery in abnormal splitting of the second heart sound. *Am Heart J* 1962;63:501.
49. Shaver JA, et al. Sound pressure correlates of the second heart sound. *Circulation* 1974;49:316.
50. Singh SP. Unusual splitting of the second heart sound in pulmonary stenosis. *Am J Cardiol* 1970;25:28.
51. Slodki SJ, et al. The Q-II interval: A study of the second heart sound in old age. *J Am Geriatr Soc* 1969;17:673.
52. Stefanadis C, et al. Aortic distensibility in poststenotic aortic dilatation: The effect of coexisting coronary artery disease. *J Cardiol* 1983;18:189.
53. Stein PD. Frequency spectrum of the aortic component of the second heart sound in patients with normal valves and porcine xenografts. *Am J Cardiol* 1980;46:48.
54. Stock E. Auscultation and phonocardiography in acute myocardial infarction. *Med J Aust* 1966;1:1060.
55. Sutton G, et al. Second heart sound in pulmonary hypertension. *Br Heart J* 1968;30:743.
56. Tanaka C, et al. Phonocardiographic findings in adult ASD. *CV Sound Bull* 1975;5:107.
57. Tavel ME. Clinical phonocardiography. *JAMA* 1968;203:123.
58. Vana S, et al. Hegglinuv priznak u tyreotoxikosy a jeho vztah k hladine proteinoveho jodu v séru. *Vnitr Lek* 1972;23:42.

10

The Opening Snap (OS)

MECHANISM AND TIMING

1. What is usually necessary before the opening of the mitral valve becomes audible?

   ANS.: There is usually some mitral stenosis (MS) due to fibrous thickening and often to calcification of the margins of the mitral leaflets, especially the large anterior leaflet. The commissures are also fused by fibrosis or calcium. The mitral valve belly may act like a sail that billows downward into a dome in diastole as the left ventricle (LV) attempts to "suck" left atrial blood into the LV cavity. This sudden diastolic doming causes the anterior leaflet to bulge downward with a snap (Fig. 1).

2. Why must it be the anterior leaflet that is responsible for the OS of MS?

   ANS.: Not only is the anterior leaflet three times broader than the posterior leaflet, but the surface chordae tendineae of the anterior leaflet are also attached to the peripheral zone of the valve, leaving the bellies intact, whereas the surface chordae of the posterior leaflets are attached to its entire ventricular surface (21). Therefore, even though MS tends to convert the two semi-independent leaflets into a continuous funnel-like sleeve with a fish-mouth opening, the belly of the anterior leaflet contributes most to the loud S_1 and OS.

   Note: a. An OS can occur with dominant mitral regurgitation (MR) if the regurgitation is due to a thickened, rolled, immobile posterior (mural) leaflet and if the anterior (septal) leaflet still has a mobile belly (11).

   b. Torrential flow through the mitral valve on rare occasions may produce an OS in the absence of MS. It has occasionally been recorded in ventricular septal defect (VSD), persistent ductus arteriosus, tricuspid atresia, thyrotoxicosis, and after a Blalock-Taussig operation for tetralogy of Fallot.

   c. In congenital MS in infants there is rarely an OS because the congenitally abnormal leaflets usually do not have pliable bellies.

   d. An OS-like sound has been heard in patients who have a prolapsed mitral valve either with a click or with both a click and a systolic murmur (1,4). Because the sound may be simultaneous with the D point on an echocardiogram, it is probably due to recoaptation of a prolapsed posterior leaflet with the anterior leaflet when the LV pressure falls below the left atrial pressure. When, however, it is associated with a "floppy valve" (i.e., marked anterior leaflet prolapse and a severe pansystolic MR murmur), the OS is synchronous with the E point of the mitral

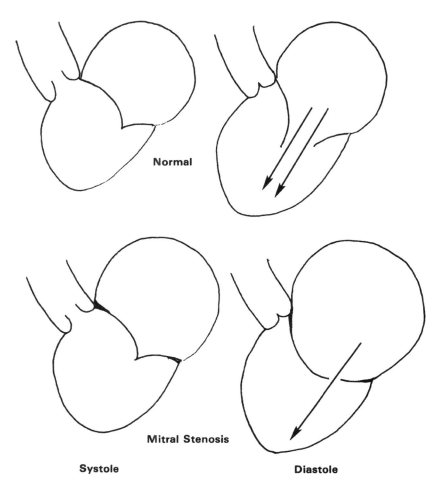

Normal

Mitral Stenosis

Systole   **Diastole**

FIG. 1. The opening snap is produced by the belly of the stenotic anterior leaflet bulging or doming downward with a jerk to produce a clicking or snapping sound. The anterior leaflet, therefore, must also close with a snap as it domes upward. The posterior leaflet has too short a ring-to-
free edge distance to produce a "belly snap."

echocardiogram and is due to marked anterior leaflet prolapse (10).
These sounds are best heard at the apex.

e. An OS-like sound has also been heard about 70 msec after the P_2 in patients with massive ascites (8). It occurs simultaneously with the onset
of mitral valve opening on echophonocardiograms and is thought to be
due to the heart striking against the high diaphragm because it disappears on inspiration and when the ascites is gone.

f. The early S_3 of left atrial myxoma (called the "tumor plop") often occurs
only 0.07 to 0.11 sec after the A_2, which is the same range as the OS
from the A_2.

g. It is customary to call the isovolumic relaxation interval between the
aortic closure sound and the OS sound the A_2OS interval or, simply, the
2OS interval.

RELATION BETWEEN THE 2OS AND THE SEVERITY OF MITRAL STENOSIS

1. What controls the duration of isovolumic relaxation, or the 2OS interval?

    ANS.: a. The pressure in the left atrium at the time the mitral valve opens.

    b. The heart rate. The more rapid the heart rate, the shorter the 2OS interval because isovolumic relaxation is faster under the influence of increased sympathetic tone or catecholamines that cause the faster rate, and left atrial pressure is higher due to the reduced atrial emptying time with the short diastoles.

    c. The stiffness of the mitral valve (due mostly to calcium) (12). (See question 5 below.)

    d. The rate and strength of relaxation of the myocardium (i.e., the state of myocardial function or inotropic state [contractility] of the myocardium).

    e. The pressure at which the aortic valve closes (near systolic pressure).

    Note: Left ventricular early expansion is not merely a relaxation or recoil phenomenon. It has an active suction effect related to the degree of cardiac function or inotropism.

2. What is the relationship between the degree of MS and the height of the V wave in the left atrium?

    ANS.: The greater the stenosis, the greater the obstruction to flow, and thus the slower and more incomplete the emptying of the left atrium. Therefore, the greater the MS, the higher the V wave.

    Note: a. This will be clear only if you recall that the V wave is built up during ventricular systole when the mitral valve is closed. If the V wave begins to build up from a high pressure, the wave rises even higher. If the left atrium did not empty well in diastole due to MS, the V wave starts to build up from an already high pressure.

    b. A high left atrial pressure makes the 2OS interval shorter because the LV pressure does not have to fall as far to open the mitral valve after closure of the aortic valve or A_2 (Fig. 2).

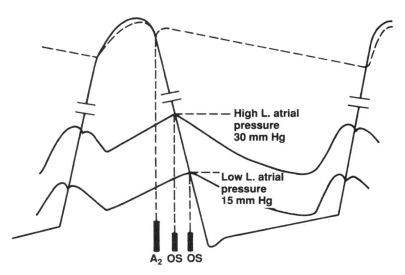

A_2 OS OS

FIG. 2. Note that the distance between the A_2 and the OS is shorter with the higher left atrial pressure.

c. The high V wave caused by concomitant MR does not necessarily cause an early OS, probably because the OS in MS occurs not at the peak but early on the Y descent, and if MR is also present, the OS may occur farther down the Y descent (16). Even though the descent of the mitral leaflets begins at the crossover of left ventricular and left atrial pressure, maximum excursion of the leaflets may take another 25 to 70 msec, and the OS occurs at the moment of maximum excursion.

3. Will the beat that follows a long diastole in atrial fibrillation produce a long or a short 2OS? Why?

ANS.: It produces a long 2OS because a long diastole gives more time to empty the left atrium, allowing its pressure to drop. The next systole begins and ends with a lower left atrial pressure, thus making a long 2OS.

4. Will a very stiff mitral valve make the OS earlier or later; that is, will the 2OS interval be shortened or lengthened? Why?

ANS.: The 2OS interval will be lengthened, because the stiffer (less mobile) the valve, the lower the LV pressure has to fall below atrial pressure before it can "suck" the valve open (12).

Note: Calcification has been shown to slow the velocity of mitral valve opening. The 2OS interval is the sum of the true isovolumic relaxation period (A_2 to the beginning of the opening of the mitral valve) plus mitral valve excursion. Therefore, even though a high left atrial pressure shortens the true isovolumic relaxation time, valve calcification and stiffness lengthen the mitral valve excursion period. The result is a longer than expected 2OS for the degree of MS (9,14). Echophonocardiographic correlations have shown that the true isovolumic relaxation period (A_2 to the onset of mitral valve opening) correlates better with MS severity than does the 2OS interval.

5. List the causes of a late OS aside from a mild degree of MS or a heavily calcified mitral valve.

ANS.: a. Bradycardia. This prolongs the isovolumic relaxation time mainly because long diastoles allow more left atrial emptying and lower left atrial pressure. (Bradycardia may also decrease the slope of fall of LV pressure.)

b. Poor myocardial function due to either damage or aging. This causes prolongation of the isovolumic relaxation time. (Isovolumic relaxation time increases strikingly with age [7].)

c. Aortic regurgitation (AR). This is presumably due to the AR jet striking the underbelly of the anterior mitral leaflet and preventing rapid downward excursion. (AR may even eliminate an OS.)

d. A low left atrial pressure due to a large left atrium and severe failure with low flow.

e. High aortic pressure. If the aortic valve closes at a high pressure, more time is required for the LV pressure to drop below left atrial pressure to open the mitral valve and create the OS.

Note: At an aortic systolic pressure of more than 130 mm Hg, the 2OS interval is unreliable in indicating the degree of MS (3) (Fig. 3).

6. Which is more reliable in predicting the degree of MS, a narrow 2OS or a wide one? Why?

ANS.: A narrow 2OS is more reliable because there is not much besides a tight MS or tachycardia that can narrow a 2OS interval, whereas there are at least five causes besides mild MS for a wide 2OS.

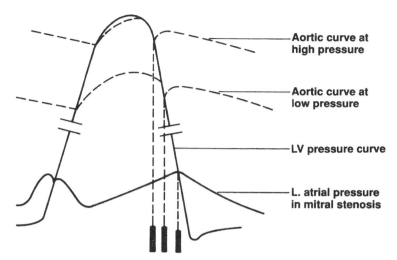

FIG. 3. Note that the higher the aortic pressure, the longer the A₂OS interval.

> *Note*: a. Unequivocally tight MS is suggested by a resting 2OS of 50 msec or less, even if only after exercise (5,19).
> b. The shortest 2OS interval with almost normal left atrial pressure is about 95 msec (the time it takes to "pa-pa" as quickly as possible).
> c. If you say "pa-da" as quickly as possible, you should be able to separate the sounds by about 50 to 70 msec (0.05 to 0.07 sec). This is a narrow 2OS and suggests moderate to tight MS.

LOUDNESS OF THE OPENING SNAP

1. Other than an obese or emphysematous chest, what can cause a soft or absent OS?
   ANS.: a. The mitral valve may be too calcified for the bellies to snap into their maximal open positions.
   > *Note*: a. An OS can be heard even with heavy calcification but it will be soft, late, and low-pitched (i.e., it loses high frequencies) (2,13). This is opposite to the degeneration of a bioprosthetic valve, which loses low frequencies when it becomes fibrotic.
   > b. Fibrosis alone is rarely responsible for a soft OS.
   > c. Congenital mitral stenosis has no opening snap due mainly to the rubbery consistency of the valve.
   > d. Although a relatively immobile calcified mitral valve may attenuate the mitral opening snap and may make it disappear, the first heart sound may still remain loud, although occasionally it also becomes soft.

   b. Extremely low flow due to exceptional severity of the stenosis, secondary pulmonary hypertension, concomitant aortic or tricuspid valve disease, or myocardial dysfunction.

   c. A large right ventricle (RV) (usually due to pulmonary hypertension or tricuspid regurgitation) that pushes the LV away from the chest wall.

   d. Moderate to severe AR that can "cushion" the mitral valve anterior leaflet as it domes downward.

Note: When a patient with both AR and MS sits up, you may hear a soft OS for the first time, probably because the decreased venous return of the sitting position reduces the amount of AR.

2. Why will severe pulmonary hypertension in a patient with MS produce a low flow and therefore a soft OS?

ANS.: Because there are then two causes of a low flow: obstruction at the mitral valve and obstruction at the pulmonary arterioles.

Note: a. A reduced flow occurs with pulmonary hypertension, probably because elevation of the RV pressure does not completely compensate for the high resistance produced by the pulmonary arteriolar constriction. (It may be that compensatory mechanisms in biological systems are rarely if ever complete.)

b. Further proof that low flow can prevent the appearance of an OS is the observation that standing can cause a soft OS to disappear, and raising the legs can make it louder.

c. A mitral commissurotomy will eliminate the OS in about half the cases.

DIFFERENTIATING A_2P_2 FROM A_2OS

Similarities Between A_2P_2 and 2OS

1. Where on the chest wall is the OS usually best heard?

ANS.: An OS is usually best heard between the apex and the left sternal border or at the left sternal border. This is not too surprising when one considers that the anterior leaflet of the mitral valve, which creates most of the sound, makes its opening motion in a line that points almost directly toward the left sternal border. A P_2 is also best heard at the left sternal border, and because the chest wall may keep the stethoscope farther away from the heart when one is listening at the upper left sternal border, the P_2 may be better heard at the third or fourth left interspace just as with an OS.

Note: a. Peculiarly, an OS can often be heard well at the second right interspace, even if it is only moderately loud at the left lower sternal border. This may be because the mitral valve is in fibrous continuity with the aortic root, which may be more anterior than usual due to the dilated left atrium. A louder than normal P_2, however, may also be heard at the second right interspace.

b. Like all sounds and murmurs, a loud OS can be heard anywhere on the chest wall. An OS may even be grade 6 in loudness.

c. Although the A_2P_2 may be as long as 100 msec and is often not different from an A_2OS, it may be as short as 20 msec, which would be unusual for a 2OS.

d. Although the quality, frequency, and duration of an OS usually do not differ much from those of a P_2, occasionally the OS may consist mostly of low frequencies, especially if the valve is heavily calcified.

Differences Between A_2P_2 and 2OS

1. Is a loud P_2 ever as loud at the apex as it is at the left sternal border?

ANS.: Only if the chest shape attenuates all sounds at the left sternal border. Then if the

P_2 is loud, it may be heard as loudly at the apex as at the left sternal border (in the left lateral decubitus position).

> *Note*: An OS is louder or as loud at the apex as it is at the left sternal border only when the LV is dilated, or if a rib has been removed in previous heart surgery.

OS VERSUS P_2 RULE NO. 1: *If the second component of a split S_2 is louder or as loud at the apex as elsewhere, it is probably an OS.*

2. How does the effect of respiration affect the loudness of the P_2 and of the OS?

ANS.: Inspiration makes the P_2 louder and the OS softer (blood is withheld from the left atrium on inspiration).

> *Note*: The P_2 can be expected to become louder on inspiration only at the left *lower* sternal border because all sounds tend to become softer on inspiration high on the chest.

OS VERSUS P_2 RULE NO. 2: *If the second component of an S_2 split becomes softer on inspiration at the left lower sternal border (in the absence of left bundle branch block [LBBB]), it is probably a mitral OS.*

3. When will a 2OS sound like a reversed split?

ANS.: A 2OS interval sometimes gives the illusion of widening on expiration but actually does not. On expiration the P_2 moves slightly toward the A_2 and, therefore, away from the OS (Fig. 4).

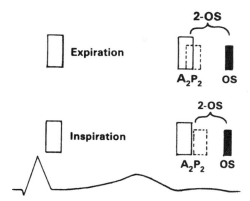

FIG. 4. Note that respiration gives the impression of a reversed split, because the P_2 moves away from the OS on expiration and toward the OS on inspiration.

> *Note*: a. Sinus arrhythmia may contribute to the widening of the 2OS on expiration by slowing the heart rate on expiration.
>
> b. Even though the left atrial pressure rises on expiration and therefore should make the 2OS shorter, the aortic pressure also rises on expiration, thereby keeping the 2OS about the same.

OS VERSUS P_2 RULE NO. 3: *A widely split S_2 on inspiration that appears to become wider on expiration is an OS, in the absence of LBBB.*

4. How can you recognize an A_2, P_2, and OS as three distinct sounds in one place?

ANS.: A triple S_2 can often be recognized along the left sternal border in MS by listening for a snare-drum effect or a tongue-rolling (Spanish r) effect with the second sound. This snare-drum triple S_2 is most likely to be heard during inspiration, when the P_2 pulls away from the A_2. But occasionally the OS is so soft that it can be heard only on expiration, and you hear the snare-drum effect only on expiration (Fig. 5).

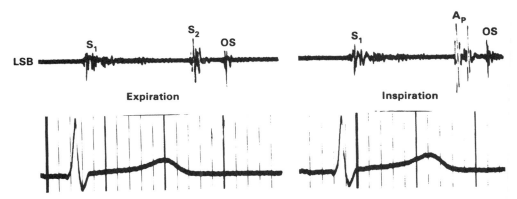

FIG. 5. On inspiration, the S_2 split opened up into its A_2 and P_2 components. Together with the OS, a triple second sound is heard that produces a snare-drum effect

OS VERSUS P_2 RULE NO. 4: *A triple second sound, in which the three sounds are close enough together to sound like a snare-drum, implies that an OS is present as the final component.*

5. What effect does standing have on the 2OS interval? Why?

    ANS.: It widens it. The pooling of blood in the legs decreases venous return to the left atrium. This lowers the pressure behind the obstructed mitral valve and makes a wider 2OS interval.

      Note: a. The A_2P_2 interval on standing either remains the same or narrows. The reason for this is that although there is a decrease in volume to both ventricles, the RV responds to the decrease more than does the LV.

        b. One proof that the RV responds to filling pressure changes to a greater extent than does the LV is seen in patients with RV pacemakers and complete atrioventricular (AV) block. When the P wave falls before the QRS to give a good atrial kick, the P_2 occurs later than the A_2; that is, the reversed splits become narrower, single, or even normal (17).

    OS VERSUS P_2 RULE NO. 5: *If a split second sound becomes wider on standing, its second component is an OS.*

6. Why should the presence of an OS imply that the first sound should have a snapping quality?

    ANS.: The stiffness and doming of the valve that produced the OS should also make a snapping S_1. In other words, a mitral valve that has an OS usually has a "closing snap."

      Note: A loud S_1 and closing snap may be present even with a mitral valve that is too stiff to produce an OS. Therefore, a loud S_1 with a closing snap suggests the presence of an OS, and a soft S_1 denies the presence of an OS.

    OS VERSUS P_2 RULE NO. 6: *If the S_1 is soft or only a low-pitched thud, the second component of the S_2 is not likely to be an OS.*

Summary of Signs Differentiating an A_2P_2 from a 2OS

1. If the second component of a split S_1 is as loud at the apex as at the left sternal border, it is probably an OS.
2. If the second component decreases with inspiration, it is an OS (in the absence of LBBB).

3. If the split tends to narrow on inspiration, it is 2OS (in the absence of LBBB).
4. If there is a triple second sound at the left sternal border, an OS is present.
5. If the split widens on standing, the second component is an OS.
6. If the S_1 is soft or muffled, the second component of the split S_2 is probably a P_2.

Differential Diagnosis of an Opening Snap

1. What can imitate a late OS?
   ANS.: a. The early S_3 of constrictive pericarditis (see p. 192). This is the "pericardial knock."
   b. The tumor plop of a left atrial myxoma (see p. 191).
   c. A vegetation on the mitral valve that moves rapidly from the left atrium into the LV and strikes the base of the ventricular septum (very rare) (20).

THE TRICUSPID OPENING SNAP

1. When will a tricuspid OS be present in the absence of tricuspid stenosis (TS)?
   ANS.: When a large volume enters the RV by way of the tricuspid valve. With an atrial septal defect (ASD) or anomalous pulmonary venous drainage into the right atrium, partial or complete, the torrential flow may cause a tricuspid OS along the left sternal border, 30 to 50 msec from the P_2. (It may be heard in more than three-quarters of patients over age 35 with an ASD [18].)
   Note: a. In one study a tricuspid OS was found only in patients with pulmonary-systemic flow ratios of 2 : 1 or more (15). The left-to-right shunt in another study was 1.5 to 2 times greater in patients with tricuspid OS than in those without (6). However, an OS can occur even with a reduced left-to-right shunt if the flow is reduced due to pulmonary hypertension, provided that tricuspid regurgitation (TR) is present to add to the volume of blood flowing through the tricuspid valve in diastole. The dilated and hypertrophied RV may stretch the ring and stiffen the leaflets enough to cause an OS.
   b. With a deformed tricuspid valve, as in Ebstein's anomaly, the second component of a widely split S_2 is synchronous with the echocardiographic maximum opening point of the tricuspid valve.

2. How does the effect of respiration on the mitral and tricuspid opening snaps differ?
   ANS.: A tricuspid OS becomes louder on inspiration because more blood flows through the tricuspid valve on inspiration. This fact is helpful because when a huge RV takes over the usual site of the apex beat, a tricuspid OS may be as loud at the apex area as at the left sternal border, thus mimicking a mitral OS.
   Note: a. A normal tricuspid valve usually opens first. In the presence of both MS and TS, however, the mitral OS usually occurs first because the MS is usually much more severe, making left atrial pressure higher than right atrial pressure. In the presence of mild MS, the tricuspid OS may occur prior to the mitral OS. This is expected in view of the fact that the isovolumic relaxation time of the RV is shorter than that of the LV by about 50 to 80 msec.
   b. In Ebstein's anomaly, the tricuspid OS occurs late, presumably because the smaller than normal RV not only contracts poorly but also expands poorly.

3. How can you distinguish a tricuspid OS from a widely split A_2P_2?
    ANS.: a. Listen for the snare-drum effect of a triple S_2 with the last sound becoming louder on inspiration.
    b. Ask the patient to stand. An A_2P_2 may remain the same or become narrower when the patient is standing but an A_2-tricuspid OS interval either remains the same or becomes wider.

REFERENCES

1. Aintablian A, et al. Opening snap in mitral valve prolapse-click syndrome. *N Y State J Med* 1978;78:1764.
2. Battaglia G, et al. Revised phonocardiographic and polygraphic findings in calcified mitral stenosis. *Folia Cardiol* 1965;24:229.
3. Bayer O, et al. The mitral opening snap in the quantitative diagnosis of mitral stenosis. *Am Heart J* 1956;2:234.
4. Bonner AJ Jr, et al. Early diastolic sound associated with mitral valve prolapse. *Arch Intern Med* 1976;136:347.
5. Delman AJ, et al. The second sound-mitral opening snap interval during exercise in the evaluation of mitral stenosis. *Circulation* 1966;33:399.
6. Funatsu T, et al. The cause of tricuspid opening snap in atrial septal defect. *CV Sound Bull* 1975;5:305.
7. Harrison TR, et al. The relation of age to the duration of contraction, ejection, and relaxation of the normal human heart. *Am Heart J* 1964;67:189.
8. Ichiyasu H, et al. Pseudo-knock sound in a patient with nephrotic syndrome and massive ascites. *Jpn Heart J* 1982;23:137.
9. Kalmanson D, et al. Opening snap and isovolumic relaxation period in mitral stenosis. *Br Heart J* 1975;38:135.
10. Matsue T, et al. Anterior mitral leaflet prolapse with mitral opening snap. *J Cardiol* 1977;7:243.
11. Nixon PGF, et al. The opening snap in mitral incompetence. *Br Heart J* 1960;22:395.
12. Rackley CE, et al. Phonocardiographic discrepancies in the assessment of mitral stenosis. *Arch Intern Med* 1968; 121:50.
13. Rahko PS, et al. Extent of mitral calcific deposits determined by cineangiography in mitral stenosis and their effect on valve motion hemodynamics and clinical signs. *Am J Cardiol* 1986;58:121.
14. Raizada V, et al. Non-invasive evaluation of normally functioning mitral bioprosthesis. *Abstracts*. Tokyo: World Congress of Cardiology, 1978, p. 1330.
15. Rees A, et al. Phonocardiographic, radiological, and hemodynamic correlation in atrial septal defect. *Br Heart J* 1972;34:781.
16. Ross RS, Criley JM. Cineangiocardiographic studies of the origin of cardiovascular physical signs. *Circulation* 1964;30:255.
17. Sakai H, et al. Relation between the atria contraction and the patterns of the splitting of the second heart sound in patients with right ventricular pacemakers. *J Cardiol* 1978;8:755.
18. Tanaka C, et al. Phonocardiographic findings in adult ASD. *CV Sound Bull* 1975;5:107.
19. Uyttenhove P, et al. Phonocardiography in mitral stenosis. *Acta Cardiol* 1963;18:24.
20. Valois R, Charuzi Y. Vegetation diastolic sound in mitral valve endocarditis. *Am Heart J* 1982;103:432.
21. Van Der Spuy JC. The functional and clinical anatomy of the mitral valve. *Br Heart J* 1958;20:471.

11

The Third Heart Sound (S₃)

NOMENCLATURE

1. What are the other names for the S_3?

   ANS.: The third heart sound, protodiastolic gallop sound, ventricular gallop, early-filling gallop sound, and early- or rapid-filling sound.

   Note: The term **protodiastole** was originally coined by Wiggers (21) to represent the time on the aortic pressure pulse between the peak pressure and the closure of the aortic valve. This interval or period of reduced ejection was assumed to represent the beginning of ventricular relaxation or diastole. However, the auscultator defines **diastole** as the period beginning with aortic valve closure as signaled by the S_2 (Fig. 1).

   Protodiastolic is used as a synonym for **early diastolic**, yet the prefix *protos* does not mean "early" but "first." Therefore, the S_4 should be called **hystidiastolic**, from the Greek *hystidos*, which means "last." Since we do

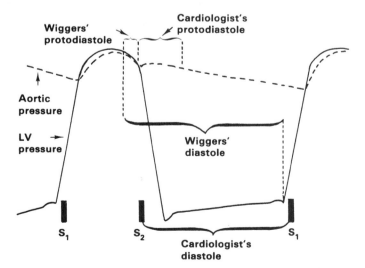

FIG. 1. The physiologist considers diastole to begin with the earliest point suggestive of ventricular relaxation or where ejection begins to slacken off. This is not so precise or useful a point as the cardiologist would like, so diastole is considered to begin with the S_2 or the incisura of the arterial pulse.

181

not use such a word for the S_4, it is inconsistent to use Greek nomenclature only for the S_3.

2. What factors besides brevity make the term S_3 preferable to the term **rapid-filling sound**?

   ANS.: a. The S_4 is also due to rapid filling of the left ventricle (LV), but this is secondary to atrial contraction.

   b. The S_3 has been produced in a vigorously contracting dog heart with no blood in it at all (20).

   c. A gallop cannot be one sound. The word **gallop** must refer to a rhythm or cadence made by at least three sounds in succession. A ventricular gallop is the triple rhythm made by the sequence of the S_1, S_2, and S_3. Therefore, the term S_3 is preferable.

   Note: The term **gallop rhythm** was originally used to describe any rapid series of three or more sounds in the presence of a tachycardia and heart failure. It included any extra sounds in systole (systolic gallop) as well as diastole. It also eliminated any S_3 with a normal heart rate or without heart failure. Therefore, the meaning of the term gallop rhythm has changed because it now refers to any series of three or more sounds in which the extra sounds occur *only in diastole* and are due to an S_3, an S_4, or both. Although it is convenient and clear to describe a rhythm as an S_3 gallop or an S_4 gallop, the general term gallop rhythm has a pathologic connotation and should not be used for the physiologic S_3 gallop.

TIMING

1. Does the ventricle fill most rapidly in early, middle, or late diastole?

   ANS.: In early diastole. The ventricle has two rates of expansion: an early, short, rapid one and a later, longer, slow one. Once the aortic valve closes, the LV expands very rapidly. During this expansion the LV first goes through the state of isovolumic expansion in about 100 msec (the time it takes to say "pa-pa" as quickly as possible) and then, when the mitral valve opens, through the stage of rapid filling while the ventricle continues its rapid expansion phase for about another 60 msec (0.06 sec). At the end of the rapid filling phase rapid expansion is suddenly checked by unknown forces, and the slow expansion phase takes over.

   Note: About 80% of ventricular filling occurs in the early rapid-filling phase of diastole in comparison with the later slow-filling phase of diastole. After the initial rapid filling, the volume of the ventricle changes very little until atrial contraction squeezes the last 20% of blood into the ventricle.

2. At what point during the rapid-filling phase of the LV pressure curve does the S_3 occur?

   ANS.: Near the end of the rapid pressure drop in the LV (i.e., near the point at which rapid expansion changes to the slow expansion phase).

   Note: Some rapid filling continues to occur after the S_3.

3. Which conditions shorten the A_2S_3 interval?

   ANS.: Anything that shortens isovolumic relaxation times such as

   a. Restrictive cardiomyopathies or constrictive pericarditis, both of which limit the extent of early expansion.

   b. Heart rates of more than 100 beats per minute. Presumably, sympathetic stimulation causes ventricular expansion to complete its early rapid filling phase more rapidly.

Note: The time between the opening of the mitral valve and the S$_3$ remains relatively constant for all heart rates under 100 beats per minute.

MECHANISM OF PRODUCTION

1. How is the S$_3$ produced?
   ANS.: There are two theories: an internal and an external production theory.

The Internal Production Theory of the S$_3$

1. What is the internal production theory?
   ANS.: In the internal production theory the S$_3$ is due to a sudden "pulling short" of the rapidly expanding ventricle by unknown myocardial forces at the end of the rapid expansion phase in early diastole (2). At the moment of the S$_3$, the ventricle has stopped rapid expansion, and pressure in the ventricle is no longer falling but is relatively stable for about 40 msec, despite continued rapid filling due to the inertia of the blood mass. The continued rapid increase in blood volume in the ventricle at the time of the sudden transition may act as a sudden distending force that causes the sound.
   Note: The following facts are evidence that the S$_3$ is not caused by a sudden stretch of the papillary muscles and chordae attached to mitral leaflets.
   a. An S$_3$ can occur with homograft (human cadaver), heterograft (porcine), or prosthetic ball valve replacement of the mitral valve where chordae tendineae are absent (5,8).
   b. On an echocardiogram the S$_3$ occurs when the anterior mitral leaflet is between its maximum opening position and the nadir of its early partial closure position (see Fig. 2). There is no evidence here that the mitral valve apparatus plays any important role in the production of the S$_3$.

The External Production Theory of the S$_3$

1. Why is an external production theory necessary to account for the S$_3$?
   ANS.: a. An S$_3$ often cannot be recorded inside the LV in patients or dogs in whom it can be recorded on the chest wall (1,3).
   b. No sound was produced when one end of a piece of ventricle was fixed and the other end was pulled by various amounts of sudden force (6).
   c. A sound is produced by the heart striking the chest wall in rare instances of pericardial effusion, when a systolic thrust of the heart against the chest wall coincides with a loud systolic sound (12).
   d. The apex cardiogram shows a peak of rapid early outward movement at the time of the S$_3$. When marked, this peak is palpable and is then accompanied by a loud S$_3$ (Fig. 3).
   e. There is no feature of the LV pressure curve that corresponds to the rapid filling wave of an apex cardiogram or to the S$_3$ (16).
   f. The loudness of the S$_3$ is very dependent on how well the apex beat comes out between the ribs and how close the heart is to the chest wall.
   g. In dogs with empty hearts, an S$_3$ can be recorded as long as the heart is beating vigorously (21).

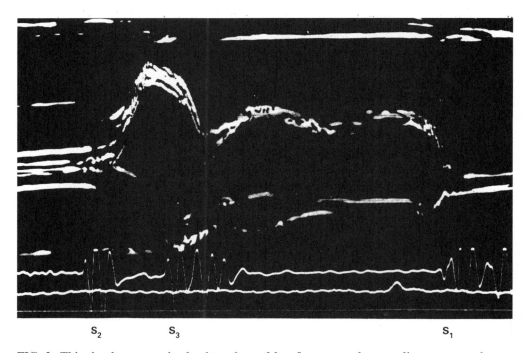

S_2 S_3 S_1

FIG. 2. This simultaneous mitral valve echo and low-frequency phonocardiogram was taken at very fast film speed from a 20-year-old man with heart failure and atrial fibrillation due to a severe idiopathic cardiomyopathy. The apical phonocardiogram shows the loud S_3 beginning just before the change of slope in the first closing movement of mitral valve. This man had at times a double S_3 (very rare). However, on the day of this tracing the S_3 was more like a prolonged S_3 or an S_3 followed by a short rumble. (The cause of a split S_3 is unknown, but the split S_3 has been attributed to a transient opening and closing movement of the mitral valve.)

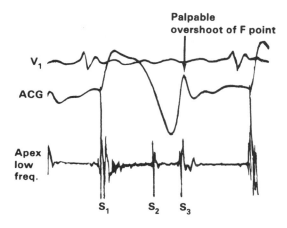

FIG. 3. The apex cardiogram and simultaneous apex phonocardiogram are from the same 20-year-old man as in the echocardiogram above. The pathologic S_3 was extremely loud and could be heard anywhere on his chest. It is difficult to say whether it was the overshoot of the rapid filling wave (F point) or the vibrations of the S_3 that was palpable.

2. What is the external production theory for the S₃?

ANS.: During contraction the heart rotates counterclockwise, as viewed from the apex. The momentum of its rotation keeps it rotating in the same direction until the time of early diastole. Its rotation also twists the great vessels and stretches the restraining elastic structures that work to limit its rotation. If the heart rotates with enough energy, its momentum may stretch the restraining structures to such an extent that there is a strong recoil at the end of its rotation in early diastole. This recoil may throw the heart against the chest wall hard enough to produce a sound.

THE PHYSIOLOGIC S₃

1. How common is the physiologic S₃ in normal subjects?

ANS.: In one study it was recorded on a phonocardiogram near the apex in one-third of normal subjects under age 15 (18). (This is not to say that it was audible in all cases in which it was recorded.) It is rarely audible or recordable in normal subjects over age 30. However, it may persist into the fifth decade in some women.

2. What cardiovascular conditions tend to produce an audible S₃ in the normal heart?

ANS.: Anything that increases the velocity of ventricular expansion and recoil, such as an increase in flow or sympathetic stimulation (e.g., tachycardias).

Note: a. There is some physiologic proof that the more energetic the expansion of the LV, the more likely the presence of an S₃. The S₃ usually occurs only if atrial pressure is *more than slightly* higher than ventricular pressure near the end of rapid ventricular filling. The more vigorously the ventricle expands, the greater the pressure gradient between the left atrium and the LV, and the more likely the occurrence of an S₃ (Fig. 4).

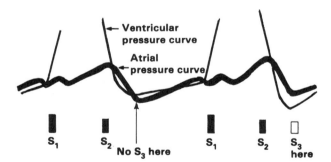

FIG. 4. When the LV expands with enough energy to create a gradient between it and the left atrium, an S₃ occurs.

b. The presence of a physiologic S₃ tells you that at least a normal circulation time is present. The sympathetic tone and catecholamines that produce the rapid early expansion necessary for the S₃ also increase the cardiac output and accelerate the circulation time. A venous hum in the neck implies a normal or rapid circulation time, and its presence helps confirm that the S₃ is physiologic and is not associated with heart failure. (See p. 273 for a method of eliciting a venous hum.)

3. When will a tachycardia produce a loud physiologic S_3 in a normal patient over age 30?
    ANS.: There will be a loud S_3 if the rapid filling phase of ventricular expansion is augmented by atrial contraction. The gallop rhythm that results is then known as a summation gallop. This occurs when atrial contraction occurs in the early part of diastole, as with marked tachycardia or with a moderate tachycardia together with a first-degree atrioventricular (AV) block.
        Note: It has been calculated that with a PR of 0.14 sec, a tachycardia of 120 beats per minute may produce a summation gallop; with a PR of 0.16 sec, the summation rate is 115 beats per minute, with a PR of 0.18, it is 110, and with a PR of 0.20, it is 105 (10) (Fig. 5).

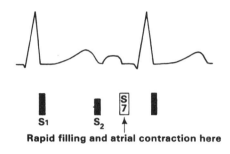

FIG. 5. Simultaneous occurrence of atrial contraction and early rapid filling produces a summation sound facetiously called the "S_7" (S_3 + S_4). This usually requires a prolonged PR interval.

4. How can you tell whether or not a triple rhythm is due to a summation gallop?
    ANS.: If you can slow the heart rate by carotid sinus pressure, diastole is lengthened, and the gallop disappears. Slowing the heart rate separates the later atrial contraction from the earlier rapid filling phase (Fig. 6).
        Note: a. The summation sound is nearly always very loud.
             b. If an S_4 is made louder by occurring during the early rapid filling phase, or if a pathologic S_3 is made louder by an early atrial contraction, that triple rhythm is called an augmented gallop. (See Fig. 206.)

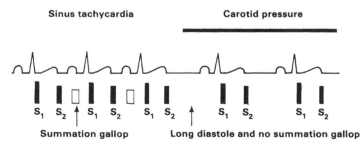

FIG. 6. Carotid pressure slows the heart rate and separates the time of atrial contraction from the time of early rapid ventricular filling, thus eliminating a summation gallop. (See also Figure on p. 206.)

LOUDNESS OF THE S$_3$

1. Which chestpiece and what degree of stethoscope pressure best brings out the S$_3$?
   ANS.: The bell, applied with light to moderate pressure so that the low frequencies are not dampened out.
2. What increases the loudness of the S$_3$, inspiration or expiration?
   ANS.: Either. Although expiration can make the S$_3$ louder by squeezing blood out of the lungs into the left atrium and ventricle and by bringing the stethoscope closer to the heart, inspiration can make it louder by increasing sympathetic tone if there is sinus arrhythmia and the heart speeds up during inspiration. However, either inspiration or expiration can make the S$_3$ louder by causing the apex beat to emerge between the ribs in any particular patient. In some patients, the apex beat comes out between the ribs on inspiration and in others it does so on expiration. The S$_3$ is very sensitive to the proximity of the stethoscope to the apex beat.
   Note: You can bring the apex beat closer to the stethoscope by turning the patient into the left lateral decubitus position (Fig. 7).

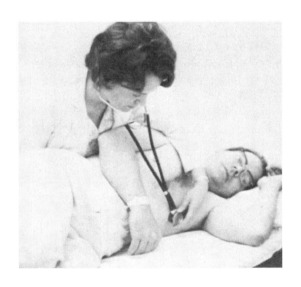

FIG. 7. In the left lateral decubitus position shown, the apex of the heart is brought as close to the stethoscope as possible. This is an absolute necessity for hearing a soft S$_3$, because it is sensitive to proximity.

3. What proof is there that ventricular volume and flow control the audibility of the S$_3$?
   ANS.: a. Conditions that increase the volume of flow make the S$_3$ louder (e.g., exercise or mitral regurgitation).
   b. Conditions that decrease flow to the heart and decrease ventricular volume cause decreased audibility of the S$_3$ (e.g., standing up, venous tourniquets, or the water-loss effect of diuretics).
   Note: a.   One of the characteristics that is most confusing to the beginner when listening to a soft S$_3$ is its intermittent audibility; that is, it waxes and wanes in and out of one's hearing threshold. This probably occurs because S$_3$ loudness is very sensitive to slight changes in proximity and volume caused by respiration.
   b.   In a study of interobserver agreement on the presence of an S$_3$, if a board

certified internist, a board-certified cardiologist, a trainee in cardiology, or a trainee internist heard an S_3, there was only a 35% chance that a second observer of the group would also hear the S_3 (11).

THE EXAGGERATED PHYSIOLOGIC S_3

1. What can exaggerate the physiologic S_3?

    ANS.: Any condition that causes excessive blood flow through the mitral valve. Excessive flow through the mitral valve brings back the physiologic S_3, as in

    a. The two left-to-right shunts, ventricular septal defect (VSD), and persistent ductus arteriosus (PDA).

    b. An incompetent mitral valve (i.e., mitral regurgitation [MR]) (Fig. 8).

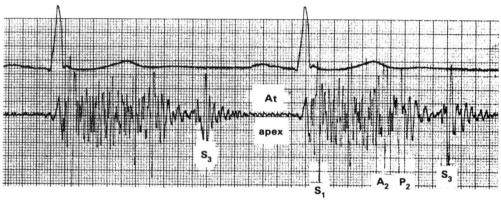

FIG. 8. Low-frequency phonocardiogram from a 15-year-old girl with severe rheumatic MR. Besides the loud MR murmur and S_3, note the following: (a) The widely split S_2 (A_2P_2) expected if moderate to severe MR is present; (b) the P_2 is well heard at the apex and should make you suspect some pulmonary hypertension. The patient's pulmonary artery systolic pressure was 35 mm Hg (upper normal is 25 mm Hg).

Note: Excessive flow through a tricuspid valve does not usually cause a right-sided S_3; that is, there is no physiologic right-sided S_3. The right ventricular S_3 requires not only a large right ventricle (RV) but also a high right atrial pressure. For example, in an uncomplicated ASD with a very large flow through the tricuspid valve, there is usually no S_3. It seems that the right ventricular S_3 occurs only when there is an abnormal relationship between the rate of rapid filling and the ventricle's ability to accommodate its increasing diastolic volume; that is, only when there is reduced compliance (9). The normal RV is more compliant than the LV, and it expands easily to accommodate increased flow unless it is also pressure-overloaded.

2. How can the detection of an apical S_3 tell you whether the pulmonary hypertension in a patient with a VSD or PDA is due to an increased flow (hyperkinetic) or to a fixed irreversible resistance?

    ANS.: The presence of an S_3 from the LV signifies that there is increased flow through the pulmonary circuit and that, therefore, the pulmonary hypertension is hyperkinetic and not fixed. This means that surgical closure of the VSD or PDA may lower the pulmonary artery pressure to normal (23). (You will learn later that a diastolic flow murmur at the apex also signifies reversible pulmonary hypertension; see p. 309.)

THE PATHOLOGIC S₃

1. What are the most common associated cardiac findings in subjects with a pathologic S₃?

    ANS.: A high mean left atrial pressure (due to a high V wave), a noncompliant LV, and a large ventricle associated with a poor ejection fraction.

    Note: Noncompliance of the distended ventricle is part of the mechanism that produces an S₃. This fact is suggested by its occurrence in a considerable proportion of patients with diastolic dysfunction and normal systolic function, especially if they have clinical congestive heart failure (22). An S₃ is heard even without congestive heart failure in patients with hypertrophic subaortic stenosis (HSS, or HOCM) who have very thick ventricles. Low as well as high filling rates have been found in patients with a pathologic S₃ (16).

2. What pathologic cardiac condition is generally present when an S₃ occurs in the presence of a high left atrial pressure due to a low ejection fraction?

    ANS.: A cardiomyopathy, most often idiopathic or due to extensive ischemic heart disease. Much more rarely, it is due to an infiltrate such as amyloid or sarcoid.

    Note: a. An S₃ in a patient with AR usually means LV dysfunction. An S₃ in a patient with AR correlates with an increased LV residual systolic volume and not with the severity of AR (1).

    b. In the presence of sudden severe AR, LV pressure may rise so rapidly and steeply in diastole that it produces a middiastolic closure of the mitral valve with a middiastolic S₁, which could be mistaken for an S₃. If the first heart sound is very loud, it may be entirely due to tricuspid closure (17).

    c. Some patients with a pathologic S₃ secondary to a past infarction are relatively asymptomatic; that is, they do not have the decreased exercise tolerance that is the usual consequence of a high left atrial V wave. The S₃ in these patients is often associated with a **ventricular aneurysm** or a large akinetic area. The mechanism for this S₃ is unknown.

3. Does a high filling pressure always mean LV dysfunction and low ejection fraction?

    ANS.: Not if it is caused primarily by a high A wave, because a strong left atrial contraction can produce a high A wave at the end of diastole and so cause a high filling pressure despite a normal ejection fraction. This occurs because it is the *mean* and not the *end-diastolic* filling pressure that best correlates with cardiac dysfunction. For example, in severe aortic stenosis there may be a 20-mm Hg LV end-diastolic pressure but a mean left atrial pressure of 10 mm Hg and therefore no decreased function.

THE PHYSIOLOGIC VERSUS THE PATHOLOGIC S₃

1. What is the difference in timing, quality, and loudness between the physiologic and the pathologic S₃?

    ANS.: None, except that the S₃ found in constrictive pericarditis may occur earlier than usual.

Note: You can tell a physiologic S_3 from a pathologic S_3 only by knowing the circumstances under which it occurs; that is, by finding the reason for the pathologic S_3, such as symptoms and signs of heart failure or myocardial abnormalities.

2. What is the difference between the physiologic S_3 and the pathologic S_3 in the response to pooling of blood in the legs caused by standing?

ANS.: Because pooling of blood in the legs is much more difficult to achieve in the patient who has congestive failure with edema and high venous pressure, standing will have less of an attenuating effect on the S_3 than is usual in such patients.

Note: A short diastolic rumble is often heard following the pathologic S_3. It is also heard with the torrential flow through the mitral valve that occurs when the physiologic S_3 is exaggerated either by MR or by a PDA. It is also sometimes heard in young children following their normal S_3. This low-frequency diastolic murmur following the S_3 occurs while the mitral valve leaflets are being rapidly swung into their semiclosed position by eddy currents under the mitral leaflets (Fig. 9).

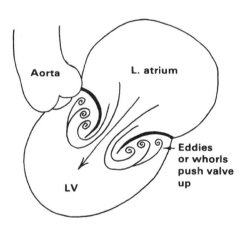

FIG. 9. If the flow is fast, eddy currents may push the valve up enough to create a partial obstruction and so produce turbulent flow and a short diastolic murmur.

The flow under high pressure through the semiclosed AV valve presumably produces this rumble because rapid ventricular filling continues for a short time after the S_3 (16). This short diastolic flow murmur following the S_3 should not be mistaken for the much longer murmur of mitral stenosis. (See p. 296 for method of distinguishing this murmur from the murmur of mitral stenosis.)

THE RIGHT VERSUS THE LEFT VENTRICULAR S_3

1. How can you tell the RV from the LV S_3?

ANS.: a. An S_3 generated by the RV is louder over the RV area (i.e., near the lower sternal area or epigastrium, unless the ventricle is markedly enlarged, in which case it may be loud anywhere over those parts of the precordium usually occupied by the LV).

b. The RV S₃ is usually louder on inspiration. The LV S₃ may be louder on either inspiration or expiration. (See p. 187 for explanation.) Auscultation with the bell in the subxiphoid region improves the sensitivity of the inspiratory maneuver by avoiding the dampening effect of inspiration at the left sternal edge as the chest dimension increases.

c. An S₃ from the RV is usually associated with a RV heave or rock (see p. 104 for explanation), a large jugular V wave, and a rapid Y descent.

2. List some of the common causes of an S₃ generated by the RV.

ANS.: The common causes are right ventricular dilatation and high right atrial pressure secondary to

a. Severe tricuspid regurgitation due to pulmonary hypertension.

b. Sudden RV outflow obstruction, as in massive pulmonary embolism.

Note: Although pulmonary stenosis is also an outflow obstruction, it requires chronic stenosis that is severe enough to produce RV failure before the RV will dilate and cause an S₃. This occurs rarely, because the compensatory mechanism for a chronic obstruction to outflow from birth is hyperplasia as well as hypertrophy, both of which are able to overcome all but the most severe obstruction.

THE S₃ VERSUS THE OPENING SNAP AND TUMOR PLOP

1. What is the difference between the A₂OS interval and the A₂S₃ interval?

ANS.: The A₂OS interval is rarely more than 100 msec (0.10 sec), whereas the shortest A₂S₃ interval is usually 120 msec (0.12 sec). The difference between 100 and 120 msec is merely the difference between saying "pa-pa" as quickly as possible and saying it at a normal speaking rate.

Note: There are rare exceptions to both these figures (e.g., by phonocardiogram the A₂OS has been seen to be as long as 120 msec, and the S₂ in constrictive pericarditis or the "tumor plop" of left atrial myxoma may occur as early as 100 msec after the S₂.

2. How does a "tumor plop" differ from an OS or an S₃?

ANS.: A "tumor plop" is the early diastolic sound produced when a left (or right) atrial myxoma attached to a stalk prolapses through the mitral (or tricuspid) valve in diastole. This early diastolic sound can occur at the time one would expect either an OS or an S₃. However, it may be intermittent or may vary in loudness and may even vary its time relationship to the second sound (9). It may differ from an S₃, even if it occurs at the same interval from the A₂ as the usual S₃, by being more easily heard at the left lower sternal border than expected. An S₃ is not usually heard at the left lower sternal border unless it is extremely loud or is a right-sided S₃. An S₃ is almost always loudest at the apex.

3. How does the quality or pitch of the S₃ help to distinguish it from the OS?

ANS.: The S₃ differs from the OS because it is usually low in pitch, sounds like a thud or boom, and is best heard with the bell. The OS, on the other hand, is usually a high-frequency, short clicking sound best recognized with the diaphragm. Occasionally, the OS is atypical and deceptively low in pitch. This occurs when the mitral valve is very calcified or if early ventricular expansion is poor due to severe myocardial damage.

Note: a. If there is a large LV, the OS may be as loud at the apical area as at the left sternal border.

      b. An OS is almost always associated with a loud, snapping first sound (the "closing snap"). Therefore, a soft or muffled first sound tends to deny the presence of an OS. Unfortunately, constrictive pericarditis and also the "tumor plop" are frequently associated with a loud S_1, thus causing the early pericardial knock or "tumor plop" to seem like an OS.

4. When can both an OS and an S_3 be present in the same person?

    ANS.: If a mobile anterior leaflet is associated with severe MR and the posterior leaflet is even slightly fibrosed and fixes the edges of the anterior leaflet, the normal anterior leaflet belly produces a snap as it opens, and the severe MR produces the exaggerated physiologic S_3.

5. What is the rhythm of an S_1 followed by an S_2, OS, and S_3? Can you make a rhythmic phrase that fits?

    ANS.:   Tum   tu-du-boom   Tum   tu-du-boom
            1   2 OS 3   1   2 OS 3

Summary of Signs Differentiating an S_3 from an OS

1. The OS is not usually more than 100 msec (0.10 sec, a rapid "pa-pa") from the S_2. The S_3 is rarely less than 120 msec (0.12 sec) from the A_2 (usually 140 msec).
2. The OS is usually a short, sharp click, best heard with the diaphragm near the left sternal border. The S_3 is a thud or boom, best heard by applying light or moderate pressure with the bell near the apex.
3. The OS is associated with a sharp, loud S_1. The S_3 may or may not have loud S_1.
4. An OS separates further from the A_2 when the patient stands. An S_3 does not change its distance from the A_2 on standing.

THE S_3 AND PERICARDIAL KNOCK

1. Why will pericardial constriction produce an early and loud S_3?

    ANS.: Pericardial constriction is the only condition besides tamponade in which, despite normal AV valves, there is a high-pressure V wave in the atrium proximal to a ventricle that may be normal in size and function. Because the ventricle is restricted in the extent to which it can expand, it compensates by reaching a maximum state of expansion early and rapidly, because of a high filling pressure that causes it to expand with more energy, generating a loud sound known as a pericardial knock. There is also some suggestion from systolic time interval studies that in constrictive pericarditis there is an excessive effect of catecholamines on the LV.

        Note: a. Cineangiograms of patients with constrictive pericarditis show that this early filling of the LV is accomplished with exceptional rapidity.

            b. The early S_3 of constriction may occasionally be very faint or absent. It may be brought out by squatting or increasing the afterload, as with phenylephrine. It may be obliterated by decreasing venous return, as with nitroglycerin (15).

            c. In restrictive cardiomyopathy the hemodynamic picture is quite similar to that seen in constriction, and the S_3 is usually loud and is best heard at the apex (4).

2. Why is the pericardial knock not present in tamponade?

    ANS.: The pericardial knock is not present in tamponade because early rapid expansion of the ventricles is markedly blunted by the fluid (7). However, in patients with effusive-constrictive-type pericarditis, the pericardial knock is usually present.

> *Note*: a. If a pericardial knock occurs early enough, as with severe constriction, it can come at the end of maximum opening of the mitral valve (i.e., at the time of the E point of the mitral echo), which is analogous to the timing of the OS. Although the usual pericardial knock occurs early (i.e., 60 to 110 msec after the A$_2$), it may occur at the usual S$_3$ time (i.e., 120 msec after the A$_2$ [19]).
>
> b. In constrictive pericarditis the pericardial knock may be loudest at the left sternal border, possibly because the RV also produces the sound in this condition (13). The first sound may be loud, suggesting further similarity to MS (14).
>
> c. Just as with the usual S$_3$, the knock is sensitive to blood volume. Therefore, diuretics may eliminate the knock and squatting can bring out a knock that is absent recumbent.

THE S$_3$ AND MITRAL STENOSIS

1. Why is a left ventricular S$_3$ not to be expected in significant mitral stenosis (MS)?

   ANS.: Mitral valve obstruction tends to prevent rapid filling of the LV in early diastole, despite a high left atrial pressure. Without rapid early filling, an S$_3$ is an unexpected finding. However, if the mitral diastolic murmur begins with a loud sound, that sound is probably an S$_3$. One recent study showed that when the S$_3$ was recorded in MS, its presence and intensity were independent of the severity of the MS. The S$_3$ varied only with the intensity of LV expansion and recoil in early diastole and could be present even in severe MS with reduced flow. The S$_3$ probably reflects good LV function (i.e., the LV can expand rapidly).

   > *Note*: In the French literature, the loud S$_3$-like beginning of the diastolic murmur has been called the "initial jerk" of the MS murmur.

2. When may a right ventricular S$_3$ be heard in MS?

   ANS.: If the right atrial pressure is high and the RV is dilated due to pulmonary hypertension and congestive failure. If the enlarged RV usurps the apex area, the S$_3$ may be heard well into the middle of the left thorax and may be mistaken for an LV S$_3$.

REFERENCES

1. Abdulla AM, et al. Clinical significance and hemodynamic correlates of the third heart sound in aortic regurgitation. *Circulation* 1981;64:464.
2. Arevalo F, et al. Hemodynamic correlates of the third heart sound. *Am J Physiol* 1964;207:319.
3. Aubert AE, et al. Investigation of genesis of gallop sounds using quantitative phonocardiography and digital frequency analysis. *Circulation* (Abst) 1983;68:240.
4. Chew CYC, et al. Primary restrictive cardiomyopathy, non-tropical endomyocardial fibrosis and hypereosinophilic heart disease. *Br Heart J* 1977;39:399.
5. Coulshed N, Epstein EJ. Third heart sound after mitral valve replacement. *Br Heart J* 1972;34:301.
6. Dock W. The forces needed to evoke sounds from cardiac tissues. *Circulation* 1959;19:376.
7. Firestein G, et al. Left ventricular function in the presence of small pericardial effusions. *Br Heart J* 1980;43:382.
8. Gianelly RE, et al. Heart sounds in patients with homograft replacement of mitral valve. *Circulation* 1970;42:309.
9. Goldschlager A, et al. Right atrial myxoma with right to left shunt and polycythemia. *Am J Cardiol* 1972;30:82.
10. Grayzel J. Gallop rhythm of the heart. *Circulation* 1959;20:1053.
11. Ishmail AA, et al. Interobserver agreement by auscultation in the presence of a third heart sound in patients with congestive heart failure. *Chest* 1987;91:870.

12. Kay CF, et al. The "late systolic heartbeat" of pericardial effusion. *Am Heart J* 1966;72:7.
13. Matsuzaki M, et. al. A study of abnormal interventricular septal motion. *J Cardiol* 1977;7:153.
14. Moreyra E, et al. Constrictive pericarditis masquerading as mitral stenosis. *Chest* 1970;57:245.
15. Nicholson WJ, et al. Early diastolic sound of constrictive pericarditis. *Am J Cardiol* 1980;45:378.
16. Prewitt T, et al. The "rapid filling wave" of the apex cardiogram. *Br Heart J* 1975;37:1256.
17. Rothbaum DA, et al. Diastolic heart sound produced by mid-diastolic closure of the mitral valve. *Am J Cardiol* 1974;34:367.
18. Schwartze D. Frequency of the normal third heart sound in childhood. *Z Kreislaufforsch* 1966;55:306.
19. Shah PM, Yu PN. Gallop rhythm: Hemodynamic and clinical correlation. *Am Heart J* 1969;78:823.
20. Smith JR. Observations on the mechanisms of the physiologic third heart sound. *Am Heart J* 1944;28:661.
21. Wiggers CJ. Studies on the consecutive phase of the cardiac cycle. *Am J Physiol* 1921;56:415.
22. Wohlgelernter D, et al. Third heart sound in patients with clinical congestive heart failure and normal left ventricular systolic performance. *J Am Coll Cardiol* (Abst) 1984;3:543.
23. Wood P. The Eisenmenger syndrome. *Br Med J* 1958;2:701. (Classic article)

12

The Fourth Heart Sound (S₄)

NOMENCLATURE

1. What has the triple rhythm produced by the sequence of a fourth heart sound, the S_1, and the S_2 been called?

   ANS.: An atrial gallop, a presystolic gallop, or an S_4 gallop.

   > *Note*: a. The term **atrial gallop** implies that the atrium itself is the source of the extra sound. Atrial contraction itself is not audible with the stethoscope.
   >
   > b. The term **presystolic gallop** is misleading because the gallop sound produced by an S_3 may also be "presystolic" during a tachycardia when the first sound follows very shortly after the S_3.
   >
   > c. The term S_4 specifies exactly which extra sound is thought to be producing the triple rhythm, regardless of diastolic length and without reference to exact mechanisms. It enables you to refer to the single sound S_4 without the necessity of always using the term **gallop**, which by definition implies at least three sounds.

THE INAUDIBLE S₄ COMPONENT

1. Does the atrial muscle itself produce vibrations as it contracts?

   ANS.: Yes, but such vibrations are usually inaudible because they are too low in frequency and amplitude. They can be picked up by placing a phonocatheter inside the atrium or in the esophagus. However, contractions of the atrium may cause an audible sound in complete atrioventricular (AV) block or junctional rhythm. These vibrations can sometimes be recorded at the apex during systole as the atrium contracts against the closed AV valves. In some cases of atrial flutter in patients in heart failure, clicking sounds, which are loudest at the base of the heart, occur after each F wave (10). They can be heard during both systole and diastole and may become louder during diastole.

   Since the only chamber in which such sounds can be recorded by intracardiac phonocatheter is the atrium, they appear to represent the effect of atrial contraction itself (22). They have also been heard during atrial fibrillation. Echocardiograms have shown simultaneous fluttering motions of both mitral and tricuspid leaflets in patients with atrial fibrillation.

THE AUDIBLE PHYSIOLOGIC AND PATHOLOGIC S_4

Mode of Production

1. Where is the S_4 best recorded by an intracardiac phonocatheter, in the atrium or in the ventricle?

    ANS.: In the ventricle.

    > *Note*: a. An apex cardiogram shows a hump just before the systolic outward impulse. This presystolic hump or A wave is often large enough to be palpable. The peak of the atrial hump coincides with the largest vibrations of the S_4 (Fig. 1).

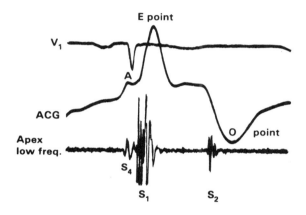

FIG. 1. Apex cardiogram and phono-cardiogram from a 50-year-old man with a previous infarction. The S_4 is simultaneous with a large palpable atrial hump (A wave) on the apex cardiogram. The A wave is 15% of the total apex pulse amplitude, or vertical E to O distance. Atrial humps of 15% or more of the E–O amplitude are usually palpable.

The A wave or end-diastolic outward movement of the apex impulse is the effect of left atrial contraction, causing a slight increase in the volume of the LV at the end of diastole. This slight increase in volume before the ventricle contracts can be seen on a cineangiogram, even in normal subjects.

An apical A wave may be palpable even when the S_4 is too low in frequency to be audible. On the other hand, a pathologic S_4 may be heard in the absence of a palpable A wave. This is obvious when you realize that only a chest that allows an apex beat to be easily palpated will allow you to palpate the A wave, yet the S_4 sound may still be heard. There are cardiologists who believe that you should never call an S_4 pathologic unless you can find a palpable A wave with it (29). If you follow this school of thought, you will misinterpret every pathologic S_4 in which the apex beat is difficult to palpate.

    b. An S_4 cannot be produced by an atrium that is contracting against a stenotic AV valve as in mitral stenosis (MS). The atrium must be able to transmit its pressure freely to the left ventricle (LV); otherwise, only a presystolic murmur will be heard.

2. What theory could account for the production of an audible S_4 if it (a) occurs at the peak of atrial contraction, (b) causes such an increase in LV end-diastolic volume that it produces a recordable and often palpable systolic outward movement, (c) occurs when atrial

pressure is higher than ventricular pressure, (d) sounds the same as an S_3, and (e) cannot occur if the AV valves are closed or stenotic?

ANS.:   Atrial contraction, by causing eddy currents on the undersurface of the AV valves, tends to hold them upward. However, since atrial contraction also raises the volume in the ventricle, the chordae tendineae and papillary muscles are stretched at exactly the same time the AV valves are being pulled up or held in the opposite direction. If it has enough energy, this tug on the chordae and papillary muscles could account for the sound.

> *Note*: Since the atria are within the restricting envelope in constrictive pericarditis, their function is reduced. In addition, it is difficult for a contracting left atrium to expand the constricted LV. Therefore, an S_4 tends to deny the presence of constriction (28).

RECOGNIZING THE RHYTHM OF THE S₄ GALLOP

If you remember that the P wave indirectly produces the S_4 and the QRS is responsible for the S_1, and if you know that the S_2 occurs at the end of the T, then you know the rhythm of S_4, S_1, and S_2 is the same as that of P, QRS, and end of T (Fig. 2).

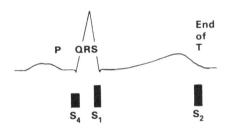

FIG. 2. **If you realize that the T wave is a systolic event, it will be easy to remember that the S_2 comes at the end of the T wave. Thus, the rhythm of an S_4 gallop is the rhythm symbolized by P,R–T, where R represents the QRS complex and T represents the end of the T.**

Because the P is closer to the QRS than the QRS is to the end of the T, the rhythm or cadence is a pair of sounds close together followed by a pause, then the second sound. Therefore, the rhythm of the two cycles is as follows: 4-1—2, 4-1—2. Vocal imitations of the heart sounds can help in perceiving the actual phenomena. Because the S_4 is low-pitched, you should practice imitating the S_4-S_1—S_2 by saying "huh-one—two." Place the "huh" as close as possible to the "one" so that they are practically one word, "huh-one." Also, say the "huh" as softly as possible, because the S_4 is often just within the realm of audibility and, in fact, like the S_3, tends to range in and out of audibility from beat to beat when it is soft.

The Physiologic S₄

1. Can an S_4 be heard in normal subjects?

   ANS.:   It occasionally can be heard in normal subjects in all age groups. It is so rarely normal, however, that unless it is heard in a young person with a concomitant physiologic S_3 or in an athlete with physiologic hypertrophy, you should suspect it is an abnormal finding.

   > *Note*: About 50% of tall athletes (e.g., basketball players) have a physiologic S_4. Almost all those with an S_4 show some electrocardiogram (ECG) or vectorcardiographic evidence of left ventricular hypertrophy (LVH) (25). Although it can be recorded in almost two-thirds of young boys with a

high-gain, low-frequency phonocardiogram, and in 35% to 70% of apparently normal subjects over age 40, this does not mean that these vibrations are audible (2,5,24). In one study, asymptomatic patients over age 40 with a recorded S_4 had positive treadmill tests. Therefore, it is questionable how often a physiologic S_4 is heard in perfectly normal hearts in persons over age 40 (2).

2. Why is the physiologic S_4 so rarely heard?
   ANS.: a. It is usually too soft and too low-pitched.
   b. It is often too close to the S_1 to be separated from it by ear. It is then called the atrial component of the S_1.
3. What is the mechanism of the physiologic S_4?
   ANS.: The normal atrium may contract in a peristaltic fashion toward the ventricle. Therefore, by the time atrial contraction has caused the ventricle to reach its peak presystolic pressure, most of the atrium is relaxed and has a lower pressure (X descent). At this time, however, the ventricle is not relaxing, and there is a momentary reversal of the pressure gradient. This reversal of pressure tends to close the mitral leaflets, pulls up on the chordae tendineae, and produces a sound (16). This peristaltic atrial movement is probably not present in a hypertrophied, strongly contracting atrium and is probably not the mechanism for the pathologic S_4.
   Note: a. The physiologic S_4 has been correlated with echocardiographic closure of the mitral valve at the completion of atrial relaxation in patients with AV block (6).
   b. This method of AV valve closure for the physiologic S_4 is probably a different mechanism than that for the pathologic S_4, as suggested by the following factors.
      1. In complete AV block with myocardial damage, split S_4 sounds are frequently audible. The first component of the split occurs at the usual distance of an S_4 after the P wave, and the second one occurs 200 msec or more from the P wave. (The pathologic S_4 is rarely more than 140 msec from the beginning of the P wave.)
      2. The atrial pressure is higher than the ventricular pressure at the time of the usual pathologic S_4 but is lower than ventricular pressure at the time of the second S_4 component in complete AV block, in both animals and humans. (See Fig. 3.)

The Pathologic S_4

Causes and Associated Conditions

1. After what age is an S_4 most likely to be pathologic?
   ANS.: You should consider any S_4 likely to be pathologic if the patient does not have the physiologic hypertrophy of an athlete or of a person with the daily activity that requires much exertion, especially isometric. Before you call an S_4 physiologic in a young person (i.e., under age 20), however, you should probably hear a physiologic S_3, hear a physiologically split S_2, feel a normal apex beat, hear a venous hum in the neck, and obtain a normal ECG and chest x-ray. An ECG should also be done to rule out a hypertrophic cardiomyopathy.
2. What kind of atrial contraction is necessary for the production of an audible S_4?
   ANS.: A strong atrial contraction is the most important requirement for an audible S_4. Any condition in which the ventricle is "stiffer" than normal (i.e., in which the

ventricle has decreased distensibility or compliance) generates a strong atrial contraction.

> *Note*: In hypertension the left atrial contraction is increased not only because of a Starling effect but also because of an enhanced inotropic state of the left atrium (30).

3. What conditions may cause a decreased compliance of the ventricle besides hypertrophy?

ANS.: Those in which the ventricle is stiffened by replacement of the myocardium by fibrous tissue or infiltrate (e.g., as with an old myocardial infarction or Duchenne muscular dystrophy) or stiffened by acute infarction or ischemia due to angina. (Subtotal or total acute coronary occlusion in dogs can be shown to increase the stiffness of the LV [29].)

> *Note*: a. The stretch of the LV produced by forcing blood into the ventricle just before it contracts is often called the "atrial kick" effect.
>
> b. A patient whose filling pressure is elevated only by a strong atrial contraction or A wave is less dyspneic than one who has the same high filling pressure due to a high V wave because a high A wave starting from a low left atrial pressure results in a lower mean left atrial pressure than does a high V wave falling to a high left atrial pressure (Fig. 3).

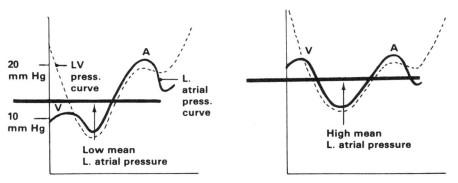

FIG. 3. A low V wave and a disproportionately high A wave are seen on the left. These give a lower mean left atrial pressure and therefore less dyspnea than do both a high V wave and a relatively poor atrial contraction, as seen on the right.

> c. Although mitral stenosis can prevent even a strong atrial contraction from being transmitted to the LV, if the mitral obstruction is due to a left atrial myxoma, an S₄ can occur, presumably because either the atrial contraction has some effect on the tumor or the atrial contraction can transmit its pressure to the LV by way of the atrial tumor.

4. What causes an atrium in sinus rhythm to be too weak to help out a ventricle?

ANS.: a. If the atrium is too large, as in chronic severe rheumatic mitral regurgitation (MR), the atrium may be overstretched and may, therefore, contract less efficiently. This can also occur when the left atrium is severely damaged by myocarditis, infarction, or infiltrate.

> b. The atrium may also be weak if there is excess vagal stimulation (15).
>
> c. Too little blood in the atrium (i.e., decreased venous return due to either diuresis or having the patient stand) also weakens the atrial contraction.

5. How can the S_4 assist in the diagnosis of constriction or tamponade?

   ANS.: An S_4 is not heard in constriction or tamponade. This seems surprising at first because in tamponade the pressure rises quickly to a high point in the "atrioventricle" during diastole, and you would think that the stretch of the atrium would stimulate it to contract strongly. On the other hand,

   a. The inability of the ventricle to expand at the end of diastole due to the con-
      striction could account for the loss of the forces necessary to produce an S_4.

   b. The LV pressure rises so high at the end of diastole that the left atrium may not
      be able to open the mitral valve well. Indeed, reversed end-diastolic flow across
      the mitral valve has been shown in constrictive pericarditis (33).

   c. The atrium may be so tethered by the constrictive process that it cannot con-
      tract well.

The S_4 in Myocardial Infarction and Angina

1. What proportion of patients with acute myocardial infarction have an S_4?

   ANS.: Although almost all patients with acute infarction have a phonocardiographic S_4,
   it is heard by auscultation in only about half of the patients during the first few
   days following an infarction (29). Although this hyperacute S_4 may disappear, it
   rarely does so if it remains beyond the first few days.

   Note: a. The frequent S_4 heard in the first few days following infarction is partly
   explained by one study that claims that the infarcted area, whether dys-
   kinetic (bulges out like an aneurysm in systole) or akinetic (no movement during systole), causes loss of compliance of the LV (17). It has
   also been shown that ischemia or the presence of excess catecholamines
   in the first few days of infarction can cause a loss of compliance of the
   LV (8).

   b. An S_4 may occur only during an attack of angina because there is a
   marked increase in stiffness of the LV during angina (3).

The S_4 in Volume Overload

1. When is ventricular enlargement usually associated with a normally compliant ventricle
   and, therefore, with an absent S_4?

   ANS.: When the volume overload is chronic due to regurgitant or shunt flows (e.g., in
   ventricular septal defect [VSD], persistent ductus arteriosus [PDA], chronic aortic
   regurgitation [AR], or chronic MR), especially if there is rheumatic damage to the
   left atrium.

   Note: An S_4 can, however, occur with the volume overload that occurs in severe
   anemia (1).

2. When will there be an S_4 in a subject with MR?

   ANS.: When the MR is

   a. Secondary to papillary muscle dysfunction or LV dilatation due to fibrosis or is-
      chemia.

   b. Sudden and severe due to ruptured chordae. In this case, the left atrium and ven-
      tricle are enlarged only moderately despite the massive volume overload because
      the pericardium resists acute stretching.

LOUDNESS AND AUDIBILITY OF THE S₄

1. Where is the LV S_4 usually best heard?

   ANS.: At the apex, when the patient is in the left lateral decubitus position.

   Note: The LV S_4 is occasionally better heard at the left lower sternal border than at the apex. The reason for this is unknown, but it occurs most often in patients with angina or a history of infarction (31).

2. Why should you usually use the stethoscope bell to bring out the S_4?

   ANS.: Most of the energy of the S_4 (as of the S_3) is in the low-frequency range.

   Note: An S_3 or S_4 may occasionally be heard better with the firm bell pressure because

   a. When the S_3 or S_4 is loud, high frequencies develop, and attenuating the low frequencies by firm bell pressure can sharpen the perception of the extra sounds by helping to separate them from the S_1 or S_2, especially during tachycardia.

   b. With heavy bell pressure, the volume inside the bell is reduced. It may be that volume displacement by the A wave into a smaller total volume produces a greater effect on the eardrum.

3. What are the pitfalls of using held expiration as a means of bringing the stethoscope closer to the heart to help hear the S_4?

   ANS.: Held respiration (apnea) will decrease venous return because with respiration the lungs act like a pump and help speed up the circulation time. The soft S_4 is very sensitive to blood volume.

4. How can the S_4 be made louder?

   ANS.: a. By increasing blood flow to the atrium.

   b. By increasing the pressure in the left atrium so that there is a greater stretch force on the atrial walls.

   c. By bringing ventricular movements closer to the stethoscope.

5. Besides having the patient exercise, how can you increase the flow to the atrium?

   ANS.: By asking the patient to

   a. Release a Valsalva strain that has been maintained for at least 10 sec. This causes a sudden rush of blood to the right ventricle (RV) and a few seconds later to the LV, which then also must pump against an increased resistance for several seconds after the Valsalva.

   b. Cough several times. This is really another form of exercise as well as a mini-Valsalva maneuver.

   c. Take four or five deep, rapid breaths. This activates the lung pump and thus increases flow to the heart.

   d. Squat. This can increase cardiac output for a few beats.

   e. Do isometric contraction through handgrip (see below for hemodynamics). This increases cardiac output as well as blood pressure.

   Note: These maneuvers also cause the S_4 to occur farther from the S_1, and so make the gallop rhythm more apparent.

6. How can you bring ventricular movements closer to the stethoscope?

   ANS.: Turn the patient into the left lateral decubitus position. If you listen immediately afterward, the effect of the exertion is also operative for a few beats.

   Note: When this maneuver fails to produce an S_4 that is suspected, have the patient change from a standing to a sudden left lateral decubitus position. This often produces an S_4 for a few beats.

HANDGRIP AND THE S_4

1. When does isometric handgrip contraction, such as when one squeezes a folded towel with one hand, bring out an S_4?

   ANS.: A handgrip has this effect only if it raises blood pressure.

2. When and how does handgrip contraction increase blood pressure?

   ANS.: A strong handgrip produces local ischemia, which generates reflexes whose apparent purpose is to supply more blood flow to the ischemic area. In most subjects, cardiac output increases through increased heart rate and contractility (14). Handgrip also increases peripheral resistance in hypertensive patients, in patients with a reduction in cardiac reserve (23), and in patients with significant obstructive lesions, as in MS.

   Note: a. Handgrip has been widely recommended to bring out an S_4. It does not always help for this purpose, probably because the increased contractility of the LV reduces the need for an S_4. If, however, the patient has angina or a pressure-loaded LV, as in aortic stenosis or elevated blood pressure, the end-diastolic pressure is usually elevated by handgrip, and an S_4 is brought out (7).

   b. The strength of the handgrip does not control the peak heart rate and blood pressure rise as much as does the degree of fatigue produced. The strength of the handgrip controls only the rate of development of the peak heart rate and blood pressure. For example, a 75% maximum voluntary contraction for 1 minute achieves about the same effect as a 25% effort for 5 minutes.

DIFFERENTIATING THE S_4 FROM THE S_3

1. How does the quality or the pitch of the S_4 differ from that of the S_3?

   ANS.: They do not differ. They both may be described as a low-pitched thud or boom. Because of the very low frequency of vibration, they often feel more like a physical movement felt by the eardrum than a sound heard by the auditory system.

   It is difficult to differentiate an S_3 from an S_4 during tachycardia. Therefore, you should try to slow the rate with carotid pressure. If the extra sound maintains a constant relationship with the S_1, it is an S_4.

   Wait for a pause following a premature beat. An S_4 will obviously precede the S_1 that ends the pause.

   Note: a. The long diastole after a premature ventricular contraction does not always allow you to hear an S_4. Often the S_4 disappears at the end of a long diastole, possibly because of the reduced afterload.

   b. When both an S_3 and an S_4 are present, the rhythm is called quadruple rhythm, train-wheel rhythm, or double gallop (Fig. 4).

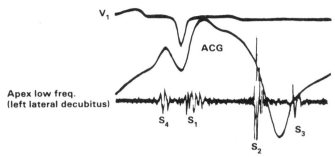

FIG. 4. Apex cardiogram and phonocardiogram from a 55-year-old male with two previous infarctions. Surprisingly, despite his S_3 and S_4, or double gallop, he was almost asymptomatic without treatment. His atrial hump was easily palpable.

DIFFERENTIATING AN S_4S_1 FROM A SPLIT S_1 (M_1A_1)

1. When is an S_4S_1 difficult to distinguish from a split S_1 due to an M_1-ejection sound?
   ANS.: When the S_4 is very close to the S_1.
      Note: Even experienced auscultators can mistake a split S_1 for an S_4S_1 as shown by a study in which they were asked to record whether or not an S_4 was heard in 200 consecutive patients over age 50. Among 34 patients without an S_4 on phonocardiogram, there were 56% false-positive answers (24).
2. What is the general principle that allows quick distinction between an S_4S_1 and an M_1A_1, or M_1 ejection sound?
   ANS.: It is easy to get rid of an S_4 but difficult to eliminate an M_1.
3. List the ways of attenuating an S_4 that have little effect on the M_1.
   ANS.: a. Firm pressure with the diaphragm often eliminates an S_4 (Fig. 5).

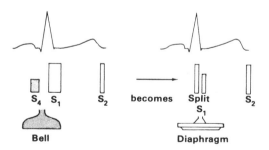

FIG. 5. Pressure with the bell or the use of a diaphragm will eliminate most soft S_4s and may bring out the narrow, sharp, clicking physiologic split of S_1.

   b. Listening at sites away from the apex beat eliminates an S_4.
   c. Listening with the patient supine may make the apex beat impalpable and eliminate an S_4.
   d. Listening with the patient sitting or standing to decrease blood volume to the heart often eliminates an S_4.
      Note: a. A soft S_4 tends to disappear from perception from beat to beat; an M_1

does not characteristically do this. The change from beat to beat is due to the fact that the S_4 is very sensitive to changes in volume in the LV as well as to proximity of the LV to the stethoscope. Both of these parameters are affected by respiration.

    b. If the S_4 is so loud that none of the preceding maneuvers eliminate it, it is usually palpable as an atrial hump or A wave on the apex beat's pulse contour, in the left lateral decubitus position.

SEVERITY OF CARDIAC DYSFUNCTION AND PRESENCE OF AN S_4

1. When does an S_4 occur with the pressure overloads caused by *mild* aortic stenosis (AS) or *mild* systemic hypertension?

    ANS.: Only when enough myocardial damage has resulted from some other disease, such as ischemic heart disease, so that the additional loss of LV compliance is sufficient to cause an S_4.

2. When is a right-sided S_4 not expected despite severe pulmonary hypertension?

    ANS.: When the contraction of the right atrium can decompress itself through a large atrial septal defect (ASD) or VSD.

        Note: In the occasional ASD a presystolic murmur instead of an S_4 may be produced by atrial contraction.

3. What does the presence of an S_4 indicate about the gradient in AS and in pulmonary stenosis (PS)?

    ANS.: In valvular AS or in PS it suggests a severe gradient of at least 70 mm Hg across the valve (32). (This should refer to an audible and not just a phonocardiographic S_4.) This is not valid in either subjects with angina in whom ischemic heart disease may be an additional cause of an S_4 or subjects with hypertrophic subaortic stenosis (HSS, or HOCM) who may have an S_4 with any gradient (13).

        Note: In severe PS a strong right atrial contraction may actually open the pulmonary valve and produce a presystolic murmur or even a presystolic pulmonary valve opening click. The presystolic click often occurs between the S_4 and the S_1 and signifies severe PS, just as the S_4 does.

4. Which is a more serious sign of heart disease, the pathologic left-sided S_3 or the S_4?

    ANS.: A pathologic S_3 is more serious because it is associated with both a stiff LV as well as an increase in left atrial V wave pressure, which is a sign of decompensation at rest. An S_4, on the other hand, merely means that a poorly compliant ventricle is "calling on the atrium for help" and has only a high A wave pressure. The help it receives may be enough to keep the output adequate, even with moderate exercise.

5. What happens to the S_4 when failure becomes severe and an S_3 develops?

    ANS.: After a stage in which both an S_3 and an S_4 may be present, the S_4 tends to soften and then disappear, and the patient with severe failure may be left with only an S_3 (4).

6. When is an S_4 heard in the neck? Why?

    ANS.: When a right atrial contraction is so strong (as in PS or pulmonary hypertension) that it produces a forceful jugular A wave that strikes the stethoscope chestpiece, producing a sound with the timing of an S_4. It is not surprising that the effect of a strong right atrial contraction can be heard in the neck because sudden tensing of strips of various tissues has shown that the superior vena cava produces the loudest sounds among all cardiac tissues that have been tested (i.e., pulmonary artery, aorta, valves, and the walls of the ventricles) (9).

Note: Right-sided S$_4$s are heard under the same circumstances at the right side of
the heart as are left-sided S$_4$s at the left side. Therefore, they are heard in
the presence of right ventricle (RV) overloads that cause loss of compliance of the RV, such as severe PS and pulmonary hypertension. They are
also heard in sudden, severe tricuspid regurgitation or endocarditis. (Right-
sided endocarditis is usually seen only in heroin addicts.)

7. Which myocardial diseases does the presence of an audible S$_4$ tend to rule out?

ANS.: Those with poor left atrial contractility and poor ability of the left ventricle to
stretch easily (i.e., restrictive or constrictive myocardial disease due to such things
as amyloid, tamponade, and constrictive pericarditis).

SEVERITY OF CARDIAC DYSFUNCTION AND TIMING AND AMPLITUDE OF THE S$_4$

1. When is the relation between the PS$_4$ interval and the severity of the loss of compliance?

ANS.: The shorter the PS$_4$ interval, the more severe the loss of compliance (11). If the
PS$_4$ interval is short, the S$_4$S$_1$ interval will be long (i.e., the greater the stiffness of
the LV, the earlier the S$_4$) (Fig. 6).

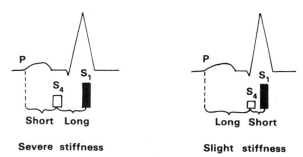

**FIG. 6. The longer the S$_4$S$_1$ interval, the greater the loss of compliance of the left ventricle (pro-
vided the PR interval is not prolonged) and usually the louder the S$_4$.**

2. What will happen to the S$_4$S$_1$ interval in a patient who is hypertensive and either is made
normotensive with an antihypertensive agent or has the flow to the heart decreased by
standing up?

ANS.: Both of these maneuvers cause a narrow S$_4$S$_1$ interval; that is, the S$_4$ moves toward
the S$_1$ and may join with it, becoming indistinguishable (18).

Note: a. The earlier the S$_4$, the louder it becomes. By electrical pacing of dogs'
atria it has been shown that the earlier in diastole the atrium contracts,
the more powerfully it contracts. It has also been shown that long S$_4$S$_1$
intervals result in more energetic ventricular contractions than do short
S$_4$S$_1$ intervals.

b. As the S$_4$ moves farther from the S$_1$, the S$_1$ becomes softer (21). If the
atrium reaches its peak pressure early, it may allow left atrial relaxation
(X descent) to reach low levels early, and left atrial pressure is then relatively low when the ventricle starts to contract. Therefore, the LV

closes the mitral valve at the slowest part of its acceleration curve. (See Fig. 139.)

   c. The S_4S_1 interval in hypertensive patients with LVH should be well separated even if the PS_4 interval is not shortened, because in LVH the QM_1 interval is prolonged due to prolongation of the electromechanical interval (4).

   d. Catecholamines that reach a high level in acute infarction tend to shorten the QM_1 interval and therefore narrow the S_4S_1 interval.

   e. Right-sided S_4S_1 intervals are usually relatively long.

3. How can you best diagnose the presence of a summation gallop?

   ANS.: If the heart rate of a patient with a summation gallop is slowed by carotid sinus pressure, you may hear either nothing or a pathologic S_3, a pathologic S_4, a physiologic S_3, or both a pathologic S_3 and a pathologic S_4 (i.e., a double gallop) (Fig. 7).

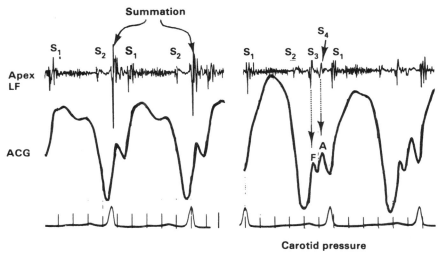

FIG. 7. In this patient with heart failure and AS, a tachycardia of 115 with a PR of 150 msec (0.15 sec) causes a summation gallop. When the rate is slowed by carotid pressure, both an S_3 and an S_4 appear. Therefore, this is an augmented type of summation gallop. (LF = low frequency.)

THE PACEMAKER S_4-LIKE CLICK

1. When can an electronic pacemaker produce an extra sound? When does the extra sound occur?

   ANS.: When it causes intercostal skeletal muscle contraction, an electronic pacemaker can produce a high-pitched clicking sound just preceding the M_1, so that it sounds like a widely split S_1 (19,20). It is accentuated by inspiration and occurs about 6 msec after the pacing stimulus.

   Although perforation of the myocardium should be suspected when the pacemaker-induced sound occurs, this is not a necessary concomitant.

   Note: Pacemaker sounds are occasionally audible only in the left lateral decubitus position.

2. Where has the pacemaker been situated when it produced a click plus diaphragmatic contraction with each click, without perforation of the heart?

ANS.: a. In the coronary sinus, where it stimulated the left hemidiaphragm, according to one report (27).

b. In the RV posteroinferior apical region close to the left hemidiaphragm or at the apex of the RV anteriorly (12).

Note: An atrial click also occurs (100 to 200 msec after a P wave) in patients with many different cardiac conditions such as ASD, thoracic deformities, hyperthyroidism, idiopathic cardiomyopathies, pericardiectomy, and pericarditis (26).

REFERENCES

1. Argano BJ. Phonocardiographic findings in anemia. *Chest* 1971;60:599.
2. Aronow WS, et al. Effects of position on the resting and postexercise phonocardiogram. *Chest* 1972; 61:439.
3. Barry WH, et al. Changes in diastolic stiffness and tone of the left ventricle in angina. *Circulation* 1974;49:255.
4. Bethell HJN, Nixon PGF. Understanding the atrial sound. *Br Heart J* 1973;35:229.
5. Bridgman EW. Notes on a presystolic sound. *Arch Intern Med* 1914;14:474.
6. Brockman SK. Dynamic function of atrial contraction in regulation of cardiac performance. *Am J Physiol* 1961; 204:597.
7. Cohn PF, et al. Diastolic heart sounds during static exercise in patients with chest pain. *Circulation* 1973; 47:1217.
8. Diamond G, Forrester JS. Effect of coronary artery disease and acute myocardial infarction on left ventricular compliance. *Circulation* 1972;45:11.
9. Dock W. The genesis of diastolic heart sounds. *Am J Med* 1971;50:178.
10. Dolara A, Tardini B. Atrial flutter sounds: Report of a case. *Am Heart J* 1969;78:369.
11. Duchosal P. A study of gallop rhythm. *Am Heart J* 1932;7:613.
12. Gaidula JJ, Barold SS. Diaphragmatic origin of the pacemaker sound. *Chest* 1972;61:195.
13. Goldblatt A, et al. Hemodynamic phonocardiographic correlations of the fourth heart sound in aortic stenosis. *Circulation* 1962;26:92.
14. Grossman W, et al. Changes in the inotropic state of the left ventricle during isometric exercise. *Br Heart J* 1973; 35:697.
15. Harris WS, et al. Modification of the atrial sound by the cold pressure test, carotid sinus massage, and the Valsalva maneuver. *Circulation* 1963;28:1128.
16. Herbert WH. Basis for effects of atrial dynamics on ventricular function. *NY State J Med* 1967;67:675.
17. Hood WB Jr, et al. Experimental myocardial infarction, reduction of left ventricular compliance in healing phase. *J Clin Invest* 1970;49:1316.
18. Kincaid-Smith P, Barlow J. The atrial sound in hypertension and ischaemic heart disease. *Br Heart J* 1959; 21:479.
19. Kluge WF. Pacemaker sound and its origin. *Am J Cardiol* 1970;25:362.
20. Kramer DH, et al. Mechanisms and significance of pacemaker-induced extracardiac sound. *Am J Cardiol* 1970; 25:367.
21. Leonard JJ, et al. Observations on the mechanism of atrial gallop rhythm. *Circulation* 1958;42:1007.
22. Massumi RA, et al. The audible sound of atrial tachyarrhythmia. *Circulation* 1966;33:607.
23. Matthews OA, et al. Left ventricular function during isometric exercise (handgrip): Significance of an atrial gallop. *Am Heart J* 1974;88:686.
24. Rectra EH, et al. Audibility of the fourth heart sound: A perspective "blind" auscultatory and polygraphic investigation. *JAMA* 1972;221:36.
25. Roeske WB, et al. Noninvasive study of athletes' hearts. *Circulation* 1976;53:287.
26. Sakamoto T, et al. Clinical observations of atrial click. *CV Sound Bull* 1975;5:275.
27. Schluger J, Wolf RE. Sound caused by diaphragmatic contraction resulting from transvenous cardiac pacemaker. *Chest* 1972;61:693.
28. Shah KD, et al. Echo-phono-apexcardiography in constrictive pericarditis. *J Cardiography* 1984;14:89.
29. Stock E. Auscultation and phonocardiography in acute myocardial infarction. *Med J Aust* 1966;1:1060.
30. Tamitani M, et al. Studies on systolic performance of the left atrium. *J Cardiol* 1983;13:587.
31. Turner PP, Hunter J. The atrial sound in ischaemic heart disease. *Br Heart J* 1973;35:657.
32. Vogelpoel L, Schrire V. Auscultatory and phonocardiographic assessment of pulmonary stenosis with intact ventricular septum. *Circulation* 1960;22:55.
33. Yazaki Y, et al. Transmitral reversed flow during mid- and end-diastole in constrictive pericarditis. *Am Heart J* 1986;112:855.

<h1 style="text-align:center">13</h1>

<h1 style="text-align:center">Ejection Murmurs</h1>

PHYSICAL CAUSES

1. What anatomic situations tend to produce high enough energy turbulence to produce sounds?
    ANS.: a. Obstruction to blood flow, caused either by circumferential narrowing or by a local protrusion into the bloodstream.
    b. Flow into a distal chamber of larger diameter than the proximal one (Fig. 1).

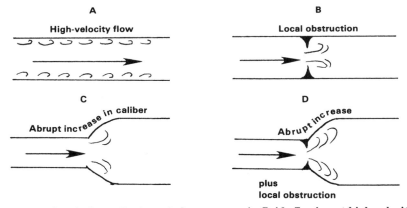

FIG. 1. Causes of turbulence. In A, turbulence occurs in fluids flowing at high velocity through tubes of uniform caliber, according to the formula for Reynolds numbers. In B and C, either a local obstruction or fluid flowing into a channel of larger diameter can produce turbulence at much less flow velocity. In D, a combined effect of obstruction and abrupt increase in caliber, as in poststenotic dilatation, produces turbulence at relatively low flow velocity.

2. How does the area of an orifice affect the rate of flow across it, and the loudness of the murmur?
    ANS.: With a decrease in orifice area and given enough time, the volume of flow tends to be maintained by a compensatory increase in pressure upstream from the stenotic area. The smaller the orifice, the greater the velocity of flow at the orifice and the greater the turbulence and the loudness of the murmur.
    Note: Turbulence is also affected by the following factors.
    a. Viscosity. The greater the viscosity, the less the turbulence. It is to be expected, then, that the high hematocrit present in patients with cyan-

otic congenital heart disease can increase blood viscosity enough to attenuate murmurs.

   b. The irregularity and sharpness of the edge of the orifice. The greater
      the irregularity and sharpness at the orifice edges, the louder the mur-
      mur.

3. What is the vortex or eddy theory of the cause of murmurs?

   ANS.: Turbulence sets up vortices or eddies, and these can strike the walls of the vascu-
      lar system to produce vibrations that have frequencies and amplitudes compatible
      with actual murmurs.

      Note: A good analogy for eddies is that they are like smoke rings.

4. How does the frequency or pitch of a murmur relate to the gradient and flow?

   ANS.: a. The greater the gradient, the higher the frequency and pitch produced. High gra-
      dients with little flow volume produce "blowing" murmurs.

      b. The greater the flow, the more frequently are low and medium frequencies pro-
         duced; that is, "the greater the flow, the more the low." When low gradients pro-
         duce murmurs that are highly dependent on flow, the result is a "rumbling" mur-
         mur.

      c. A combination of high gradient and high flow produces mixed frequencies that,
         if loud, can result in harsh murmurs.

CHARACTERISTICS

1. What valvular flow event is implied by the term **ejection** murmur?

   ANS.: The term implies a murmur produced by blood flowing forward through a **semilu-
      nar valve** during systole.

2. What is characteristic of ejection murmurs on a phonocardiogram?

   ANS.: They start with the final component of the first heart sound (S_1), are crescendo-de-
      crescendo, and finish before the second sound of the side of the heart from which
      the murmur originates. This means that a left-sided ejection murmur finishes be-
      fore the A_2, and a right-sided ejection murmur finishes before the P_2 (Fig. 2).

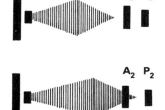

**FIG. 2. This murmur could be either pulmonary or aortic, since
it ends before both components of the second sound.**

A_2 P_2

**This murmur can be a pulmonary ejection murmur, since al-
though it extends beyond the A_2, it finishes before the P_2.**

3. Why must an ejection murmur be crescendo-decrescendo in loudness?

   ANS.: The configuration of the loudness of a murmur across a valve is controlled mainly
      by the shape of the gradient. This gradient is controlled by the velocity and accel-
      eration of flow; that is, the greater the velocity and acceleration of flow, the greater
      the gradient and the louder the murmur.

      In aortic stenosis (AS), as the pressure in the left ventricle (LV) rises to just
      above diastolic pressure in the aorta, it takes a short time to overcome the inertia
      of the aortic blood and walls. Therefore, the initial gradient across the aortic ori-

fice is slight, and the murmur starts softly. The pressure gradient and velocity of flow then increases toward midsystole, as does the murmur. As soon as the ventricle begins the state of reduced ejection, just past the middle of systole, the flow decreases, the gradient decreases, and the murmur decreases (Fig. 3).

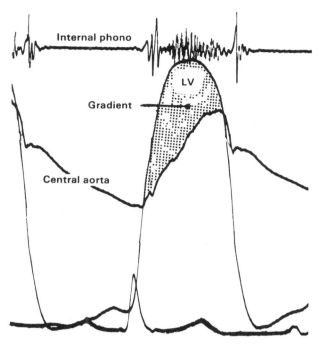

FIG. 3. A simultaneous aortic and LV pressure (taken with a catheter-tip micromanometer to eliminate time delays through tubes) in a subject with valvular AS. The shape of the murmur follows the shape of the gradient (*shaded area*).

> *Note*: Ejection murmurs seem to end with a slight pause before the S_2 because the decrescendo is so steep that the ear cannot hear the very end, even though the second sound is reached on a phonocardiogram. Since regurgitant murmurs go over the second sound and would eliminate any S_2 that was softer than or the same loudness as the murmur, you can sometimes use this to diagnose the presence of an ejection murmur; that is, if the murmur is louder or as loud as the S_2 and you can hear the S_2, it must be an ejection murmur.

4. What happens to the loudness of an ejection murmur after a long diastole, as in the long pause after a premature ventricular contraction or after the long diastoles of atrial fibrillation? Why?

   ANS.: It increases (i.e., becomes louder). The main reason may be because the long period of diastole allows a large volume to collect in the LV and stretch its walls. This increased volume is ejected during the next systole with increased energy by means of the Starling effect.

   > *Note*: One study could not show by ventriculography that the long diastole after a premature beat actually causes an increased volume in the ventricle (56). This study suggests the following reasons for an accentuated ejection murmur after a sudden long diastole.

a. The **postextrasystolic potentiation** following an early ventricular depolarization (as with a premature ectopic beat) produces a positive inotropic effect on the ventricle (believed to be due to a calcium flux effect) and contributes to the loudness of the ejection murmur after a long
diastole produced by a premature ventricular contraction (PVC). It has
been shown in one study that the worse the myocardial function, the
greater the postextrasystolic potentiation effect. This suggests that the
greater the increase in loudness after a sudden long pause, the worse
may be the myocardial function (46,63).

b. A long diastole allows more peripheral runoff and, therefore, a reduction in afterload. This causes an increase in the velocity of myocardial
shortening and an increase in the volume of forward flow (Fig. 4).

5. Why do the pitch or frequency characteristics of an ejection murmur not change even
when the murmur is soft?

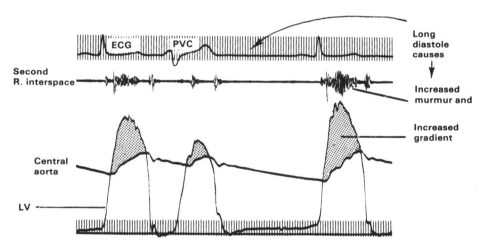

**FIG. 4. A phonocardiogram and simultaneous aortic and LV pressure tracing from a 16-year-old
boy with valvular AS. Not only did the murmur and gradient increase after the long diastole, but
the ejection sound also increased. Note that the small gradient of the premature ventricular contraction (PVC) itself produced only a short early systolic murmur.**

ANS.: The ejection murmur retains the low (and medium) frequencies because ejection
murmurs are produced by the entire stroke volume passing through the aortic or
pulmonary valve with each systole. Therefore, there is always enough flow to produce low and medium frequencies, even when the obstruction or gradient across
the valve is trivial. Soft regurgitant murmurs are purely high-frequency.

6. How can you best define an ejection murmur?

ANS.: It is best defined as an ejection murmur complex; that is, a murmur that begins at
the end of the S_1 is crescendo-decrescendo, ends before the second sound of its
side, can be heard even if it is the same loudness or softer than the murmur, becomes louder after a sudden long diastole, and retains low and medium frequencies even when soft.

Note: The original meaning of the term **ejection murmur** was a "midsystolic"
crescendo-decrescendo murmur that ended before the second sound of its
side (34). This definition ignores the following facts.

a. On phonocardiograms, most ejection murmurs can usually be seen to start without any pause after the S_1. This makes the term **midsystolic murmur** a poor substitute for **ejection murmur**.

b. A regurgitant murmur may also be slightly crescendo-decrescendo and may occasionally end before the S_2 of its side.

7. How can you tell by auscultation alone that a murmur is crescendo-decrescendo (diamond- or kite-shaped on a phonocardiogram)?

ANS.: A rhythmic cadence is created by the sequence of S_1 followed by the peak of the crescendo, followed by S_2.

huh-huh-duh
S_1 peak S_2
of
diamond

Note: If an S_2 is missing, "huh-huh" tells you that the murmur is crescendo-de-crescendo. If the S_1 is missing, the rhythm of "huh-duh" also tells you that the murmur is crescendo-decrescendo. With mild to moderate gradients, the peak of the crescendo-decrescendo is usually early in systole and not in midsystole, so that it is best imitated by "huh-huh" close together, then " . . . duh." This is another reason to avoid the substitute term **midsystolic** for ejection murmurs (Fig. 5).

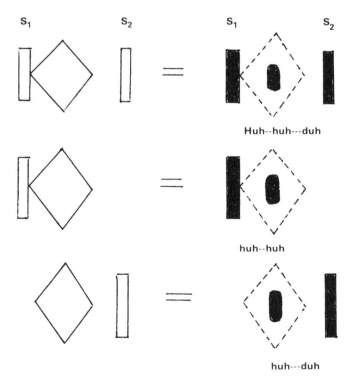

FIG. 5. If you imagine the string section of an orchestra playing a long note during systole and the drums playing a rhythm of two or three notes, you will have the impression given by the peak of an ejection murmur plus either an S_1, an S_2, or both.

8. How can the loudness of an ejection murmur tell you whether or not there is a significant gradient across a valve?

ANS.: A soft murmur (i.e., grade 2 or less) is likely to occur with an unimportant gradient, provided that artifactual reasons for the softness, such as obesity or heart failure, are absent. If the murmur is very loud (i.e., grade 4/6 or more), the gradient is likely to be at least 20 mm Hg. Unfortunately, a loud murmur does not tell you how much over 20 mm Hg the gradient may be.

Note: A spurious increase in loudness of the ejection murmur may be due to a thin chest wall and any cause of increased flow, such as a shunt or a regurgitant-induced volume. Also, systolic expansion of a markedly dilated pulmonary artery can create loud artifactual crunches by pressure against surrounding lung tissue.

TYPES

1. What are the two most common types of ejection murmurs?

ANS.: The aortic or pulmonary stenosis ejection murmur and the systolic flow murmur (i.e., a murmur due to causes other than obstruction to flow).

2. List the six types of systolic flow murmurs.

ANS.: a. The murmur due to the normal "impulse gradient," which is perceivable only because of a thin chest or a quiet room. A normal impulse gradient is the gradient produced by the normal acceleration of ventricular blood across a nonobstructed semilunar valve.

b. The flow murmur due to increased stroke volume or rate of ejection.

c. The murmur due to unknown anatomic causes of turbulence, namely, the innocent humming ejection murmur of childhood.

d. The murmur due to aortic sclerosis.

e. The murmur due to increased septal-aortic angulation.

f. The murmur due to ejection into a dilated artery.

Note: When flow suddenly enters a dilated chamber (i.e., a dilated pulmonary artery or aorta), it can produce turbulence that results in a murmur. The two major examples of this type of murmur are idiopathic dilatation of the pulmonary artery or of the ascending aorta (as with an aneurysm) and the pulmonary ejection murmur occurring in patients with severe pulmonary hypertension. These murmurs are very short, finishing at about midsystole. It is possible that when these murmurs go beyond midsystole they are artifactually produced by adhesions between a dilated ascending aorta or main pulmonary artery and the surrounding pleura. (See p. 216, Question 2.)

SYSTOLIC FLOW MURMURS

The Normal Impulse Gradient Murmur and the Increased Flow Murmur

1. What is the relationship between the gradient across a semilunar valve and the shape of the murmur?

ANS.: The greater the gradient across a semilunar valve, the louder and longer the murmur and the later the peak of the crescendo-decrescendo.

Note: a. Across a normal valve, however, the shape of the murmur is controlled entirely by the velocity of flow, not by the shape of the gradient. The velocity of flow across a normal semilunar valve is crescendo-decrescendo with an early peak. The normal peak gradient across a normal aortic valve (the impulse gradient) is earlier than the peak of velocity of flow because gradient is related to acceleration of flow, and acceleration peaks earlier than velocity of flow, in the absence of stenosis (Fig. 6).

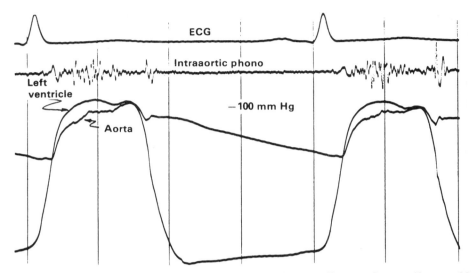

FIG. 6. Aortic and LV pressure tracings together with a phonocardiogram from a 40-year-old man with an innocent aortic ejection murmur. Note the early systolic gradient between the LV and aorta, which is the normal impulse gradient found not only in normal left-sided chambers but also normally seen between the right ventricle and pulmonary artery. This tracing is taken by a single catheter with two end holes, to obtain absolutely accurate timing and pressure differences across the aortic valve.

     b. In a soundproof room, the normal impulse gradient ejection murmur is heard in 100% of normal subjects along the left sternal border, often only after elevation of the legs, hyperventilation, or mild exercise (23). About 90% of healthy children and about 15% of adults have innocent ejection murmurs at the left sternal border on ordinary clinical examination in a quiet room (10,35).

2. Why are young patients most likely to have an easily audible flow murmur, other than their thinner chests?

    ANS.: Because of their more rapid circulation time.

        Note: Young patients with innocent murmurs have been shown in one study to have lower blood viscosity and lower hematocrits than patients without murmurs (49).

Ejection Murmurs Due to Increased Flow

1. What is meant by an innocent murmur?

    ANS.: A murmur without any demonstrable evidence of cardiovascular disease.

2. What are the preferred terms for an easily audible ejection murmur produced by an increase in flow across a valve rather than by valve narrowing?

    ANS.: An **innocent flow murmur** is the preferred term when you are speaking to patients. This is a reassuring term because it implies that the prognosis is such that it will give the patient no trouble.

Note: a. The term **relative stenosis** does not aptly explain the flow murmur shape across a normal valve because such a shape is more related to changes in velocity (acceleration) than to gradient. Therefore, the flow murmur is different from a stenosis murmur, in which the gradient, flow velocity, and murmur have the same shape.

b. The terms **benign** or **functional** are not desirable because benign implies that an abnormality is present but is not malignant. Functional may have no meaning to a layman, although to a physician it may mean "due to increased flow."

3. List the most common causes of ejection flow murmurs due to increased stroke volume.

ANS.: Shunt flows, regurgitant flows, bradycardia, and increased cardiac output.

Note: a. Cardiac output is not significantly increased in anemia until the hemoglobin and hematocrit drop to about 50% of normal. Patients with anemia may have a lower viscosity than normal, and this may also increase turbulence.

b. About 90% of pregnant women have ejection murmurs due to increased blood volume (22).

c. Flow murmurs are more likely to occur across an aortic than across a pulmonary valve because peak velocity and turbulence intensity are higher across the normal aortic orifice than across the pulmonic valve, presumably because of the larger cross-sectional area of the pulmonic valve and the slightly longer duration of ejection through the pulmonic valve (54,55).

d. Supraclavicular arterial murmurs (arterial murmurs are usually called bruits) are ejection in type, of brief duration, in early or midsystole. These patients have signs of a hyperkinetic circulation (i.e., an S_3) and a venous hum (see p. 272).

4. What is meant by a "hemic" murmur?

ANS.: A hemic murmur is any murmur that is present in the anemic state and disappears when the anemia is corrected. For example, mitral regurgitation (MR) may be heard only with the increased heart size, blood volume, and need for coronary flow caused by severe anemia (13).

Atrial Septal Defect Systolic Flow Murmurs

1. What causes a systolic murmur in patients with an uncomplicated atrial septal defect (ASD)?

ANS.: Increased flow through the dilated main pulmonary artery.

Note: a. There is no murmur through the defect in the atrial septum because there is almost no gradient across the defect. If the defect is large, the two atria act as a single chamber, so that the pressures on each side of the defect are almost equal.

b. A soft murmur through an ASD might be inaudible even if one occurred at that site, because an acoustic signal produced artificially by a mechanical sound generator in the right atrium is almost completely dissipated before it reaches the chest wall (16).

c. A continuous murmur may be produced across an ASD in the presence of a small defect plus MR or mitral stenosis (MS), which raises the pressure in the left atrium considerably higher than in the right atrium. An ASD plus MS is called the "Lutembacher syndrome."

d. Although the ejection murmur of ASD is best heard at the second or third left interspace, there is frequent transmission to the apex even when the murmur is soft, probably because the dilated right ventricle (RV) transmits RV and pulmonary artery events to the apex.

2. What suggests that part of the pulmonary flow murmur of ASD is extracardiac; that is, probably due to adhesions between the dilated pulmonary artery and the pleura?

ANS.: a. It is often crackly, crunchy, or scratchy (34).

b. Other causes of marked pulmonary artery dilatation sometimes produce this crackling or crunchy type of murmur (e.g., idiopathic dilatation of the pulmonary artery).

c. It is often louder and longer than a mere flow murmur should be, despite the absence of pulmonary stenosis (PS).

d. In some ASDs there is no ejection murmur, despite a moderate shunt and normal pulmonary artery pressure.

3. How can you tell by auscultation that the ASD shunt flow-to-systemic flow ratio is more than 3:1?

ANS.: Sinus arrhythmia disappears.

Straight Back (Narrow Chest) Syndrome Ejection Murmur

1. What is meant by the straight back syndrome?

ANS.: Compression of the heart by a narrow chest due to loss of the normal dorsal curvature of the spine, resulting in a pulmonary ejection murmur that is usually mistaken for that of either PS or ASD (Fig. 7) .

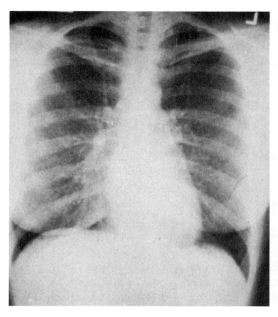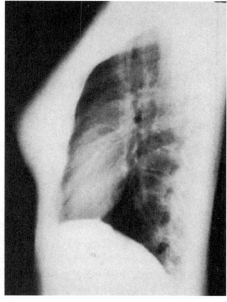

FIG. 7. In this patient, with the loss of dorsal curvature, the anteroposterior diameter is one-third of the transverse diameter. The "straight front," plus the slight anterior bowing of the lower thoracic spine, probably contributed to the compression effect on the heart. (Courtesy of Dr. Antonio C. deLeon, Jr.)

2. What other palpatory and auscultatory findings in the straight back syndrome mimic ASDs?

ANS.: a. An exaggerated left parasternal movement may be present.

   b. The split of the S_2 may be wide and the second component of the split S_1 may be accentuated (15).

   c. The systolic murmur is often scratchy or crunchy.

   Note: a. The ejection murmur of the straight back syndrome may range from grade 1/6 to grade 4/6. Even without a pectus excavatum, a markedly narrowed anteroposterior diameter can occasionally cause a murmur loud enough to have a thrill (11). The murmur has occasionally been noted to change markedly in intensity by as much as two grades with increasing stethoscope pressure.

   b. A short, early, grade 1/6 scratchy diastolic murmur along the left sternal border that increases with inspiration is present in many patients with the straight back syndrome.

   c. The narrow posteroanterior diameter compresses upper mediastinal structures, including the pulmonary artery, against the sternum, thus creating murmurs. In a small percentage of such patients there is actually a gradient of 5 to 15 mm Hg in the pulmonary outflow tract, apparently created by this compression.

   d. An anteroposterior chest diameter (back of sternum to front of vertebrae) that is one-third or less of the transverse diameter (from the inside of the ribs measured at just above the right dome of the diaphragm) is almost diagnostic of the straight back syndrome (11).

3. What are the objections to the term **straight back syndrome**?

ANS.: a. Although many subjects with straight backs also have rather straight sternums and even a pectus excavatum that makes a narrow PA diameter, there are some with straight backs who have anteriorly bowed sternums that provide ample space for the heart and thus have no pseudocardiac disease (12).

   b. Scoliosis is commonly found with a straight back syndrome.

Humming Systolic Ejection Murmur of Childhood

1. What adjectives have been used to describe the quality, or timbre, of the humming (innocent) ejection murmur found in children? What eponym has been used for it?

ANS.: It has been described as a humming, buzzing, vibratory, moaning, or groaning murmur. It has also been called Still's murmur, after the British author of a pediatric textbook published in 1918, who described it as "a twanging string" murmur (Fig. 8) .

2. What does the humming character of an ejection murmur in childhood tell you about the gradient across the semilunar valve?

ANS.: It means that there is only a slight gradient across the valve producing the murmur. It also strongly suggests that the murmur is innocent and will either disappear after puberty or sound the same 15 years later (13).

3. What appears to be the source of the humming murmur?

ANS.: The aortic outflow tract. A fine *thrill* can be recorded on the carotid tracings of some children with this murmur. Also, it has been suggested that the aortic root is relatively narrow in subjects with this murmur.

   Note: a. Almost 1% of children have false tendons on echocardiograms, and

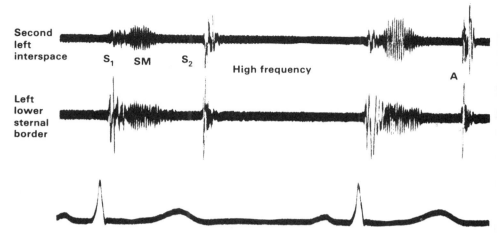

FIG. 8. The regular vibrations on this phonocardiogram of a humming systolic murmur (SM) tell you that the murmur has a musical quality. The peak of the crescendo occurring in the first third of systole tells you that the gradient across the semilunar valve is probably trivial.

more than 90% of those with false tendons have this type of murmur, often loudest over the left lower sternal border and associated with premature ventricular contractions (PVCs) that disappear with tachycardias (44). In the presence of a slightly hyperkinetic contractility, as often found in young children, it is possible that a "twanging string" effect may actually be present, and this may account for why the humming murmur is often best heard between the apex and the left sternal border.

Further support for the possibility of a twanging string or Aeolian harp effect of flow across an anomalous left ventricular band is found in a report of a 68-year-old man who had a grade 2 musical murmur when his heart was large but that disappeared when his heart decreased in size with treatment for heart failure (47). Most children with this murmur have a false tendon over 60% of which stretches across the outflow tract of the LV.

It is surprising how widespread and difficult it is to localize this innocent murmur. When the systolic musical murmur is present in older age groups and is maximum at the left lower sternal border, the murmur may be caused by a false tendon that was stretched as the heart became larger. It, therefore, may be present only with congestive heart failure (47).

   b. It was once proposed that a taut pulmonary valve fibrous ring could cause vibrations as blood passed through it. However, pulmonary hypertension or pulmonary artery dilatation from any cause that tenses the valve ring does not cause a humming murmur. Also, intracardiac phonocardiograms from the pulmonary artery in patients who have this murmur do not show a vibratory murmur (62).

4. What suggests that the humming murmur of childhood depends on increased flow and is not due to actual obstruction?

   ANS.: a. The murmur is never louder than grade 3/6.

      b. The murmur is usually short and reaches its peak early.

c. Children with this murmur tend to have shorter isovolumic contraction times than those without (12).

d. It is often associated with a loud venous hum (7).

e. It consists of low and medium frequencies (i.e., between 75 and 160 cycles per second). A murmur that is relatively low in pitch suggests that it is due mostly to flow with very little gradient.

    Note: These humming murmurs may become as long as important murmurs in the presence of further increased blood flow, such as that occurring with high fever or severe anemia.

f. The murmur is louder supine than sitting.

Aortic Sclerosis Murmur

1. What percentage of patients over age 50 have an easily audible aortic ejection murmur without valvular stenosis?

  ANS.: About 50%. Therefore, we have called this the "50 over 50" (50/50) murmur. However, if you eliminate patients with previous infarction or elevated blood pressure with electrocardiogram (ECG) evidence of LV hypertrophy, then only about 30% have an aortic sclerosis murmur (43).

2. What is the cause of this aortic ejection murmur?

  ANS.: There are several theories.

    a. It may be due to fibrosis, thickening, and often some calcification involving the bases of the aortic cusps. The cusps do not open fully because of stiffness (aortic valve sclerosis), but they do open enough to prevent any significant gradient across the orifice. However, there is enough narrowing to cause turbulence and an ejection murmur.

    b. It may be due to calcific spurs on the aortic ring, which may protrude into the bloodstream when calcium is laid down at the roots of the cusps.

    c. It may be due to atherosclerotic plaques in the ascending aorta that may cause turbulence as the aortic stream strikes the roughened endocardium.

    Note: a. The general condition alluded to by these theories is called aortic sclerosis.

        b. If calcification caused the sclerosis murmur, and the calcium becomes excessive, severe aortic valve obstruction may occur; this is known as calcific aortic stenosis (Fig. 9) .

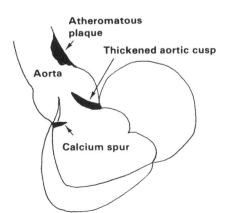

FIG. 9. A slight but abrupt protuberance (e.g., a calcium spur) is capable of producing a murmur of considerable intensity.

      c. It may be due to septal turbulence caused by an unusually acute angle of the septum to the aorta, which is well seen on the long axis view of an echocardiogram. A color Doppler mosaic of turbulence is seen exactly at the septal bulge (18).

3. What factors in the elderly are known to increase the incidence of the 50/50 murmur?

    ANS.: a. Hypertension. The higher the blood pressure, the more likely the murmur.

        Note: In one series of severely hypertensive patients, everyone was found to have an ejection murmur (26).

      b. Sex. The incidence of this murmur is almost twice as high in women as in men.

      c. A tendency to calcification. A high percentage of patients with the 50/50 murmur have mitral ring calcification on echocardiogram (42).

      d. An increase in aortic septal angulation (18), often with a sigmoid septum.

AORTIC STENOSIS EJECTION MURMURS

Valvular Aortic Stenosis Murmurs

Murmur Shape, Duration, and Quality

1. How can you tell the severity of aortic stenosis by the shape and length of the murmur?

    ANS.: In general, the later the peak of the crescendo and the longer the murmur, the more severe the stenosis.

        Note: Even though the peak of the crescendo in valvular AS extends only very slightly beyond midsystole, no matter how severe the stenosis, a rough correlation can be found between the Q-peak interval and the presence of either mild or severe AS. If the Q-peak interval is less than 200 msec, severe stenosis (valve area less than 0.75 cm^2) is very unlikely. If the Q-peak interval is more than 240 msec, severe stenosis is likely (4). In another study, a Q-peak interval of less than 220 msec excluded severe AS in the elderly (19). If the patient is hypertensive, the peak may occur falsely early (21). The Doppler point of maximal systolic velocity can also be used as a substitute for the phonocardiographic peak (57).

2. How may the pitch and quality of an aortic ejection murmur create confusion when listening at the apex? What is this phenomenon called?

    ANS.: The highest-frequency components tend to radiate to the apex and may even sound musical at this site. Therefore, a murmur of MR is suggested. This is the Gallavardin phenomenon (6).

        Note: In the elderly patient, the murmur of calcific AS often sounds musical or cooing at the apex. Commissural fusion is commonly absent in these valves, allowing the cusps to vibrate and produce pure frequencies (48).

3. What is the characteristic quality of the loud murmur of moderate to severe AS?

    ANS.: The harsh, rasping, grunting, and coarse murmur, which sounds like a person clearing his throat, can be imitated by placing your palm on the diaphragm of a stethoscope while you scratch the dorsal surface of the hand with your fingernail.

Loudness and Site

1. Where can you hear the aortic systolic murmur of valvular AS?

    ANS.: Although it is loudest as a rule in the second right interspace, it may be heard anywhere in a line from the second right interspace to the apex. (If the patient is obese or has emphysema, the murmur may be loudest on or above the clavicle.)

2. What is usually meant by the aortic area?

    ANS.: The second right interspace.

3. Why should the second right interspace *not* be called the aortic area?

    ANS.: All aortic events can be heard anywhere in a "sash" or "shoulder harness" area from the second right interspace to the apex. Terms such as **aortic, pulmonary,** and **tricuspid areas** assume situs solitus in all patients (Fig. 10) .

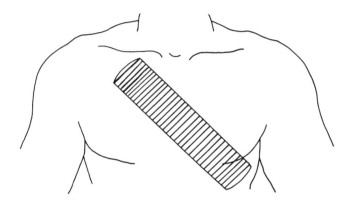

Aortic area

FIG. 10. Since aortic ejection murmurs and clicks are often best heard at the apex area, and aortic regurgitation murmurs are usually best heard along the left lower sternal border or midsternum, it should no longer be taught that the "aortic area" is the second right interspace.

> *Note*: It is confusing to the student to be told that aortic regurgitation murmurs are best heard at the left sternal border or sternum, aortic ejection sounds or clicks are best heard near the apex, murmurs of hypertrophic subaortic stenosis (HSS, or HOCM) are best heard either at the apex or medial to it, and the A_2 is louder than the P_2 at the second and third left interspace, while being told that the second right interspace is the aortic area. Therefore, the second right interspace may be called the "traditional" or "classic" aortic area, but it is best to simply say **second right interspace**.

4. What is characteristic of the upward radiation of an aortic valvular murmur?

    ANS.: a. It tends to radiate into the neck bilaterally, but often radiates well along the innominate vein, making the murmur slightly louder over the *left* carotid. If the murmur radiates better to the right carotid than to the left, you should suspect supravalvular AS. (See p. 227.)

    b. It not only radiates well to the clavicle but is usually amplified there. Because the aortic ejection murmur is usually louder over the clavicle than over the carotid, any murmur louder over the carotid than the clavicle should be considered a local arterial murmur (52).

    > *Note*: a. Innocent aortic ejection murmurs are characteristically maximal along the left sternal border near the anatomic aortic valve area. With significant aortic valvular obstruction, however, the maximum turbulence occurs further downstream from the orifice and tends to be loudest at the second right interspace (55).

      b. Occasionally, an aortic ejection murmur sounds louder near the carotid bifurcation than lower in the neck, presumably because the bifurcation is closer to the skin than the common carotid and subclavian arteries (32).

5. Is a very loud ejection murmur (at least grade 4/6) ever associated with mild AS?

    ANS.: Yes. A small percentage of such murmurs occurs with moderate and even mild AS (1). If, however, the loud murmur is associated with an absent or very soft A_2, it almost always indicates severe AS because the soft A_2 implies heavy calcification. Conversely, if heart failure develops with resultant reduced stroke volume, the murmur of even severe AS may almost disappear. Concomitant MS also decreases the loudness of the AS murmur, but unless the MS is very severe, the AS murmur dominates the picture and can even cause the MS murmur to be absent. This occurs because the loss of compliance caused by left ventricular hypertrophy (LVH) can result in slow diastolic expansion of the LV and attenuate the MS murmur (58).

        Note: A low flow due to heart failure or severe MS may result in almost no murmur across a moderately obstructed aortic valve because the physiologic cross-sectional area of the aortic valve opening during systole is always smaller than the potential anatomic area, and the lower the flow, the smaller the physiologic cross-sectional area used by the forward stream (54).

6. Why may the murmur of severe AS be soft in the elderly in the absence of heart failure?

    ANS.: a. There is commonly an increased anteroposterior chest diameter in the elderly, especially at the base of the heart.

      b. The stiff cusp bases and lack of commissural fusion may cause some of the blood to be ejected between the cusps and, therefore, to form a "spray" rather than a jet. This may make the murmur not only more musical but also less loud and harsh (48).

Summary of Auscultatory Clues to the Diagnosis of Severe Valvular Aortic Stenosis

The AS is probably severe; that is, the gradient is at least 70 mm Hg or, in the presence of congestive heart failure, at least 50 mm Hg, if

1. An S_4 is present in a patient under age 40 (8).
2. The murmur is long, its peak is in midsystole, it is at least grade 4/6, and it is associated with a soft or absent A_2. (Such a murmur may be only grade 2 to 3/6 if the patient has a large, thick chest, heart failure, or significant MS or MR.)
3. The presence of any of the triad of dyspnea, angina, or syncope plus an LVH strain pattern on electrocardiography implies a gradient of more than 80 mm Hg, unless the patient has decreased myocardial function (30).

Hypertrophic Subaortic Stenosis or Hypertrophic Obstructive Cardiomyopathy Murmurs

1. What causes the outflow obstruction in HSS or HOCM (hypertrophic obstructive cardiomyopathy)?

    ANS.: A hypertrophied septum bulging into the outflow tract, approximating abnormal anterior or posterior (or both) mitral leaflets or, rarely, redundant chordae. The outflow tract, which is the space between the septum and the anterior leaflet of the mitral valve, becomes narrowed when a freely mobile distal portion of the mitral valve is pulled toward the septum by a Bernoulli or Venturi effect.[1] The systolic anterior motion (SAM) of mitral leaflets is readily visible on an echocardiogram (Fig. 11).

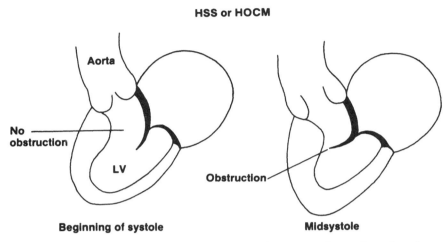

FIG. 11. The asymmetric septal hypertrophy (ASH) of the LV causes obstruction when the upper part of the septum meets a mobile part of the septal leaflet that is "sucked anteriorly." It is made mobile by an abnormal apposition of the anterior to the posterior leaflet.

Note: a. Although almost all HOCM patients have some MR due to constriction of the mitral valve ring caused by the hyperdynamic contraction characteristic of HSS, the MR is usually trivial and not responsible for the typical ejection murmur found in these patients.

b. The portion of the leaflets abutting the septum shows SAM on echocardiography. Often there is a fine fluttering of the leaflet manifesting the SAM, and this has been correlated with the musical quality of the murmur (28) (Fig. 12).

Note: The term **asymmetric septal hypertrophy** (ASH) of the heart is often used in describing the heart in HOCM because the septum is disproportionately hypertrophied relative to hypertrophy of the free wall. The hypertrophied ventricle may so distort the mitral valve apparatus that it sometimes causes inflow obstruction of the LV and even of the RV, and can cause occasional mitral or tricuspid inflow gradients. Although the dominant obstruction is almost always on the left side, occasionally the highest gradients and obstructions are in the outflow tract of the RV (39).

---

[1]The Bernoulli or Venturi effect is characterized by a drop in pressure on the surface of any structure caused by blood flow over that surface, which pulls the structure toward the stream. An instrument utilizing the Bernoulli effect to measure flow is called a Venturi meter.

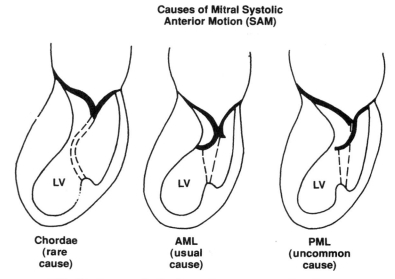

**Causes of Mitral Systolic
Anterior Motion (SAM)**

Chordae
(rare
cause)

AML
(usual
cause)

PML
(uncommon
cause)

FIG. 12. Causes of mitral systolic anterior motion (SAM).

Not all patients with ASH have enough SAM of the mitral leaflets to cause obstruction, in which case HOCM becomes simply HCM. One of the reasons for an absence of SAM is that the direction of flow in the outflow tract can be directed partly medially toward the under surface of the anterior leaflets, thus pushing it upward and preventing SAM (51).

2. When in systole does the obstruction begin in HSS or HOCM? How does this relate to the onset of the ejection murmur?

ANS.: The obstruction begins just prior to midsystole but the murmur usually begins at the same time as it does in valvular stenosis (i.e., at the beginning of systole). (This is contrary to statements in the literature that are probably based either on very mild cases or on phonocardiograms that are too well filtered or too hastily examined.) The murmur usually begins early because even though the obstruction is delayed to slightly beyond the time of onset of aortic valve opening, the tremendously rapid early ejection characteristic of HOCM can cause early turbulence. In the normal heart only about 50% of ventricular volume is ejected during the first half of systole, but in HOCM, 80% or more is ejected during this period (45). This rapid flow can produce a murmur in early systole. However, if the obstruction is mild, there may not be an early flow murmur, and only the delayed murmur due to the midsystolic obstruction may be present.

Note: Occasionally, a low-amplitude ejection sound can be seen on a phonocardiogram preceding the murmur. The rapid ejection in early systole can set up the necessary conditions for an ejection sound.

Differentiating the Ejection Murmur of HOCM from that of Valvular Aortic Stenosis

1. How can raising the blood pressure by a vasopressor agent or by having the patient squat help differentiate between the ejection murmur of valvular AS and that of HSS?

ANS.: In valvular AS, if an inotropic vasopressor such as metaraminol is used to raise the blood pressure, it also stimulates contractility, increases the gradient, and makes the murmur louder. Even if a noninotropic vasopressor agent produces a bradycardia by the vagal effect of suddenly raising the blood pressure, there may be more time for diastolic filling, and in valvular AS, the greater stroke volume may also increase the loudness of the murmur.

In patients with HSS or HOCM, on the other hand, any vasopressor decreases the murmur because the increased resistance to outflow tends to hold the outflow tract open by pushing the mitral leaflets away from the septum.

Note: Maximum handgrip for 30 sec, by raising the blood pressure, also causes the HOCM murmur to diminish (Fig. 13). (You may ask the patient to squeeze steadily on a rolled-up towel.)

Normal mean pressure   **High mean pressure**

120 mm Hg   150 mm Hg

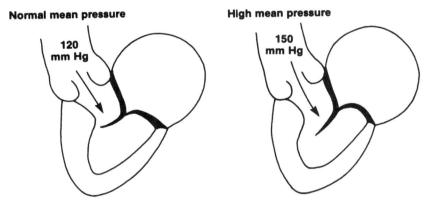

FIG. 13. A high pressure in the aorta during ejection is transmitted to the mobile portion of the mitral valve leaflet and pushes it away from the septum and decreases the outflow obstruction.

2. What tends to make an HSS or HOCM obstruction worse, making the LV cavity smaller, or making it larger? Why?

ANS.: Making it smaller allows the hypertrophied septum to obliterate the outflow tract space more easily.

Note: Many patients with HOCM do not have an increase in their ejection murmur after the pause following a PVC. This implies that in these patients, the increase in left ventricular volume can have a stronger effect on the obstruction than the decreased afterload effect (33).

3. How can a Valsalva maneuver help differentiate the ejection murmur of valvular AS from that of HSS?

ANS.: During a strain, the venous return is decreased. Thus, the stroke volume is decreased, and the ejection murmur of valvular AS is decreased. However, in a patient with HOCM, the decreased venous return produces a smaller LV and, therefore, more obstruction and a louder murmur.

Note: a. The Valsalva maneuver may not always work because

1. It may produce such a rise in systemic and aortic resistance and pressure that it overcomes the effect of reduced heart size.

2. If the patient is in heart failure, the LV volume may not change during the strain (37).

3. The obstruction may already be so severe that a Valsalva would produce too much obstruction so there would be too little flow across the outflow tract to make the murmur louder.

    b. A Müller maneuver (inspiration against a closed glottis) shifts the septum to the left and could theoretically cause more obstruction (24). However, this maneuver surprisingly causes the HOCM murmur to decrease and is reliable enough to be used at the bedside to help diagnose HOCM.

4. How can amyl nitrite inhalation differentiate the ejection murmur of valvular AS from that of HOCM?

    ANS.: The blood pressure drops immediately with amyl nitrite inhalation, but flow does not increase until about 20 sec later. Therefore, the murmur of valvular AS, which is dependent on flow, does not begin to increase for about 20 sec. The murmur of HOCM, on the other hand, becomes louder within a few beats after inhalation because as soon as the blood pressure drops (which occurs almost immediately), the loss of resistance to outflow causes a loss of pressure against the anterior leaflet of the mitral valve as the ventricle contracts. (See p. 250 for hemodynamic effects of amyl nitrite.)

5. How will squatting differentiate between the murmur of HOCM and that of valvular AS?

    ANS.: Squatting, especially for the first few beats, diminishes the murmur of HOCM because it causes both increased venous return for a few beats and a persistent increase in peripheral arterial resistance. In the presence of valvular AS, the increase in venous return tends to increase the murmur.

        Note: a. Squatting is the most reliable maneuver for diagnosing HOCM because it results in two mechanisms for diminishing the murmur.

            b. Auscultation should be in the order of squatting first then prompt standing. During squatting the patient should use the right hand for support, holding the edge of the bed or a chair.

6. What is the effect of carotid sinus pressure on the murmur of HOCM?

    ANS.: The bradycardia and decreased aortic resistance cause an increased force of contractions and loudness. This sign is 100% specific for HOCM but only 60% sensitive.

7. How can the site of maximum loudness of the HOCM murmur help differentiate it from the murmur of valvular AS?

    ANS.: It is usually louder near the apex, but occasionally it is loudest at the left lower sternal border.

        Note: When septal hypertrophy is so great that it also produces RV outflow (infundibular) obstruction (rare), the infundibular obstruction may cause the murmur to be louder at the base than elsewhere (as in other forms of pulmonary stenosis).

8. Why is an HOCM murmur often mistaken for an MR murmur?

    ANS.: Because the HOCM murmur often tends to be loudest at the apex.

        Note: a. Some MR is usually present. Two explanations are offered for the presence of MR, which is usually trivial.

            1. The hypertrophied septum may distort the direction in which the papillary muscles pull on the valve cusps, so that a Bernoulli or Venturi effect can pull an unsupported free edge of an anterior

leaflet toward the septum. This SAM can cause not only outflow obstruction but also some MR.
2. Mitral valve prolapse may occur in as many as 75% of patients with HOCM. This may be due to the cavity obliteration that often occurs with HOCM, causing the mitral ring to become too small for the area of valve tissue.
3. A pansystolic apical murmur of MR in a patient with HOCM probably will not disappear after corrective surgery for HOCM.

Supravalvular Aortic Stenosis Murmurs

1. Where in the aorta is the stenosis of supravalvular AS?
   ANS.: Above the sinus of Valsalva.
     Note: It may be focal (hourglass), discrete membranous, or diffusely hypo-plastic.
2. At what unusual site might the murmur be loudest in supravalvular AS? Does this help differentiate it from valvular AS?
   ANS.: It may be loudest in the suprasternal notch, the first right intercostal space, or over the manubrium (3,50). (However, it also may be loudest in the second right intercostal space, the best site for a valvular AS murmur.)
     Note: Supravalvular AS is often found with the murmurs of stenosis of the pulmonary arteries, termed **pulmonary branch stenosis**. AR murmurs are also heard because the aortic valve is frequently abnormal. The AR murmur is unusual in that often it is unexpectedly intensified with amyl nitrite (50).

Summary of Clinical Findings in Supravalvular Aortic Stenosis

1. Peculiar "elfin" facies in nonfamilial type. (See p. 19 for facies of supravalvular AS.)
2. Pulse volume greater and murmur louder in the right than in the left carotid. (See p. 34 for explanation.)
3. Blood pressure higher in the right arm.
4. No ejection sound.
5. Slight AR murmur.

Discrete Subvalvular Aortic Stenosis

1. Where may the obstructive ridge in discrete subvalvular AS be located, and of what may it consist?
   ANS.: It is either a thin membrane on the ventricular septum just below the aortic valve or a fibrous ring about 1 cm below the aortic valve and is associated with muscular hypertrophy of the outflow tract.
     Note: Heavy mitral annular ring calcification can protrude into the left ventricular outflow and produce mild to moderate subaortic stenosis.
2. What other murmur is common in patients with discrete subvalvular stenosis?
   ANS.: Aortic regurgitation may occur in as many as one-third of such patients (31).
     Note: If the murmur is preceded by an ejection sound, it is not likely to be due to discrete subvalvular AS unless it happens to be associated with a bicuspid aortic valve.

PULMONARY STENOSIS EJECTION MURMURS

1. Where is the classic "pulmonary area"? What is wrong with this term?

    ANS.: The classic pulmonary area is the second left interspace. Pulmonary events, how-
    ever, can be best heard *anywhere* along the left sternal border (or even in the epi-
    gastrium in patients with chronic obstructive pulmonary disease.)

    Note: If you ask physicians which component is louder at the second left inter-
    space, the aortic or pulmonary, they automatically say the pulmonary
    component, because they are told that this is the pulmonary area. Since this
    is wrong (i.e., the aortic component is always louder than the pulmonary
    component under normal circumstances), we must avoid teaching the term
    pulmonary area when referring to the second left interspace.

2. Where is the best place for hearing the murmur of (a) valvular PS and (b) infundibular PS?

    ANS.: a. The murmur of valvular PS is heard best at the second left interspace.

    b. The murmur of infundibular PS is best heard at the third or fourth left inter-
    space.

    Note: The third left interspace parasternally often has been called Erb point.
    This name seems unnecessary and confusing; first, because some authors
    include the fourth left interspace, and second, because medical dictionar-
    ies often do not give a definition of Erb point on the chest but describe
    one on the neck over the brachial plexus.

3. What is the relation between the peak of the crescendo of the PS murmur and the severity
    of the obstruction?

    ANS.: The later the peak, the more severe the obstruction. It may occur as late as four-
    fifths of the way through RV systole.

    Note: PS may be imitated by coarctation with a bicuspid aortic valve, because
    this combination may produce an ejection sound followed by a murmur
    with a late peak (5). The murmur with the late peak in coarctation is prob-
    ably due to flow through the intercostal collaterals or possibly through the
    coarcted segment itself.

4. Why is it that in severe AS the murmur rarely peaks much beyond midsystole, yet in PS
    it may easily go beyond midsystole?

    ANS.: The RV is shaped like a teapot, with a main chamber, namely, the inflow tract (also
    known as the RV sinus), and a thick, high spout, which is the outflow tract or in-
    fundibulum.

    The inflow and outflow tracts contract asynchronously in a peristaltic fashion—
    the inflow tract first, then the infundibulum or outflow tract. The worse the ob-
    struction at the valve, the more hypertrophied is the muscle of the outflow tract and
    the later it contracts relative to the inflow tract. It is the late contraction of this RV
    outflow tract that apparently produces the late peak of the crescendo (Fig. 14) .

    The LV, on the other hand, has no distinct muscular outflow tract. The anterior
    mitral leaflet and its chordae and papillary muscles form the posterolateral wall of
    a merely functional outflow tract, which is probably seldom anatomically inde-
    pendent enough to contract more than slightly late on the left side (Fig. 15) .

5. How does infundibular PS affect the length of the murmur? Why?

    ANS.: If the stenosis is due to hypertrophy of the outflow tract (infundibulum), the mur-
    mur tends to be slightly longer than it is in valvular stenosis of similar severity. In
    this type of pulmonic stenosis, the RV outflow is also reduced by the abnormal in-
    fundibulum contracting excessively during systole. The delay in contraction of the

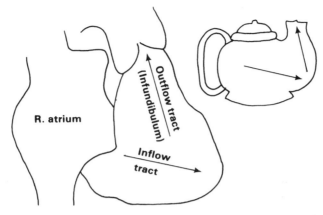

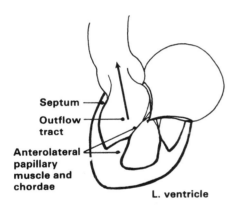

FIG. 14. The outflow tract of the RV is a tubular structure made up mostly of muscle, called the crista supraventricularis, which separates the tricuspid from the pulmonary valves.

FIG. 15. There is no infundibulum in the LV because the mitral and aortic valves are in direct continuity.

infundibulum is often so exaggerated that the infundibulum (and pulmonary artery) pressures are higher than those in the body of the RV for about 100 msec before the pulmonary valve closes (27). This causes a wide splitting of the A_2P_2 interval, even if the stenosis is mild.

    Note: a. Infundibular stenosis can be imitated by a RV anomalous muscle bundle that traverses the RV cavity just below the infundibulum. It is most commonly found together with a ventricular septal defect (VSD).

        b. Pulmonary valve or branch stenosis can be imitated by a partially obstructing pulmonary embolus.

        c. Pulmonary arterial stenosis can present with a pulmonary ejection murmur. However, the P_2 will not be delayed (in the absence of right ventricular failure).

6. How can analysis of the phonocardiogram suggest the severity of the gradient across the pulmonary valve in PS with an intact septum?

    ANS.: By the length of the murmur, the site of the peak of the crescendo, the presence or absence of an ejection click, and the width of the split of the S_2 (59) (Fig. 16) .

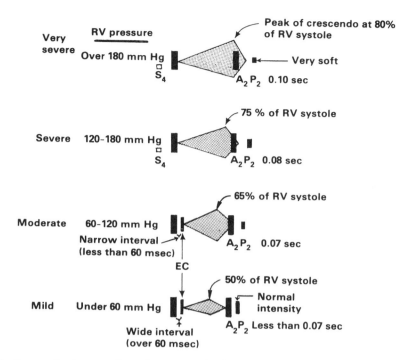

FIG. 16. As the gradient across the pulmonary valve increases, the murmur peaks later and lasts longer, and the P₂ becomes further separated from the A₂ and softer. The ejection click (EC) may be absent above 60 mm Hg of pressure in the RV, but may reappear on sitting or standing.

Murmur in Pulmonary Stenosis with an Intact Ventricular Septum Versus Murmur of Tetralogy of Fallot

1. Will the PS murmur of severe tetralogy be short or long?

    ANS.: The more severe the PS, the shorter the murmur, because the greater the obstruction at the pulmonary valve, the more the RV blood is diverted into the aorta; (i.e., the right-to-left shunt increases, and so less blood goes through the pulmonary valve). This makes sense only if you know that the murmur of a tetralogy of Fallot with cyanosis is solely due to the PS. *Right-to-left shunts do not usually produce murmurs.*

    Note: This introduces the concept of two outlets for systole, which is important in the understanding of murmur changes with maneuvers and drugs. If a ventricle has two outlets for systole, increased resistance to flow through one of the outlets causes more blood to go through the other outlet. If, on the other hand, resistance is *decreased* beyond an outlet, more blood moves through that outlet and less through the other. In tetralogy, the RV has two outlets, the pulmonary artery and the aorta that overrides the VSD. In cyanotic tetralogy you should think of the RV as pumping directly into the aorta and not into the LV first.

2. Why will the degree of cyanosis tend to correlate with the softness of the murmur?

    ANS.: Increased cyanosis means increased polycythemia, which in turn means increased blood viscosity. The greater the viscosity, the less the turbulence across an obstruction and, therefore, the softer the murmur (20). In very severe tetralogy the systolic murmur is usually no louder than grade 2/6 (60).

> *Note*: The greater the right-to-left shunt into the overriding aorta, the softer the murmur, because less blood is flowing through the pulmonary valve.

3. How can amyl nitrite differentiate between the murmur of PS in tetralogy and that occurring when the ventricular septum is intact?

   ANS.: In tetralogy the immediate decrease in peripheral resistance, with no effect on pulmonary resistance, causes an increased flow into the overriding aorta, resulting in a softer pulmonary murmur. If, on the other hand, there is PS with an intact ventricular septum, lowering the systemic resistance causes no immediate change in the PS murmur, but the increase in venous return after about 20 seconds causes the PS murmur to become louder.

   > *Note*: a. The murmur of severe PS with a "muscle-bound" RV may also diminish with amyl nitrite, presumably because the nitrite dilates the infundibulum. Therefore, amyl nitrite cannot be used to distinguish *severe* PS from tetralogy (61). It can still be used, however, to distinguish mild or moderate PS (which are never "muscle-bound") from tetralogy. A muscle-bound RV is one with such an excessive degree of outflow tract hypertrophy that RV systolic pressure fails to fall to less than 100 mm Hg immediately after valvotomy. It can be suspected by the paradoxical effect of amyl nitrite.
   >
   > b. Methoxamine is a pure alpha constrictor and produces little change in a PS murmur if the septum is intact. It will increase the loudness of the PS murmur in tetralogy of Fallot, however, because the increase in peripheral resistance raises aortic systolic pressure and "forces" more blood across the stenotic pulmonary valve.

4. How does the effect of a long diastole following a premature beat help distinguish pure PS from tetralogy of Fallot?

   ANS.: If the postextrasystolic beat has a significantly louder murmur than the normal beat, the septum is probably intact. This reflects the fact that in pure PS the pressure in the RV for the beat ending the compensatory pause usually rises more than 15 mm Hg above its regular pressure, whereas in tetralogy of Fallot the pressure rises only slightly above control levels because the pressure in the aorta falls more than the pressure in the pulmonary artery during the long diastole (25).

SUMMARY OF HOW TO DISTINGUISH A PULMONARY FROM AN AORTIC STENOSIS MURMUR BY AUSCULTATION

1. The AS murmur decreases slightly on inspiration. The PS murmur increases on inspiration, especially on standing and if you listen low on the chest posteriorly.
2. An AS murmur may be maximal in the second right intercostal space or at the apex. The PS murmur is maximal only somewhere along the left sternal border.
3. The post-Valsalva effect causes an immediate return of loudness of the PS murmur but a delay in the return of loudness of the AS murmur.
4. If an ejection click is present, it decreases or disappears on inspiration only with PS.
5. A wide, normally moving split S_2 following the murmur indicates a murmur of PS rather than of AS.
6. A right-sided S_4 (i.e., one heard at the left lower sternal border or epigastric area that in-

creases on inspiration) is due to PS, whereas an S_4 heard only at the apex that increases or becomes audible only on expiration suggests the murmur is due to AS.

THE EFFECT OF RESPIRATION ON EJECTION MURMURS

1. Which phase of respiration can increase a gradient across (a) a pulmonary valve, and (b) an aortic valve? How should this affect their murmurs?
   ANS.: a. Inspiration increases the filling of the RV, which in turn increases flow across the pulmonary valve. Therefore, inspiration increases the gradient and the loudness of the murmur. A gradient increases by the square of the increased flow.
   b. Conversely, inspiration decreases flow into the LV and across the aortic valve and, therefore, decreases both the gradient and the murmur.
   Note: a. A pulmonary flow murmur, such as that heard in an ASD, in which there is only a slight gradient across the pulmonary valve may not become louder on inspiration because the slight increase in velocity of flow due to inspiration is overcome by the increase in distance from the stethoscope caused by chest expansion. Even on intracardiac phonocardiograms, only two-thirds of ASDs show an increased amplitude of murmurs in the pulmonary artery on inspiration (17).
   b. Inspiration may not increase the PS murmur in the upper chest (base area of the heart) because it may place too much lung between the stethoscope and the heart. Therefore, listen low on the chest or even posteriorly for the effect of inspiration. Also, sinus arrhythmia in a young person may cause shorter diastoles during inspiration. This decreases stroke volume during inspiration and softens the murmur.
   c. If the murmur is due to the rare type of hypertrophic cardiomyopathy in which the septum bulges into the RV outflow tract, the murmur actually increases on expiration because any maneuver that makes the RV smaller causes more obstruction at the infundibulum (40).

2. Why does standing tend to exaggerate the increase in a PS murmur caused by inspiration?
   ANS.: The increase in pulmonary flow caused by inspiration is about 15 ml whether the subject is lying down or standing. The total stroke volume, however, is decreased on standing by about 25%, so that the same 15-ml increase in stroke volume on inspiration comprises a proportionately larger amount of stroke volume ejected (36). Therefore, on standing, there is a proportionately greater increase in gradient across the pulmonary valve.

3. How can a Valsalva maneuver distinguish a pulmonary ejection murmur from an aortic ejection murmur?
   ANS.: During the strain phase, the decreased venous return causes all ejection murmurs (with the rare exception of the HOCM murmur) to diminish. When the strain is released, the maximum loudness of the pulmonary ejection murmur returns immediately (i.e., within two or three beats). The maximum loudness of the aortic murmur is, however, delayed for about six to 10 beats due to the time needed for the dammed-up venous blood to pass through the lungs to the LV and aorta.

THORACIC, SUBCLAVIAN, CAROTID, AND THYROID ARTERY FLOW MURMURS

1. What is characteristic of the timing and duration of a physiologic (nonobstructive) vascular murmur?

ANS.: When you hear the heart sounds or, if not, when related to the pulse, the murmurs are early in systole and increase after sudden long diastoles, exercise, or the administration of amyl nitrite.

2. What are the characteristics of an arterial murmur due to obstruction?

ANS.: If a pressure difference proximal and distal to the obstruction is present in both systole and diastole, the murmur is continuous, and the systolic component is always louder than the diastolic. The murmur has either a midsystolic or a late systolic peak if the obstruction is severe.

>   *Note*: If the collateral circulation is good, a gradient steep enough to create turbulence is present only during systole. However, a continuous murmur over an artery indicates the artery is markedly narrowed and that the collateral circulation is unable to maintain diastolic pressure (53).

3. What is the difference between a bruit and a murmur?

ANS.: The word **bruit** (pronounced "brooee") is French for "noise" or "sound." In France, the first and second heart sounds are the first and second bruits. Our S_1 and S_2 are their B_1 and B_2. We tend to misuse the word to mean an arterial murmur.

4. Which arterial flow murmur may cause an ejection type of murmur at the second right or left interspace?

ANS.: Rapid flow through the proximal branches of the aorta in young people. This is often mistaken for an aortic ejection murmur.

>   *Note*: A carotid murmur is present in about 80% of children up to 4 years old but is found in only 10% of those in older age groups.

5. How can you differentiate the supraclavicular arterial murmur of childhood from a basal valvular murmur?

ANS.: a. If, as you inch gradually toward the supraclavicular area with your stethoscope, a short early murmur becomes louder, it is an arterial murmur unless it is louder over the clavicle than above it. Aortic valvular murmurs tend to be amplified over the clavicle.

>   b. If the arm flow is increased by hand-clenching exercise, the arterial murmur may become louder, but a valvular murmur does not.

>   c. If the arm is stretched downward and backward, the subclavian artery is compressed between the clavicle and the first rib. The arterial murmur gradually diminishes as the subclavian artery is compressed.

>   d. Compress the subclavian artery with your finger, and note how the murmur changes with varying degrees of obstruction.

>   >   *Note*: Listen also for a venous hum and an S_3 to confirm the presence of a hyperkinetic circulation. (See p. 273 for a method of eliciting a venous hum.)

>   e. Contralateral carotid compression will make the carotid murmur louder or continuous.

6. What kind of peripheral arterial murmurs are heard in coarctation?

ANS.: Systolic flow murmurs with delayed onset (due to the time required for the systolic flow to reach the vessel and therefore continuing beyond the S_2) can be heard over the large collateral vessels of the back. These murmurs may become softer or disappear if the arteries are compressed.

>   *Note*: a. If the systolic delayed murmur is heard between the left scapula and spine, it is questionable whether it is caused by flow through the coarctation itself or through the collaterals. Systolic delayed murmurs have been heard there when there is complete occlusion of the coarcted segment. It has generally been taught that the more severe the coarctation,

the longer the murmur over the coarcted site. Thus, if the narrowed segment is severely narrowed, the murmur crescendos in late systole and goes into diastole (continuous murmur). A mild coarctation is said to have a short, early murmur.

    b. Patients with coarctation have murmurs over the intercostal arteries because when the intercostals are collaterals, they become tortuous, and tortuosity creates turbulence (Fig. 17) .

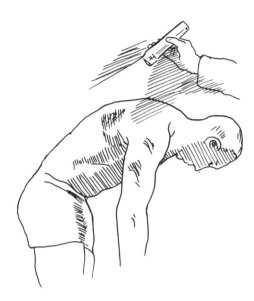

FIG. 17. In the proper light, the dilated subcostal collateral arteries can be seen to pulsate.

7. What kind of murmurs over the thyroid are heard in hyperthyroid patients?
    ANS.: The arterial murmur is systolic. If a continuous murmur is heard, it is a venous hum.
8. What are the auscultatory findings occasionally heard over arterial aneurysms?
    ANS.: Sometimes there is a dull, pistol-shot sound over an abdominal aortic aneurysm. Rarely, there is a double murmur over a large saccular aneurysm or over a dissecting aneurysm, presumably due to distention during systole and emptying during diastole.

Aortic-Coronary Artery Bypass Surgery Vascular Murmurs

1. How common is a new vascular systolic murmur after coronary bypass graft surgery?
    ANS.: Up to one-half of bypass procedures to the anterior descending artery have produced such a murmur.
2. What factors suggest that the systolic vascular murmur heard after coronary bypass surgery is indeed due to the bypass?
    ANS.: a. It is often noted in patients who did not have the murmur prior to surgery, and when it disappears the bypass has often been found to be occluded.
       b. In one study, when the murmur was present, the graft was invariably found to be patent (29).
       c. It has been heard only when the anterior descending artery has been bypassed.

3. What suggests that the mechanism for the production of a coronary bypass graft murmur is probably retrograde flow across the native coronary artery stenosis that prompted the operation?

ANS.: a. The bypass graft has no aortic valve covering it at its aortic junction as does the normal coronary ostium; that is, the native coronary ostium is "protected" by the aortic valve leaflet in systole, whereas the graft ostium is open to the full pressure of systole. This mechanism also explains why the bypass graft murmur is louder in systole than in diastole, even though we know that coronary flow is greater in diastole.

b. In no patient with a completely occluded native stenosis has the murmur developed, and if the native stenosis was later found to be completely occluded, the murmur had disappeared.

Note: a. The murmur does not occur with a right coronary artery bypass, presumably because the distal anastomotic site is well removed from the chest wall.

b. The murmur has not been heard on or around the aorta with a stethoscope during open heart surgery.

4. What is the timing and intensity of the bypass murmur? How is it brought out?

ANS.: It is a short, early ejection murmur, not much more than grade 2/6 in loudness. It is best heard at the second to fourth left parasternal areas when the patient is sitting up and leaning forward, with held expiration (2). It can be intensified by an injection of dipyridamole (at 0.14 mg/kg/min), which can even bring out a diastolic component of the murmur (41).

Note: A disappearing murmur has no significance because many become softer after a few months, and by 1 year, almost all are either soft or have disappeared.

A persistent murmur strongly suggests that the bypass graft is open.

Pulmonary Artery Stenosis Murmurs

1. What types of pulmonary arterial stenosis are there?

ANS.: Multiple peripheral stenosis or stenosis of only the right or left pulmonary artery.

Note: Pulmonary artery branch stenosis is commonly seen with rubella syndrome, other features of which may be cataracts, deafness, mental retardation, or poor growth.

2. What murmurs may be produced by peripheral pulmonary branch stenosis?

ANS.: If the stenosis is unilateral, an ejection murmur may be present. If it is bilateral, however, either an ejection murmur or a continuous murmur may be produced (14). It requires bilateral pulmonary branch stenosis or some other cause of pulmonary hypertension to produce a continuous gradient and murmur.

Note: a. A pulmonary artery branch may be stenosed and produce no murmur at all if the distal segment is supplied by enough bronchial collaterals to reduce the gradient across the stenosed segment (38).

b. A pulmonary artery stenosis murmur begins, peaks, and ends later in systole than a proximal stenosis or flow murmur. It is only rarely louder than grade 3/6.

3. Where are the murmurs of unilateral pulmonary branch stenosis heard? What can mimic them?

ANS.: These murmurs are heard anywhere on the chest. Wide radiation with equal loudness throughout (i.e., to the axillae and back) is the hallmark of a pulmonary artery branch stenosis murmur.

> *Note*: a. The pulmonary artery flow murmur found in some patients with an ASD can mimic this murmur. It also can be heard anywhere on the chest wall and disappears with closure of the ASD.
>
> b. A partially obstructing pulmonary embolism can produce a similar murmur. These murmurs can even be continuous, just as in pulmonary branch stenosis, if there are repeated bilateral pulmonary emboli with pulmonary hypertension. The pulmonary embolus murmur also increases with inspiration and may disappear with anticoagulation and resolution of the embolus (9).

REFERENCES

1. Bergeron J, et al. Aortic stenosis: Clinical manifestations and course of the disease. *Arch Intern Med* 1954; 94:911.
2. Bertrand CA, et al. A study of heart sounds by direct recordings. *Circulation* 1956;13:49.
3. Beuren AJ, et al. Supravalvular aortic stenosis in association with mental retardation and certain facial appearance. *Circulation* 1962;26:1235.
4. Bonner AJ, et al. Assessing the severity of aortic stenosis by phonocardiography and external carotid pulse recordings. *Circulation* 1973;48:247.
5. Bousvaros GA. Diagnostic auscultatory complex in coarctation of the aorta. *Br Heart J* 1967;29:443.
6. Bruns DL. A general theory of the causes of murmurs in the cardiovascular system. *Am J Med* 1959;27:360. (Classic article.)
7. Bujack W, et al. An innocent thrill. A common finding with an innocent murmur. *JAMA* 1976;235:2417.
8. Caulfield WH, et al. The clinical significance of the fourth heart sound in aortic stenosis. *Am J Cardiol* 1971; 28:179.
9. Cohen SI, et al. Flow murmur associated with partial occlusion of the right pulmonary artery. *Am Heart J* 1975; 90:376.
10. Cotter L, et al. Innocent systolic murmurs in healthy 40-year-old men. *J R Coll Physicians Lond* 1980;14:128.
11. Datey KK, et al. Straight back syndrome. *Br Heart J* 1964;26:614.
12. Daves MI. Cardiovascular anachronisms. *JAMA* 1973;224:879.
13. Dawson AA, Palmer KNV. The significance of cardiac murmurs in anemia. *Am J Med Sci* 1966;25:554.
14. D'Cruz IA, et al. Stenotic lesions of the pulmonary arteries. *Am J Cardiol* 1964;13:441.
15. DeLeon AC Jr, et al. The straight back syndrome. *Circulation* 1965;32:193.
16. Feruglio GA. An intracardiac sound generator for the study of transmission of heart murmurs. *Am Heart J* 1962; 63:232.
17. Feruglio GA, Steenivasan A. Intracardiac cardiogram in 30 cases of atrial septal defect. *Circulation* 1959; 20:1087.
18. Finkelstein M, et al. Septal turbulence: An important source of systolic murmurs. *J Am Coll Cardiol* 1988; 11:83A.
19. Flohr KH, et al. Diagnosis of aortic stenosis in older age groups using external carotid pulse recordings. *Br Heart J* 1981;45:577.
20. Garb S. The relationship of blood viscosity to the intensity of heart murmurs. *Am Heart J* 1944;25:568.
21. Genovese B, et al. Effect of hypertension on the clinical assessment of severity in aortic stenosis. *Circulation* 1977;55 & 56(Suppl):69.
22. Goldberg LM, Unland H. Heart murmurs in pregnancy. *Dis Chest* 1967;52:381.
23. Groom D, et al. The normal systolic murmur. *Ann Intern Med* 1960;52:134.
24. Guzman PA, et al. Transseptal pressure gradient with leftward septal movement during the Mueller manoeuvre in man. *Br Heart J* 1981;46:657.
25. Hoffman JIE, et al. Physiological differentiation of pulmonic stenosis with and without an intact septum. *Circulation* 1960;22:385.
26. Humerfelt SB. An epidemiological study of high blood pressure. *Acta Med Scand* 1963;173(Suppl 406):64.
27. Johnson AM. Functional infundibular stenosis, its differentiation from structural stenosis and its importance in atrial septal defect. *Guys Hosp Rep* 1959;108:373.
28. Kagawa T, et al. Genesis of the low-pitched aortic ejection sound. *J Cardiol* 1988;18:217.
29. Karpman L. The murmur of aortocoronary bypass. *Am Heart J* 1972;83:179.
30. Katz NM, et al. Discrete membranous aortic stenosis. *Circulation* 1977;56:1034.
31. Kelly DT, et al. Discrete subaortic stenosis *Circulation* 1972;46:309.

32. Kistler JP, et al. The bruit of carotid stenosis versus basal heart murmurs. *Circulation* 1978;5:975.
33. Kramer DS, et al. The postextrasystolic murmur response in hypertrophic cardiomyopathy and aortic stenosis. *J Am Coll Cardiol* (Abstr) 1985;5:394.
34. Leatham A, Gray I. Auscultatory and phonocardiographic signs of atrial septal defect. *Br Heart J* 1956;18:193.
35. Lessof M, Brigden W. Systolic murmurs in healthy children and in children with rheumatic fever. *Lancet* 1967; 2:673.
36. Lewis ML, Christianson LC. Effects of posture on lung blood volume. *Circulation* (Abstr) 1977;55 & 56(Suppl. III):74.
37. Little WC, et al. Altered effect of the Valsalva maneuver on left ventricular volume in patients with cardiomyopathy. *Circulation* 1985;71:227.
38. Massumi R, et al. Acoustically silent stenosis of a branch of the pulmonary artery. *Am J Med* 1966;40:773.
39. Matsunaga S, et al. Marked right ventricular outflow obstruction in two children with hypertrophic cardiomyopathy. *J Cardiol* 1985;15:931.
40. Mills P, et al. Non-invasive diagnosis of subpulmonary outflow tract obstruction. *Br Heart J* 1980;43:276.
41. Nozawa T, et al. Two cases with the heart murmur originated from aortocoronary bypass. *J Cardiol* 1981; 11:825.
42. Okimoto T, et al. Echo- and phonocardiographic studies of mitral ring calcification. *J Cardiol* 1986;5:707.
43. Perez GL, et al. Incidence of murmurs in the aging heart. *J Am Geriatr Soc* 1976;24:29.
44. Perry LW, et al. Left ventricular false tendons in children: Prevalence as detected by 2-dimensional echocardiography and clinical significance. *Am J Cardiol* 1983;52:1264.
45. Pierce GE, et al. Idiopathic hypertrophic subaortic stenosis. *Circulation* 1964;30(Suppl 4):152.
46. Ranganathan N, et al. Effects of postextrasystolic potentiation on systolic time intervals. *Am J Cardiol* 1978; 41:14.
47. Roberts WC. Anomalous left ventricular band: An unemphasized cause of a precordial musical murmur. *J Cardiol* 1969;23:735.
48. Roberts WC, et al. Severe valvular aortic stenosis in patients over 65 years of age. *Am J Cardiol* 1971;27:497.
49. Sabbah HN, et al. Role of blood viscosity in the production of innocent ejection murmurs. *Am J Cardiol* 1979; 43:753.
50. Sakamoto T, et al. Auscultatory and phonocardiographic findings in supravalvular aortic stenosis. *CV Sound Bull* 1973;3:323.
51. Simpson MS, et al. Outflow impingement on the mitral valve counteracts the Venturi effect and prevents systolic anterior motion: Flow studies. *Circulation* 1991;84(Suppl II):146.
52. Spodick DH, et al. Clavicular auscultation. *Chest* 1976;70:337.
53. Stead EA Jr. Pressures and pulses. *J Am Heart Assoc* 1965;31:481.
54. Stein PD, Munter WA. New functional concept of valvular mechanics in normal and diseased aortic valves. *Circulation* 1971;44:101.
55. Stein PD, Sabbah HN. Aortic origin of innocent murmurs. *Am J Cardiol* 1977;39:665.
56. Sung C-S, et al. Is postextrasystolic potentiation dependent on Starling's law? *Circulation* 1980;62:1032.
57. Tavel ME. Frequency content of systolic murmurs: An answer to the riddle of aortic stenosis? *J Am Coll Cardiol* 1985;1:64.
58. Uricchio JF, et al. Combined mitral and aortic stenosis. *Am J Cardiol* 1959;4:479.
59. Vogelpoel L, Schrire V. Auscultatory and phonocardiographic assessment of pulmonary stenosis with intact ventricular septum. *Circulation* 1960;22:55.
60. Vogelpoel L, Schrire V. Auscultatory and phonocardiographic assessment of Fallot's tetralogy. *Circulation* 1960;22:73.
61. Vogelpoel L, et al. The pre-operative recognition of the "muscle-bound" right ventricle in pulmonary stenosis. *Br Heart J* 1964;26:380.
62. Wennevold A. The origin of the innocent "vibratory" murmur studied with intracardiac phonocardiography. *Acta Med Scand* 1967;181:1.
63. Yamazoe M. Response to the left ventricle in idiopathic dilated cardiomyopathy to postextrasystolic potentiation. *Am Heart J* 1987;113:1449.

14

Systolic Regurgitant Murmurs

1. What characteristics are common to all systolic regurgitant murmurs?
   ANS.: a. If there are early components, they start with the first heart sound. If there are late systolic components, they always extend to or beyond the second heart sound of the same side. However, they are most often pansystolic.
   b. If the opening is small and a high gradient is present, the murmur is usually soft, predominantly high-pitched, and blowing.
   c. They tend to remain the same after a long diastole. (For rare exceptions to this rule, see p. 239.)
   Note: You can imitate various kinds of high-pitched blowing murmurs by whispering a drawn-out "haaa," "hooo," or "shhh," or by holding the diaphragm of the stethoscope against the palm of your hand and listening through the earpieces while you run the pads of your fingers across the back of your hand (104).

2. What are the advantages and disadvantages of the term **pansystolic** or **holosystolic** for murmurs that stretch from S_1 to beyond S_2?
   ANS.: *Holos* is a Greek word meaning "wholly," "complete," "entire," and "all." *Pan* is a Greek word meaning "each," "every," and "all." Therefore, holosystolic has only one meaning, which well fits the timing of the murmur (from S_1 to S_2). However, *pan* is such a universally used prefix, with such a well-understood meaning, "all," that there is no point in teaching an unfamiliar prefix such as *holo* for the sake of pedantic purism. *Holo* has probably become popular in English-speaking countries because it means the same as *wholly*, which sounds enough like *holo* to be easily remembered.
   Note: If a regurgitant murmur extends far enough beyond the S_2 to be recognized as reaching into diastole by auscultation, it is called a continuous murmur.

THE EFFECT OF LONG DIASTOLES ON LEFT-SIDED REGURGITANT MURMURS

1. What will happen to the loudness of a left-sided regurgitant murmur, such as that heard in mitral regurgitation (MR) or VSD, after a sudden long diastole?
   ANS.: The loudness usually remains about the same (Fig. 1). (Listening for the effect of a long diastole is one of the best ways to differentiate an ejection from a regurgitant murmur, especially if no heart sounds are present.)
   Note: If the pause is caused by a premature ventricular contraction (PVC), compare the postextrasystolic beat not with the PVC but with the normal cycle

238

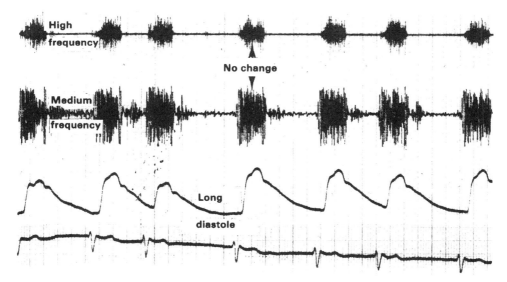

FIG. 1. A high- and medium-frequency phonocardiogram taken at the apex together with an external carotid tracing from a 45-year-old woman with moderately severe chronic rheumatic MR, with few symptoms on digitalis alone. Because of atrial fibrillation, short and long diastoles are present, demonstrating that the murmur after long diastoles does not grow louder than after short or average diastoles.

following the postextrasystolic beat. A PVC may be so premature that there is no time for any significant ventricular filling. Therefore, the loudness of a murmur produced by the premature beat itself is of no significance.

2. Why does the left-sided regurgitant murmur not usually become louder despite a larger volume in the ventricle after a long diastole?

ANS.: In MR, VSD, and PDA, the left ventricle (LV) has two outlets during systole. The amount ejected through each outlet depends on the relative resistance beyond each outlet. During the PVC, the aortic pressure is less than normal because of the small stroke volume. During the long diastole after the PVC, the pressure beyond the aortic outlet falls still more due to the long time for runoff into the periphery. Thus, by the time of the next systole, the resistance at the aortic valve has dropped so low that blood is preferentially ejected into the aorta, and relatively less is regurgitated through the other orifice. One would think at first that this would make the murmur softer. However, because there is more volume in the LV at the end of a long diastole, the absolute quantity of blood regurgitated remains about the same as that after the usual diastoles.

Note: The quantity of retrograde flow in MR and VSD actually does increase during the isovolumic contraction phase in the beat after the long pause, but this does not affect the loudness of the murmur during the major part of systole, when the amount regurgitated is not increased (57).

3. When may the MR murmur become softer after a long diastole?

ANS.: a. In the mitral valve prolapse syndrome.

b. In some papillary muscle dysfunction murmurs, when myocardial ischemia rather than fibrosis causes the MR. The long diastole may decrease myocardial

ischemia by allowing more time for coronary filling and by decreasing the afterload due to the increased time allowed for aortic pressure to fall (1).

Note: In Wolff-Parkinson-White (WPW) preexcitation, type B, in which right
ventricle (RV) contraction precedes LV contraction, the MR murmur is
made louder after a long diastole, but the reason for this is unknown (9).
This type of preexcitation has also brought out tricuspid regurgitation and
innocent ejection murmurs (9).

MITRAL REGURGITATION MURMURS

Terminology

1. Why may it be preferable to use the term **mitral regurgitation** (MR) rather than **mitral
   incompetence** or **mitral insufficiency**, even though cardiologists are about equally divided as to the preferred usage?

   ANS.: The abbreviation for mitral incompetence or insufficiency is MI, which is also
   used as an abbreviation for myocardial infarction. There is no confusion when MR
   is used.

   Note: **Regurgitation** describes the direction of flow, whereas **incompetence** or
   insufficiency describes the condition of the valve. A valve may be incompetent without being regurgitant, as when it produces a click with MVP.
   For the sake of consistency, we shall use the terms **aortic**, **pulmonary**, and
   tricuspid regurgitation, instead of **aortic**, **pulmonary**, and **tricuspid incompetence** or **insufficiency**.

Causes

1. List the four most common causes of MR murmurs in the adult.

   ANS.: Prolapse of the mitral leaflet into the left atrium, papillary muscle dysfunction,
   rheumatic valve damage, and ruptured chordae.

   Note: a. Some rare causes of MR in the adult are left atrial myxoma, calcified
   mitral annulus, and endocardial cushion defects with a cleft anterior
   leaflet. A cleft mitral valve also can occur with a secundum atrial septal
   defect (ASD), but this is rare.

   b. About 10% of patients with mitral annulus calcification have severe MR
   (36). Most of these patients also have the murmur of aortic sclerosis.

2. What are the likely causes of an MR murmur at the apex in an infant besides an endocardial cushion defect?

   ANS.: a. Papillary muscle dysfunction secondary to either an anomalous left coronary
   artery arising from the pulmonary artery or to endocardial fibroelastosis.

   b. Acute myocarditis.

   c. Myxomatous degeneration of the mitral valve with or without Marfan syndrome.

   Note: About 50% of patients with Marfan syndrome have MR (89).

   d. Ebstein's anomaly of the left atrioventricular (AV) valve (actually tricuspid
   valve) in corrected transposition of the great vessels.

3. What suggests that mitral annular dilatation is itself a rare cause of MR?

   ANS.: a. Many patients with grossly dilated hearts due to such conditions as aortic regurgitation (AR) have no MR.

    b. The surface area of the billowing mitral leaflets is more than twice the area of the mitral orifice.

    c. Severe LV dilatation may occur without any dilatation of the annulus; that is, the midportion between the apex and the base expands most.

    d. The fibromuscular portion of the annulus contracts during systole and produces a sphincter-like action. (In dogs the mitral ring decreases in area by about 10% to 50% in systole [88].) Annular calcification prevents normal contraction during systole and can cause almost any degree of MR. (Since it also prevents dilatation, a moderate degree of mitral stenosis may also be produced.)

       Note: Dilatation of the LV causes MR not by annular dilatation but by outward displacement of papillary muscles pulling the leaflets toward the apex. Left ventricular enlargement will not produce MR unless the shape changes from elliptical to spherical, which causes the papillary muscles to migrate laterally and pull the leaflets toward the apex, preventing complete closure.

4. When will corrected transposition produce a murmur that mimics MR?

    ANS.: Corrected transposition means that both the great vessels and the ventricles are transposed. Therefore, an anatomic RV on the left side of the heart feeds the aorta but receives blood through a tricuspid valve. (It should be easy to remember that the valves stay with the appropriate ventricle rather than with the atrium because the chordae tendineae and papillary muscles are attached to the valves.) If the tricuspid valve becomes regurgitant, as with an Ebstein's anomaly (downward displacement of a deformed tricuspid valve), it will *seem* to be MR. There is a high incidence of left AV (tricuspid) valve regurgitation in patients with corrected transposition (8). Anomalous insertion of chordae into the left AV valve has been found to be the cause when no Ebstein's deformity is present.

5. What are the usual causes of papillary muscle dysfunction murmurs?

    ANS.: Myocardial infarction, recent or old, with or without papillary muscle fibrosis. Infarction of the ventricle at the base of the papillary muscles or ischemia of that area with an attack of angina may cause marked MR, even with a normal papillary muscle.

       Note: a. Many patients with papillary muscle fibrosis do not have MR at all. In experiments on dogs, it has not been possible to produce significant MR by causing papillary muscle ischemia, unless it is combined with infarction of the LV at the base of the papillary muscle (77). An anomalous coronary artery arising from the pulmonary artery can cause MR in an infant, probably due to infarction of both the papillary muscle and the ventricle at the base of the papillary muscle.

            b. About 10% of papillary muscle dysfunction murmurs that are due to acute infarction disappear before the patient leaves the hospital (44).

6. How can hypertrophic subaortic stenosis (HSS) or hypertrophic obstructive cardiomyopathy (HOCM) cause MR?

    ANS.: a. The anterior leaflet may be pulled down in systole toward the septum and away from the posterior leaflet. This movement of the leaflet toward the septum is due either to the abnormal angle at which the anterolateral papillary muscle is attached to the grossly hypertrophied septum or due to the Bernoulli effect of the high-velocity stream being ejected past the anterior mitral leaflet.

            b. The obliteration of the LV cavity that takes place during systole in HSS or HOCM can cause the mitral orifice to constrict to such a degree that the mitral leaflets become redundant, and the leaflets, therefore, prolapse into the left atrium.

Papillary Muscle Dysfunction

1. How can different kinds of papillary muscle dysfunction produce MR murmurs of different shapes?

    ANS.: a. Disproportionate lengths of papillary muscle due to lack of contraction cause MR murmurs by the following mechanism. If one papillary muscle is unable to contract or is attached to infarcted muscle at its base, its muscle-plus-chordae are longer than the opposite contracting papillary muscle-plus-chordae when the ventricle and normal papillary muscle contract. As the pressure rises and the LV cavity decreases in size, the portion of the mitral leaflets with the relatively long papillary muscle plus chordae projects more and more into the left atrium, producing a crescendo murmur to the S_2.

    b. If a papillary muscle is shortened by marked fibrosis or is attached to an aneurysm or dilated akinetic area, then regurgitation is pansystolic. The shape of the murmurs may be decrescendo if dilatation was the major cause of the regurgitation. If a piece of mitral valve attached to the normal muscle loses support of the opposite leaflet in midsystole due to too short a papillary muscle-to-opposite leaflet length, it may suddenly flip upward, producing a midsystolic nonejection click or a late systolic murmur (Fig. 2).

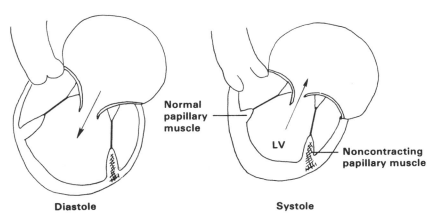

FIG. 2. A noncontracting papillary muscle may make its chordae plus papillary muscle relatively longer as the ventricle becomes smaller. This is most likely to produce a murmur that becomes progressively louder as systole proceeds (crescendo murmur to the S_2).

Note: Patients with anteroseptal myocardial infarction tend to have MR accompanied by dilatation of the mitral valve ring. This suggests that anteroseptal infarction per se does not produce papillary muscle dysfunction unless there is already a substrate for MVP. When posteroinferior myocardial infarction produces MR, the mitral ring is not dilated and the murmur is usually entirely due to the papillary muscle dynamics (85).

2. How can the shape or loudness of the MR murmur tell you whether its etiology is rheumatic fever or papillary muscle dysfunction?

ANS.: a. If the murmur is crescendo to the S_2, it is more likely to be due to papillary muscle dysfunction. Rheumatic MR is rarely crescendo to the S_2 except during the healing phase of acute rheumatic fever, usually in a patient under age 20, who has had an acute attack of rheumatic fever within a few months, during which there was also a pansystolic murmur (18).

   b. Because papillary muscle dysfunction due to HSS or HOCM almost always produces a decrescendo murmur, if a pansystolic murmur is heard at the apex in a patient with HOCM, coincidental rheumatic MR should be suspected. This murmur will probably become louder with squatting and persist after surgery for the HOCM (67).

   c. If the murmur becomes louder as the patient compensates for failure, fixed rheumatic MR is suggested. Papillary muscle dysfunction murmurs tend to become softer as the heart becomes smaller with improvement of heart failure.

   d. If an S_4 is present, it strongly suggests papillary muscle dysfunction. Rheumatic MR is rarely associated with an S_4.

   e. Papillary muscle dysfunction murmurs due to coronary disease often become softer after long diastoles. (See p. 239 for explanation.)

   f. The S_1 with papillary muscle dysfunction murmurs tends to be louder than normal, probably because of the increased sympathetic stimulation of the myocardium often seen in patients with coronary artery disease.

   Note: Papillary muscle rupture is a sequel of myocardial infarction and produces the physical finding of sudden, severe MR, mimicking the most severe case of ruptured chordae. However, the MR is so severe that, together with the myocardial damage of the myocardial infarction, the murmur of papillary muscle rupture is rarely ever louder than grade 3/6; that is, it is rare to feel a thrill with it. This finding helps to distinguish this murmur from that of ventricular septal rupture, in which 50% of such patients have murmurs of grade 4/6 or louder.

Ruptured Chordae

1. How many chordae are attached to both mitral leaflets?

   ANS.: About 120. There are about 10 chordae attached to each of about five heads of each papillary muscle, and these chordae divide about two or three times before they attach to their leaflets (97) (Fig. 3).

   Note: Spontaneous ruptures usually occur in one of the 25 major chordae closer to the papillary muscle rather than in those attached to the leaflets, thus involving at least four or five small terminal branches (92). If only a few terminal branches are torn, infective endocarditis has probably caused the rupture.

2. How can you tell if an MR murmur is due to papillary muscle dysfunction rather than to ruptured chordae?

   ANS.: a. Ruptured chordae superimposed on rheumatic heart disease produce a sudden onset of severe MR and failure (a loud S_3, a murmur of grade 3/6 or more, and an increase in symptoms). The usual papillary muscle dysfunction produces signs only of mild to moderate MR, with a murmur that is rarely more than grade 3/6, usually crescendo to the S_2. Exceptionally, however, papillary muscle dysfunction due to a large infarcted area at the base of the papillary muscle can produce severe MR. Conversely, rupture of only a few unimportant posterior chordae superimposed on a normal heart may produce few symptoms.

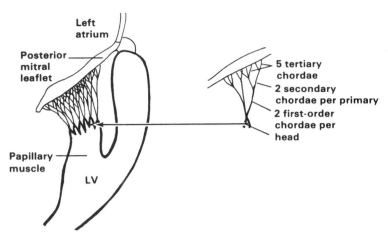

FIG. 3. Spontaneous rupture usually occurs close to a papillary muscle head and will involve at least 5 to 10 tertiary chordae. Endocarditis may rupture only a few terminal branches.

   b. A decrescendo, mixed-frequency murmur associated with symptoms of high left atrial pressure (orthopnea or paroxysmal nocturnal dyspnea) suggests ruptured chordae of recent onset. This is because the left atrium does not enlarge much with acute severe MR, probably because of the nondistensible pericardium around the atria. The poor left atrial compliance may raise the V wave pressure to a very high peak in systole (pressure as high as 70 mm Hg has been recorded). This rise in left atrial pressure plus a precipitous fall in LV pressure toward the end of systole decrease the gradient and murmur toward the end of systole (Fig. 4).

   Note: a. Chordal rupture of the posterior leaflet may cause only moderate MR. On the other hand, if one of the two chordae, larger and thicker than the rest (strut chordae), that inserts into the anterior leaflet ruptures, severe MR and a flail anterior leaflet may result (92).

   b. In sudden severe MR there may be almost no forward flow across the mitral valve during the last part of diastole because the LV resists the sudden increase in volume load, probably because of the pericardium's inability to stretch adequately in response to a sudden volume overload. The LV diastolic pressure may rise rapidly enough to momentarily exceed the left atrial pressure by mid- or late diastole, and the mitral valves may close. This makes the M_1 soft or inaudible.

3. Why may ruptured chordae imitate aortic stenosis (AS)?

   ANS.: If posterior chordae rupture, producing a flail posterior cusp, the stream of regurgitation may strike the atrial septum in such a way that murmurs with the shape and radiation (into the carotids) typical of AS are produced. To further confuse the picture, the murmur at the second right interspace may even be shorter than the one at the apex. However, only about half of posterior rupture murmurs radiate into the neck (103).

   Note: a. Radiation of a posterior rupture murmur may sometimes be better heard in the lower back than the neck. The reason is unknown.

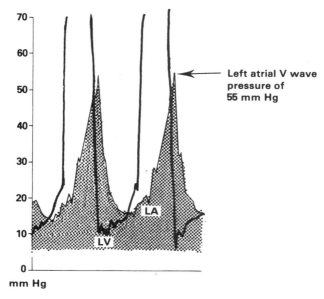

FIG. 4. This is a left atrial (wedge) and LV pressure tracing from a 23-year-old woman with rup-tured mitral chordae. The shaded area is under the left atrial (wedge) pressure curve. The slight delay in the peak wedge pressure is due to the fact that wedge pressures (taken by a catheter wedged into the distal pulmonary artery branches) always show a delay in comparison with di-rect left atrial pressure tracings. The rapid increase in V wave pressure during systole rapidly de-creases the gradient across the mitral valve and tends to cause both a decrescendo gradient and murmur. The decompressing effect on the LV of the massive loss of blood into the left atrium causes an end-systolic fall in LV pressure. This end-systolic decrease in LV pressure further de-creases the gradient across the mitral valve toward the end of systole.

         b. Despite good radiation into the second right interspace and neck, the murmur of posterior chordae rupture is still usually loudest at the apex (53).

4. What is the characteristic radiation of an MR murmur caused by a rupture of the anterior chordae?

    ANS.: It may radiate along the spine, and if loud, even to the top of the head.

        Note: There have been rare reports of patients with anterior chordal rupture who had murmurs that also imitated AS (111). The reason is unknown, but such murmurs have mixed findings such as good transmission to the back, which is also characteristic of an anterior flail leaflet (Fig. 5).

5. How do diastolic sounds tell you that a loud MR murmur is due to ruptured chordae rather than to rheumatic heart disease?

    ANS.: The atrial wall resists dilatation in patients with sudden MR (due to pericardial constraints). It responds to the stretch with a Starling effect and contracts strongly, often producing an S_4, which is rare in rheumatic MR.

        Note: a. The most common cause of ruptured chordae is infective endocarditis on an abnormal valve such as that found in patients with rheumatic heart disease or myxomatous transformation. The next most common cause is idiopathic (103). It is probable that most "idiopathic" ruptures occur on the basis of a prolapsed mitral valve with some myxomatous degenera-

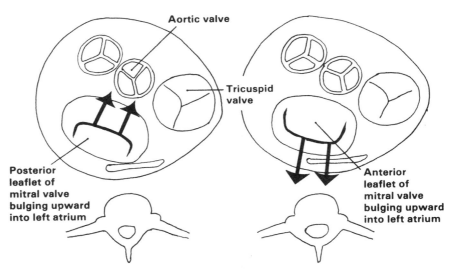

FIG. 5. These views of the valve rings from above show how posterior ruptured chordae (left) can direct the regurgitant stream against the aorta and cause the murmur to be transmitted like an aortic ejection murmur. The diagram at right shows how ruptured anterior chordae can direct the regurgitant stream posteriorly against the spine.

tion. Often a murmur of prolapse has been present for years before the rupture but has not been recognized as such (5).

b. Most patients with ruptured chordae on previously "normal" valves are males.

c. Severe myxomatous degeneration of the mitral valve most closely imitates the auscultatory findings of ruptured chordae. This is often known as the "floppy valve syndrome."

Loudness, Sites, and Radiation

1. Where are MR murmurs loudest?
   ANS.: Slightly lateral (1 to 2 cm) to the site of the maximum apex impulse.

   Note: There is at least one report of an MR murmur that was loudest at the second right interspace. This patient had only moderate MR, probably from some unusual cause (107). Another report describes two patients with probable rheumatic MR in which the murmur was just as loud at the second right interspace as at the apex area. These patients also had only mild to moderate MR. The jet in these unusual cases probably was directed anteriorly against the aortic root, which lies against the anterior atrial wall. (See Fig. 5 above.)

2. When may an MR murmur *seem* to be louder at the left sternal border than at the apex area?
   ANS.: In very long chests in which the apex area is very medially placed; that is, the LV impulse is actually near the left sternal border. You must try to shift the apex laterally either by turning the patient to the left lateral decubitus position or by having the patient sit up with legs on the bed. (In the standing position the apex area moves even more medially.)

3. What is the best radiation zone of the usual MR murmur?

ANS.: It usually radiates best to the axilla and the left posterior intrascapular area of the chest. However, if loud enough, it radiates to the right, but to a lesser degree. Distinguishing a ruptured ventricular septum VSD murmur, which is loudest near the apex, from an MR murmur is described on p. 267.

Note: a. When the murmur is due to ruptured chordae, it may have an unusual radiation zone (see p. 245).

b. If the murmur is due to an endocardial cushion defect with a cleft anterior mitral leaflet, the murmur may radiate better to the right than to the left of the apical impulse. It then may be mistaken for a VSD murmur.

c. The degree of MR after a myocardial infarction is greater for posterior than for anterior infarctions.

4. Besides an obese or emphysematous chest, what can cause silent, severe MR?

ANS.: a. Concomitant mitral stenosis (MS) can apparently direct the MR stream in such a way that the murmur is inaudible (4).

b. Prosthetic mitral valve MR due to suture breakdown may also be silent.

Note: a. Almost all adults reported with silent MR had severe regurgitation, and most had paroxysmal nocturnal dyspnea or were in atrial fibrillation (109). A widely split S_2 in the presence of a large LV and an unexpectedly large left atrium were the only clues.

b. MR may become severe and a murmur may be heard only when myocardial ischemia develops due to an attack of angina. This MR may become so severe that the patient may even develop acute pulmonary edema (73).

Shape, Pitch, and Duration

1. What are all the possible shapes of an MR murmur (Fig. 6)?

ANS.:

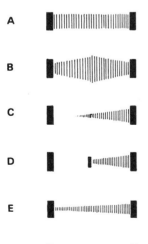

FIG. 6. Note that when the MR murmurs begin late, they always go to the second sound, and when they begin early, they always start with the first sound.

Note: Pansystolic murmurs with a slight crescendo-decrescendo (spindle shape on a phonocardiogram) are usually the loudest.

2. How does the pitch of a murmur correlate with gradient and flow?

    ANS.: A good general rule is the higher the gradient, the higher the pitch, and the more the flow, the more the low (frequencies).

3. Which MR murmurs are always associated with almost pure high frequencies (i.e., only a blowing sound)?

    ANS.: All soft murmurs with small volume flows and high gradients (e.g., those due to trivial MR).

    Note: a. The gradient between the left atrium and LV usually reaches more than 100 mm Hg during the peak of systole.

    b. All dominantly high-pitched decrescendo murmurs denote mild MR, even if loud (grade 3/6). The crescendo murmur of ruptured chordae is associated with much flow but has dominantly low and medium frequencies.

4. Why does the MR murmur extend slightly beyond the S_2?

    ANS.: Because LV pressure is higher than left atrial pressure even after the aortic valve closes (Fig. 7).

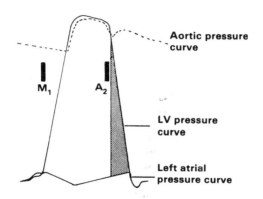

FIG. 7. Note that the LV pressure is above left atrial pressure even after the A_2.

5. Is an MR murmur louder on inspiration or expiration?

    ANS.: It is usually louder on expiration because that is when blood is pushed into the LV from the lungs.

    Note: Unusual rotations caused by inspiration may bring the heart closer to the stethoscope and cause the murmur paradoxically to sound louder on inspiration. This can often be counteracted by placing the stethoscope lateral to the apex beat. If the heart sounds also become louder on inspiration, rotation may be the cause. Unusual cardiac rotations with respiration are common after cardiac surgery.

Quantitating Degrees of MR

1. How can you tell the degree of MR by physical examination?

    ANS.: The MR is greater

    a. The larger the LV by palpation.

    b. The greater and later the left parasternal movement. (This may represent the left atrium expanding during systole.)

    c. The more palpable the early rapid filling wave at the apex (see p. 249).

    d. The louder and longer the apical systolic murmur. (Although ruptured chordae murmurs may be decrescendo, they are almost always at least grade 4/6 in loudness [5].)

  e. The more low and medium frequencies are present.
  f. The louder the S_3 (roughly proportional to the quantity of diastolic flow) and the louder and longer the diastolic flow murmur following the S_3.
  g. The wider the split of the S_2, unless the development of severe pulmonary hypertension narrows the split (Fig. 8).

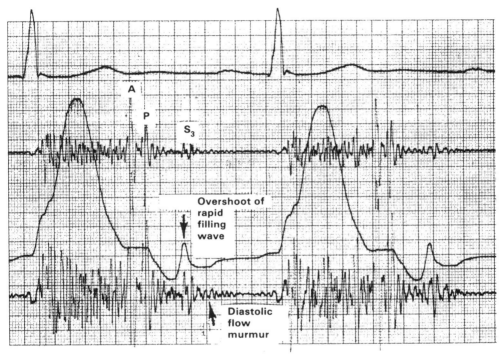

FIG. 8. This phonocardiogram and apical pulse tracing is from the same 15-year-old girl with severe rheumatic MR as in page 188. The pulse tracing was taken over the LV impulse in the supine position and is therefore an apex precordiogram instead of an apex cardiogram, which is taken to the left lateral decubitus position. The phonocardiograms are from the third left parasternal interspace. The upper one is taken at medium frequency; the lower one is a logarithmic tracing that brings out low and medium frequencies. Note the following signs of severe MR: (a) the widely split S_2 of 50 msec; (b) the diastolic flow murmur after the S_3, both of which are so loud that they can be recorded at the left sternal border (see page 188 for the same S_3 and diastolic flow murmur at the apex of this patient); (c) the exaggerated early rapid filling peak of the apical impulse (this would be palpable in the left lateral decubitus position).

Effects of Drugs and Maneuvers

Increasing Peripheral Resistance

1. What happens to left-sided regurgitant murmurs if the peripheral resistance is increased? Why?
   ANS.: They become louder, because with regurgitation there are two outlets for systole, and an increased resistance at the aortic outlet promotes more outflow through the other outlet.

2. How will raising the blood pressure with handgrip, squatting, or phenylephrine help you determine whether a long systolic murmur at the apex is due to AS or MR?

ANS.: With increased peripheral resistance aortic ejection murmurs either are unchanged or become softer, but MR murmurs become louder.

Note: a. A vasopressor drug with a strong positive inotropic effect, such as no-repinephrine, only adds a confusing variable. Phenylephrine has only weak inotropic effects. The dose of phenylephrine is 0.4 to 0.7 mg, given by slow intravenous infusion until a rise of about 20 mm Hg in systolic pressure is achieved (7).

b. Handgrip has little effect on the peripheral resistance of normal subjects or on most patients with either labile or fixed hypertension unless they have evidence of left ventricular hypertrophy or enlargement on echocardiogram (ECG) or x-ray (29). If patients are in failure, however, they cannot increase their output adequately in response to handgrip and increase instead the blood pressure by an increase in peripheral resistance (22).

Although 30% of maximum voluntary contraction produces circulatory changes, 50% of maximum voluntary contraction produces a greater elevation of blood pressure. Seventy-five percent of maximum achieves a peak response in 1 minute (29).

c. Standing to increase peripheral resistance does not necessarily increase the loudness of the murmur of MR. The smaller heart caused by the pooling effect brought about by standing and the decreased volume of regurgitation due to the diminution of venous return cause the murmur to become softer or stay the same despite the increase in resistance. (The MR murmur of the prolapsed valve syndrome becomes louder on standing. See p. 253 for details.)

d. You may bring out the type of MR murmur of papillary muscle dysfunction that is transient and is associated only with episodes of coronary insufficiency by passive leg-raising to increase the LV volume (69).

Decreasing Peripheral Resistance with Nitrites

1. Why does amyl nitrite cause an increase in cardiac output whereas nitroglycerin causes a fall in cardiac output?

ANS.: The rapid and profound drop in blood pressure produced by amyl nitrite results in a strong reflex sympathetic outflow that constricts the veins. Amyl nitrite is a volatile substance that is dissipated in the capillary system and therefore never reaches the veins. The direct effect of amyl nitrite on the capillaries may open up shunts between the dilated arterioles and venules. The increased venous return, together with reflex tachycardia, increases the cardiac output.

Nitroglycerin, on the other hand, does affect the veins and reduces venous return by causing venous pooling. The mild drop in blood pressure produced by nitroglycerin is not strong enough to result in sufficient sympathetic outflow to cause venous constriction.

2. How will amyl nitrite help separate an aortic ejection murmur from an MR murmur at the apex?

ANS.: By decreasing the peripheral resistance, it makes the MR murmur softer. By causing an increased velocity of ejection through the aortic valve, it makes the aortic ejection murmur louder.

  Note: A marked effect may be achieved with only three inhalations of amyl nitrite. The following precautions are helpful when using amyl nitrite.

  a. Wear rubber gloves. Otherwise, the odor may remain on your fingers for days. After use, flush the used capsule down the toilet; otherwise, it will impart its odor to your examining room for hours.

  b. The patient must be supine or you may produce syncope.

  c. Warn the patient that he or she will feel flushed and that the heart will pound for about 10 sec. Reassure the nervous patient by explaining that the drug was formerly used to take away "heart pain" but is no longer used because of its lingering odor.

  d. An assistant should call out the systolic blood pressures throughout the entire procedure so that you know to what degree the blood pressure is affected.

THE BALLOONED OR PROLAPSED MITRAL VALVE

Definition and Terminology

1. What is meant by a ballooned or prolapsed mitral valve? What auscultatory findings does it cause?

  ANS.: This term refers to the bulging or buckling of one or both mitral valve leaflets into the left atrium during systole, associated with systolic clicks and regurgitant murmurs.

2. What are the names given to the prolapsed mitral valve complex?

  ANS.: Mitral valve prolapse, or MVP (the most common term), ballooned valve syndrome, systolic click-murmur syndrome, Barlow syndrome, click late-systolic murmur syndrome, and billowing mitral valve syndrome.

  Note: a. The word **syndrome** is applied when there are symptoms of nonspecific chest pain, an ECG showing T wave abnormalities (negative T in aVF or the left precordium or abnormally notched T waves), and ventricular arrhythmias that occasionally lead to sudden death.

  b. It is unfortunate that **prolapsed valve** rather than **ballooned valve** became the most common term because **prolapse** suggests to the novice a downward movement into the LV when actually it is a backward and upward movement into the left atrium.

  c. **Billowing** suggests that the normal valve does not billow, which is not true. **Barlow syndrome** is not descriptive for the beginner. **Click late-systolic murmur syndrome** ignores those patients with only the click, only the murmur, or with a pansystolic murmur and multiple clicks.

  d. The term **floppy valve syndrome** has been applied by some as a synonym for MVP syndrome. This is unfortunate because this term was originally meant to describe the most marked degree of myxomatous degeneration with elongated chordae, causing severe MR (93). In the usual MVP syndrome, the MR is at most only moderate.

3. What can we call the click or sound that often precedes the delayed systolic murmur?

  ANS.: A nonejection click or sound. It may come as early as an ejection click and as late as a widely split S_2.

Note: a. The click may even come slightly after the onset of the murmur.
   b. If the etiology is primarily myocardial infarction and papillary muscle dysfunction, it is not so likely to sound like a click.

Auscultatory Findings

1. What are the most common findings on auscultation of the patient with MVP?
  ANS.: One or more crisp systolic sounds or clicks and a late systolic or pansystolic MR murmur.
    Note: a. About 6% of women between the ages of 17 and 54 in one study had either a midsystolic nonejection click, a late systolic murmur, or both. About 60% of these women had both a click and a murmur, 5% had only the late systolic murmur, and the remainder had only the click (91). In another series 30% had only a murmur, 25% had both click and murmur, and the rest had only clicks (71). In a two-dimensional echocardiographic screening study of 100 asymptomatic women ages 18 to 35, only 2% had prolapse (130).
      b. In one study about 15% of patients with prolapsed valves and MR had early systolic murmurs (86).
      c. Variability is characteristic of the systolic clicks, which from time to time may be present, absent, single, or multiple, or may be replaced by a cluster of late systolic crackles.
2. What is the usual shape of the delayed systolic murmur in the MVP syndrome?
  ANS.: To the ear, they often sound crescendo to the second sound.
    Note: a. Most of these murmurs actually are crescendo-decrescendo on a fast-paper-speed phonocardiogram (6) (Fig. 9).

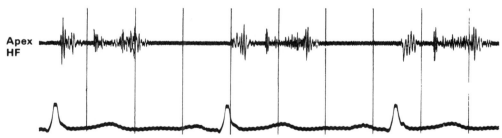

FIG. 9. The midsystolic sound was a click heard loudest at the apex in this 45-year-old woman. The murmur following it is crescendo to the S$_2$. This is the classic ballooned valve click-murmur complex by auscultation. (HF = high frequency.)

      b. A pansystolic murmur can occur even with only late systolic prolapse on echocardiogram. This is because hearts with MVP usually have varying degrees of annular dilatation and those with pansystolic murmurs have the greatest dilatation (86).

The Systolic Whoop or Honk

1. What is the loudest grade of murmur in MVP syndrome?

   ANS.: If it is not a whoop or a honk, which can be grade 6, it is almost never more than grade 3/6.

   Note: a. Systolic musical honks or whoops are not uncommon signs of a prolapsed valve. They are usually transient and disappear with different phases of respiration; when they disappear, a regurgitant murmur is almost always present. (The word **honk** refers to the similarity of this sound to the honking of a goose.) These musical honks or whoops are the loudest murmurs heard in cardiologic practice. Some murmurs can be heard even across the room (31). When a honk is associated with no prolapse on ventriculography but acquired valve disease is present instead, the honk may move freely from early to middle to late on different occasions and is rarely more than 3/6 (95).

   b. Much more rarely, a loud, musical systolic murmur may be present in the left chest when an anomalous fibrous band or cord stretches across the ventricular cavity like the string of a musical instrument. When this is stretched by cardiac dilatation, it may become taut enough to produce a murmur (96).

   c. Musical MR murmurs or honks are probably due to vibrations of the valves themselves (35). Simultaneous echophonocardiography shows valve leaflet flutter at a frequency identical to that of the musical honk or murmur (114,125). (The usual murmur is caused by turbulence around the valve rather than by the vibrations of the valves themselves.) Honks and whoops may sometimes be caused by the vibration of an elongated papillary muscle (49). A tricuspid whoop in one report was associated at autopsy with two extremely long, thin chordae that were thought to be responsible for the murmur (20).

   d. There are several reports of tricuspid whoops in patients with pulmonary hypertension, one with mild tricuspid regurgitation (TR) (124). The whoop or honk usually disappears if the pulmonary hypertension is relieved (60).

Changing the Click and Murmur with Maneuvers or Drugs

1. What happens to the nonejection click and murmur when blood volume to the LV is decreased, as occurs with standing, inspiration, or a Valsalva strain? Why?

   ANS.: They both occur earlier and they often become louder. Indeed, they may only be heard on sitting or standing. The click may actually occur so early on standing that it may fuse with the first heart sound and may seem to disappear altogether.

   Angiograms have shown that an increase in prolapse occurs in the upright position. This may occur because the redundant tissue acts like the dome of a parachute whose diameter is decreased if the edges are held down and pulled toward each other. Thus, when the ventricle becomes smaller and the diameter is reduced, the center of the "parachute" is pushed up due to the fixed length of chordae and papillary muscles (Fig. 10).

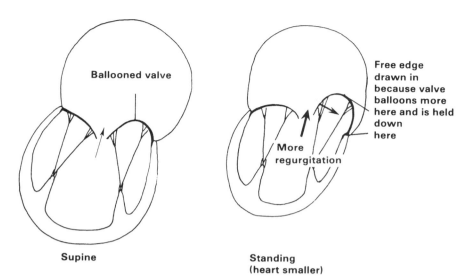

FIG. 10. One of the diagnostic characteristics of the ballooned valve murmur is that it becomes louder and begins earlier when the heart is made smaller.

    Note: a. The click may also become louder in the left lateral decubitus position, perhaps because of the change in blood pressure that occurs in some patients in that position.

     b. A premature atrial contraction or PVC can cause more severe and earlier prolapse because of the contraction that occurs with a smaller volume than normal.

     c. After the release of a Valsalva maneuver, the click may become louder because of the overshoot of blood pressure.

     d. If the heart is made larger by slowing the rate with propranolol, both the click and the murmur may diminish or disappear.

2. What happens to the (a) click and (b) murmur position and loudness with amyl nitrite?

 ANS.: a. The click occurs earlier and usually becomes softer and may even disappear. The smaller volume causes the click to come earlier, and the low systolic pressure makes it softer (101).

    b. Usually, the murmur becomes softer immediately and occurs earlier, but after about 30 sec it may become louder due to the overshoot of blood pressure. If the control murmur is only late systolic, amyl nitrite may cause it to become pansystolic (Fig. 11).

3. What effect does increasing blood pressure with phenylephrine or methoxamine have on the position and loudness of the (a) click and (b) murmur?

 ANS.: a. The click takes variable positions and usually becomes louder because of the greater force exerted on the mitral valve structure.

    b. The murmur becomes louder, and you may even bring out a late systolic murmur if only a click was present.

     Note: a. Occasionally, only a vasopressor agent can bring out any clicks or murmurs (101). Presumably, a critical systolic pressure is necessary to cause prolapse and may account for the increased incidence of these clicks and murmurs with age.

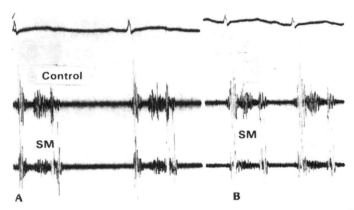

FIG. 11. A: A late systolic murmur moved toward early systole. B: The late systolic murmur became pansystolic after amyl nitrite inhalation decreased heart size.

      b. In one study of subjects with an isolated systolic nonejection click, a late systolic murmur developed with a vasopressor agent in 33% of the patients (99).

      c. There is a report of one patient with early systolic prolapse on echocardiogram who had an early systolic murmur (rare) that was made louder by methoxamine and in whom amyl nitrite elicited the late systolic component murmur of a pansystolic murmur (51).

4. How do nonejection clicks following mitral valvotomy differ from other nonejection clicks?

    ANS.: These clicks are

      a. Louder but lower in frequency and therefore have less of a clicking quality.

      b. Usually earlier in systole (more easily confused with an ejection sound) but occasionally situated late in the murmur or even at the end of an early systolic murmur.

      c. Not constant in terms of the effect of maneuvers on them.

      d. Likely to become single or multiple spontaneously.

5. How can you differentiate the late systolic murmur of papillary muscle dysfunction from the late systolic murmur of a prolapsed mitral valve (without a click) by auscultation?

    ANS.: Papillary muscle dysfunction murmurs are usually associated with an S_4 and a loud S_1, often become softer after a sudden long diastole, and increase with squatting or amyl nitrite (18,19). Prolapsed valve murmurs have no characteristic S_1, do not usually feature an S_4, and may become softer with squatting or amyl nitrite.

      Note: With severe prolapse and a pansystolic murmur, the S_1 is louder than average; with ruptured chordae the S_1 is either softer than normal or absent. When a late systolic murmur is made pansystolic by a Valsalva strain, the S_1 becomes louder and the click may disappear.

Etiology, Pathology, and Physiology

1. What is the usual mitral valve abnormality seen at surgery or necropsy when a prolapsed mitral valve is examined?

    ANS.: Myxomatous transformation. This may be recognized only on careful inspection, since the valve may appear grossly normal to casual examination by the surgeon or pathologist (Fig. 12).

> *Note*: a. The Marfan syndrome is commonly associated with myxomatous valves, and about 20% to 30% of patients with prolapsed valves have joint laxity; high, arched palates; or other skeletal abnormalities such as scoliosis, pectus excavatum, and straight backs (i.e., it may be occasionally a forme fruste of the Marfan syndrome). The Ehlers-Danlos syndrome is also commonly associated with MVP (9 of 11 patients in one series) (13).

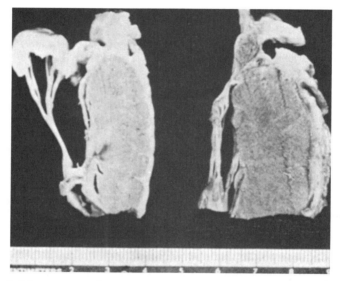

FIG. 12. On the left is a cross section of the abnormal middle scallop of the posterior leaflet. On the right is the same area from a woman with left ventricular hypertrophy but no MR. (From JK Trent, AG Adelman, ED Wigle, and MD Silver. *Am Heart J* 1970:79:539.)

> b. The tricuspid valve has also been found to prolapse in about 15% of patients with clicks and late systolic murmurs at the left lower sternal edge (72,83). Twenty percent to 50% of patients with MVP have tricuspid valve prolapse (10).
>
> Tricuspid valve prolapse with the click and murmur of TR has been reported in patients with right ventricular hypertrophy and dilatation secondary to pulmonary hypertension (116). About 5% of patients with tricuspid valve prolapse have no MVP (10).

2. List the suspected causes of MVP.

> ANS.: a. Congenital myxomatous transformation with elongated chordae (by far the most common cause).
>
> b. Papillary muscle dysfunction or ventricular asynergy due to myocardial infarction or ischemia (126).
>
> c. Dysfunction of muscle adjacent to the posterior leaflet, as in myocardial infarction or in congenital absence of the left circumflex coronary artery.

d. Effect of mitral valve surgery, probably due to unequal length of the chordae.

e. HSS or HOCM, probably because of unequal length of the chordae due to asymmetrical hypertrophy as well as the hyperkinetic contraction that obliterates the cavity and contracts the mitral valve orifice, making the mitral leaflets too large for the orifice. The small size of the cavity contracting the mitral orifice may be the reason that about one-third of patients with small hearts (cardiothoracic [C/T] ratio of less than 40%) show MVP on echocardiogram (121).

f. The occasional patient with mitral stenosis has enough free unfibrosed leaflet to buckle up into the left atrium and produce a nonejection click (21). Some believe that rheumatic fever can cause a prolapsed mitral valve, and even propose that all patients with prolapse should have rheumatic fever prophylaxis unless T wave abnormalities are present, because then the prolapse is not due to rheumatic fever (118).

g. In one study, about one-half of all patients with a history of either myocarditis or a collagen disease had MVP (76).

3. Which congenital cardiac condition has been found to be commonly associated with prolapsed mitral valves?

ANS.: ASD.

> *Note*: In the past it was thought that in a patient with an ASD, MR was present only in the primum or endocardial cushion type of ASD and that it was always due to cleft mitral valves. Now it is conceded that MR can occur in secundum ASD due not only to a cleft mitral valve (very rare) but also to myxomatous degeneration of the valve with prolapse (75). Occasionally, the MR is due to an abnormally high insertion of the chordae near the top of the ventricular septum.
>
> With ASD closure the LV enlarges and with it the mitral orifice, resulting in a decrease or disappearance of the prolapse (108). If the MR is due to a cleft mitral valve, closure of the ASD will increase the MR (64).

4. What is the cause of the nonejection click in MVP?

ANS.: The "chordal snap" theory contends that the click is due to a sudden stretch of chordae as they give way at the peak pressure in midsystole. Because the papillary muscles contract early, however, the chordae are under too much tension from the beginning of systole to "snap" during ventricular ejection (102). Therefore, this theory has been challenged by another theory that suggests the click is a *valvular* sound produced by the loss of support of one leaflet by its opposing leaflet due to redundant valve tissue or to an abnormality of chordal length. Thus, a small piece of unsupported leaflet may suddenly flip upward to its full extent to produce a click (25).

> *Note*: The click can occur at the onset or at the peak of the prolapse on M mode echocardiograms.

5. What is the "contraction ring" theory of the cause of the nonejection click?

ANS.: Often there is a posteroinferior area in the LV in which there is excessive contraction during midsystole. This area is attached mainly to the posterior papillary muscle. Since this part of the LV contracts excessively, it pushes up the posterior papillary muscle and causes the chordae to become slack. Further systole then pulls the chordae taut, producing the click (27). However, this type of contraction abnormality is not seen in most patients with MVP.

> *Note*: To support further the theory that MVP may sometimes be due to a primary myocardial abnormality, the following findings may be listed.

a. Angiograms have shown that at least 80% of patients with MVP have LV asynergy (abnormal areas of contraction or absence of contraction). At least six types of asynergy have been described (106).
1. "Ballerina foot," pattern in right anterior oblique views (vigorous posteromedial contraction and anterior convexity).
2. Reduction of the extent of shortening of the inflow tract area around the mitral valve ring (65).
3. "Hourglass-like" contraction of the middle of the ventricle.
4. Inadequate shortening of the long axis.
5. Posterior akinesis.
6. Cavity obliteration.
b. Late systolic clicks have been heard for the first time in patients during the course of their infarction.
c. A late systolic murmur and click developed in one patient after radiopaque dye was inadvertently injected directly beneath the posterior leaflet.
d. Patients with coronary disease are sometimes found to have a click and a late systolic murmur on squatting (19). This is the opposite of what happens in the usual young patient with MVP.

6. What can cause the development of heart failure in a patient with mild MR secondary to the MVP syndrome?
ANS.: a. Occasionally, chordae rupture.
b. Gradual progression from mild to severe MR can also occur, but this is rare (56).
c. Infective endocarditis on the mitral valve.

7. What are the noncardiac causes of midsystolic clicks?
ANS.: a. A small left-sided pneumothorax. When loud, it may be heard at some distance from the patient. It lasts an average of 11 days (46). One theory claims that these clicks are produced by the heart flipping the lingula against the thoracic wall (32). Another theory is that these clicks are produced by the cardiac movement displacing air bubbles between the visceral and parietal pleura. They often disappear with a change of position and reappear with a deep breath (46). (The fact that they often occur in diastole as well as in systole helps rule out a valvular etiology.)
b. Pleural-pericardial adhesions or adhesive pericarditis (68).
Note: During the first half of this century all midsystolic clicks were considered to be due to pleural-pericardial adhesions, probably because
1. Galavardin described four cases in which autopsy evidence showed pleural-pericardial adhesions (39).
2. When multiple clicks are heard with prolapsed valves, they may mimic a pericardial friction rub.
c. A very uncommon cause of a midsystolic click is the to-and-fro snapping of a floating balloon catheter against the septum in the right ventricle (RV) (52). A diastolic sound is also heard in such a case and is more common than a systolic click.
d. Complete absence of the pericardium has caused the complete syndrome of click and late systolic murmur with no prolapse on either echocardiography or angiography (74). It increases on inspiration.
e. An isolated bicuspid pulmonary valve, especially with right bundle branch block (*very rare*).

f. An aneurysm of the atrial septum may produce a midsystolic click at the time of maximal bulging of the atrial septum into the right atrium (2). (The atrial septum bulges first into the left atrium in early systole and then suddenly back into the right atrium in midsystole.)

g. In patients with aortic regurgitation a midsystolic sound that is simultaneous with the dip in the associated bisferiens pulse has been recorded. The cause is unknown (98).

h. Some very rare causes of nonejection or midsystolic clicks are a pacemaker sound, atrial myxoma either right or left, complete AV block, ventricular aneurysms, and atrial septal aneurysms.

TRICUSPID REGURGITATION MURMURS

Site, Loudness, and Shape

1. Where is the murmur of TR usually heard best? In what other places may it occasionally be heard best?

   ANS.: It is usually heard best at the left lower sternal border. It is occasionally heard best in the epigastrium, at the right sternal border, or, if the RV is very large, over the mid-left thorax at the site of the usual LV apex area, which may be taken over by the RV.

   Note: The classic method of diagnosing TR by auscultation is to listen for a pansystolic murmur that becomes louder with inspiration at the left lower sternal border or wherever a palpable RV lift is felt. This has been called the Carvallo sign (94).

2. Why does the TR murmur usually increase in loudness on inspiration?

   ANS.: Because more blood is drawn into the RV and becomes available for regurgitation. Also, since the net pulmonary artery pressure rises slightly on inspiration, there is increased resistance in that direction. (If the intrathoracic pressure fall on inspiration is not subtracted from the lesser pulmonary artery pressure fall, the pulmonary artery pressure gives a false impression of falling with inspiration.)

   Note: a. The murmur of TR remains louder on held inspiration (inspiratory apnea); that is, it does not require moving respiration, as when one is looking for movement in the S_2 split. As long as intrathoracic pressure is kept low by an expanded lung, more blood is brought into the RV on inspiration than on expiration.

   b. The TR murmur does not increase with inspiration in about two-thirds of patients with mild TR and in about one-third of patients with severe TR (70). The lack of increase with inspiration may be because

   1. The presence of RV failure or very severe TR may render the inspiratory increase in regurgitant volume incapable of increasing the murmur loudness.

   2. Inspiration may not bring much more blood into the RV because of the decreased vital capacity caused by pulmonary congestion or hypertension.

   3. Inspiration may so lower pulmonary vascular resistance that the extra blood drawn in on inspiration is ejected into the pulmonary artery rather than regurgitated.

   4. The RV may be so damaged that it is functioning on a plateau of the Starling curve, so that an increased volume and pressure in the RV cause little change in the strength of contraction.

3. How, besides by inspiration, exercise, and amyl nitrite, can you increase venous return to bring out a TR murmur?

ANS.: a. By having someone hold the patient's legs up or having the patient bend his knees up toward his chest. Sometimes this works even without deep inspiration (127).

b. By pressure below the right costal margin as with the hepatojugular reflux test (17,38). Right upper quadrant pressure can occasionally increase the murmur when inspiration fails, especially if the TR is mild, as in early endocarditis. However, right upper quadrant pressure may occasionally decrease the loudness of the murmur by obstructing inferior vena cava flow. This is especially likely if the TR is secondary to chronic obstructive pulmonary disease (COPD) (127). Pressure over or below the liver plus deep inspiration may work better than either maneuver alone.

4. When is a TR murmur decrescendo?

ANS.: In acute, severe TR due to rupture of tricuspid chordae. (See p. 244 for an explanation of a similar effect on the left side.)

Note: Occasionally, no murmur at all may be heard if free TR is present, causing the atrium and ventricle to form almost one chamber in systole. (This can also occur with a ruptured papillary muscle in the LV.) In one color and pulsed Doppler study, about 25% of patients with severe TR by ventriculography had no murmur. They were characterized by low peak velocities and laminar flow with a "candle flame" pattern by color Doppler (133). The low velocity suggests severe myocardial dysfunction and that the murmur was not secondary to pulmonary hypertension.

Differential Diagnosis of TR and MR by Auscultation

1. Why is it often difficult to tell TR from MR?

ANS.: a. The MR murmur transmitted to the left sternal border may sometimes increase on inspiration, thus mimicking TR. This is presumably due to some rotational phenomenon, which should be suspected if the heart sounds also increase with inspiration.

b. The TR murmur may be loud at the usual apex area, which may be usurped by an enlarged RV.

2. How can a Valsalva maneuver help distinguish TR from MR?

ANS.: Upon release of the strain, the TR murmur returns to the pre-Valsalva loudness within about 1 second. The MR murmur loudness returns in 3 to 4 seconds.

3. How can vasopressors and vasodilators help you distinguish between MR and TR?

ANS.: a. A pure vasopressor increases the murmur of MR without affecting a TR murmur. (Norepinephrine cannot be used for this purpose because it may raise pulmonary resistance in subjects with pulmonary hypertension and so increase the TR murmur.)

b. The administration of amyl nitrite is even more useful, because it has the opposite effect on the TR and MR murmur; that is, it usually makes the TR murmur louder by increasing venous return and the MR murmur softer by lowering peripheral resistance.

Note: If amyl nitrite causes a fall in pulmonary artery pressure because the pulmonary arteriolar constriction is vasoactive rather than fixed, the RV ejects more blood into the pulmonary artery, and therefore the TR murmur will not increase despite the increase in venous return.

Causes

1. What is necessary before secondary TR can be expected to occur (i.e., in the absence of primary tricuspid valve deformities)?

   ANS.: Both a high pressure and a large volume in the RV. The TR thus caused is **secondary** TR. The most common cause of both a high pressure and a large volume in the RV is severe pulmonary hypertension.

2. List the causes of primary TR (i.e., TR not secondary to pulmonary hypertension).

   ANS.: Trauma, Ebstein's anomaly, prolapsed tricuspid valve, papillary muscle dysfunction due to right ventricular infarction, infective endocarditis (usually in heroin addicts), carcinoid disease, and when a pacemaker distorts a tricuspid valve.

   Note: a. Systolic scratchy murmurs and crescendo-decrescendo murmurs, which may or may not increase with inspiration, have been reported with RV pacemakers, sometimes only when the pacemaker is not on.

   b. In patients over age 70, severe TR may occur due to annular dilatation, valve thickening, and malaligned coaptation (by echocardiography) associated with atrial fibrillation, all of unknown etiology (58).

   c. TR secondary to COPD is nearly always trivial (115).

   d. Almost half of asymptomatic pregnant women have trivial TR by pulsed Doppler studies, presumably due to the enlarged tricuspid annular diameter that occurs during pregnancy (66).

THE CARDIORESPIRATORY MURMUR

1. What is meant by a cardiorespiratory (or cardiopulmonary) murmur?

   ANS.: It is an extracardiac murmur, probably produced when the systolic motion of the heart compresses an expanded lung segment between the pericardium and the pleura. It is high-pitched, usually short, and may occur anywhere in systole and even in early diastole. It is heard best during deep inspiration. It tends to disappear near the end of expiration and during held inspiration. The most important differential diagnosis is with a late systolic MR murmur, a short aortic regurgitation murmur, and a TR murmur.

   Note: a. It gives the sensation of being superficial to the heart sounds. It has been described as high-pitched like vesicular breathing, blowing, or swishing. It is never harsh or rough.

   b. The xiphisternal crunch is not to be confused with a cardiorespiratory murmur. It is a crunching sound usually heard to the left and above the xiphoid process. It has been postulated to be due to the heart beating against the left seventh costal cartilage. It is usually systolic but occasionally diastolic and does not vary with respiration. It is diminished or absent in the recumbent position and increased by leaning forward.

VENTRICULAR SEPTAL DEFECT MURMURS

Shape and Duration

1. Where is the usual VSD situated?

   ANS.: In the membranous septum (i.e., in a small, translucent area extending about 1 to 2 cm below the aortic valve).

   Note: The attachment of the septal leaflet of the tricuspid valve bisects the membranous septum so that the usual VSD is below the attachment, but if the

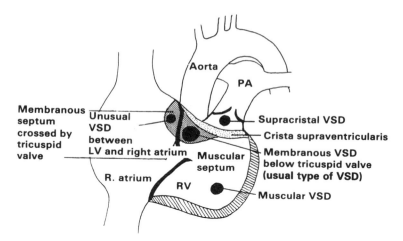

FIG. 13. Defects in the membranous septum below the tricuspid valve are the most common.

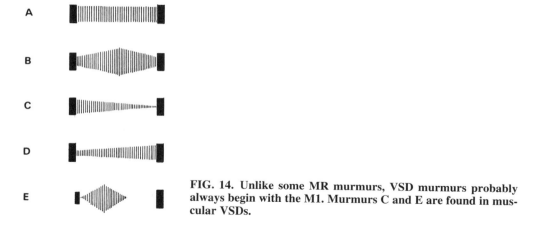

FIG. 14. Unlike some MR murmurs, VSD murmurs probably always begin with the M1. Murmurs C and E are found in muscular VSDs.

VSD is above this attachment, it may shunt blood directly into the right atrium (Figs. 13).

2. What are the various shapes of VSD murmurs?

Note: The usual shape of a murmur from a moderate or large VSD when the pulmonary artery pressure is less than 50 mm Hg is pansystolic plateau (rectangular) (45) (Figs. 14 and 15).

3. When is the VSD murmur mostly decrescendo?

ANS.: a. If it is of the muscular type (i.e., in the muscular part of the septum). Muscular contraction of the septum can close the VSD off toward the end of systole (Fig. 16).

Note: On a phonocardiogram these murmurs have a marked crescendo-decrescendo in the first third of systole (128).

b. If moderate pulmonary hypertension is present with a large VSD.

4. What does a crescendo or late systolic murmur usually imply about the size of the defect?

ANS.: They are small (Fig. 15).

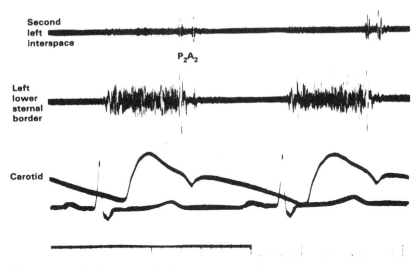

FIG. 15. This murmur is plateau in the first cycle, suggesting a pulmonary artery pressure of less than 50 mm Hg. The crescendo in the second cycle suggests that the VSD is not large, because small VSDs are the usual cause of murmurs that are crescendo to the S_2.

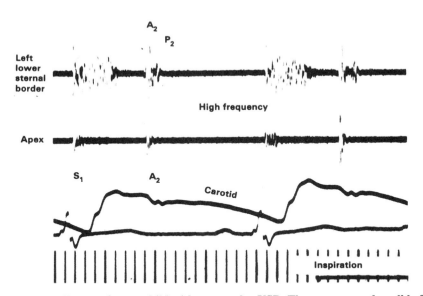

FIG. 16. Phonocardiogram from a child with a muscular VSD. The murmur ends well before the S_2. Note the normally moving split of S_2 in inspiration.

5. How can you make the short decrescendo of a muscular VSD obviously pansystolic?

ANS.: By using a vasopressor agent, which by raising the peripheral resistance to outflow causes more left-to-right shunt even during the end of systole.

Note: The murmur of a very small VSD as recorded in the RV can also be crescendo-decrescendo (129). It is as if a small VSD acts like a valvular obstruction in that it produces almost the same shape as an ejection murmur. If the crescendo-decrescendo murmur is preceded by an early none-jection click, the VSD is found on angiography to be at the apex of a mem-branous septum aneurysm that protrudes into the RV outflow tract (90). However, most VSDs associated with an aneurysm of the ventricular sep-tum produce a crescendo murmur to the S_2 (33) (Fig. 17).

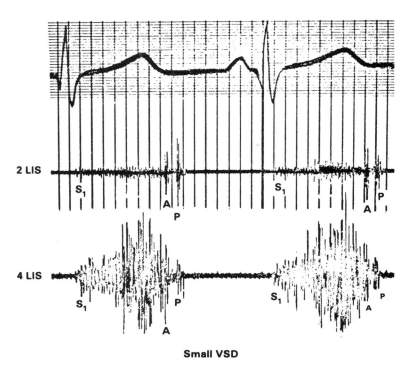

Small VSD

FIG. 17. The crescendo-decrescendo effect of this small VSD is best recorded at the fourth left interspace (4 LIS), where the A_2 is obscured by the long murmur.

6. Why may a very large VSD produce a short ejection murmur or no murmur at all?
   ANS.: It may create, in effect, a single ventricle, with the same systolic pressure in both RV and LV. When this pressure is transmitted to the pulmonary arterioles, the latter constrict reflexly in response. The raised resistance in the pulmonary circuit prevents much left-to-right flow through the VSD, and the shunt murmur may be soft or even disappear. Thus, the systolic murmur that you hear may be only an ejection murmur due to flow into a slightly dilated pulmonary artery.

Factors Controlling Loudness

1. What is the relationship between the size of the VSD and the loudness of the murmur?
   ANS.: If it is very small (pinhole VSD), the murmur may be very soft. If it is very large so that there are almost equal pressures in the RV and the LV, the murmur may also be very soft. If, however, it is moderately large, there is usually a very loud murmur (Fig. 18). (Some of the loudest murmurs observed in cardiologic practice, next to prolapsed valve honks, are caused by moderately large VSDs.)

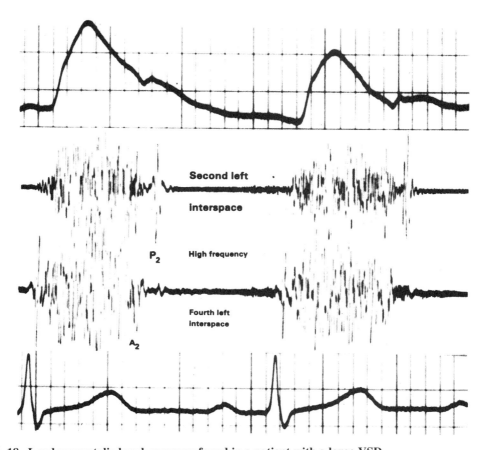

FIG. 18. Loud pansystolic harsh murmur found in a patient with a large VSD.

2. What auscultatory clues indicate that a soft VSD murmur is due to a large VSD with severe pulmonary hypertension?
   ANS.: a. The murmur is often preceded by an ejection sound when pulmonary artery
            pressure is high.
         b. The murmur is followed by a loud single S_2, which in turn may be followed by
            an early diastolic blow of pulmonary regurgitation (Graham Steell murmur).
         c. If a large flow is still present (the pulmonary hypertension is then said to be hy-
            perkinetic, vasoactive, or vasospastic), a mitral diastolic murmur due to excess
            flow through the mitral valve may be heard.

Factors Controlling Sites of Loudness

1. What is the usual site of maximum loudness of the VSD murmur in adults?
   ANS.: The left lower sternal border.
2. When may a VSD murmur be louder between the apex and the left lower sternal border
   than at the left sternal border?
   ANS.: a. When a large RV has displaced the LV to the left.

   b. When the VSD is in the muscular part of the septum near the apex. This is not
      an unusual site for a ruptured septum secondary to infarction.
         Note: If the VSD shunts directly into the right atrium, the murmur may radiate
                well into the second right interspace (100). (If the shunt into the right
                atrium is large, there may be a tricuspid inflow murmur.)
3. When can the murmur of a VSD be loudest at the second left interspace?
   ANS.: If it is supracristal (i.e., just under the pulmonary valve). The murmur is heard next
         loudest in the first rather than the third left interspace.
         Note: Because these patients have widely split second sounds and the murmur
                may be slightly crescendo-decrescendo with a late peak, their murmurs
                may be confused with the murmur of pulmonary stenosis (PS) (119).
4. When should you suspect that PS is present with a VSD on auscultation?
   ANS.: a. When the split of the S_2 is very wide and the pulmonary component (P_2) is very
            soft. The P_2 is usually of normal or increased loudness with a pure VSD.
         b. When there is an area low on the chest near the epigastrium where the murmur
            becomes louder on inspiration, especially when the patient is standing.
         c. When AR is also present; in one series, 50% of patients with VSD plus AR were
            found to have infundibular obstruction (30).
            Note: Very commonly, AR develops in patients with subpulmonic
                   (supracristal) VSDs because the right coronary cusp of the aortic valve
                   prolapses through the defect.
5. What hemodynamic problem should you suspect if a large VSD is suggested by x-ray
   signs of pulmonary plethora (shunt vascularity) and cardiomegaly yet the murmur is less
   than grade 4/6?
   ANS.: a. Another source of shunt flow through a PDA or an ASD.
         b. Pulmonary hypertension.
         c. Multiple VSDs.
            Note: The patient with multiple VSDs (Swiss cheese defect) usually has a
                   softer murmur than expected (e.g., grade 3/6 or less), even though such
                   patients usually have a large shunt (34). This softer murmur may result
                   because
                   a. These are muscular defects and thus tend to close off during the end
                      of systole.
                   b. Each individual hole may produce a moderately loud murmur, but two
                      moderately loud murmurs may not necessarily combine to make a
                      louder murmur because each one may transmit its sound to a different
                      place on the chest wall or be maximally loud at a different frequency.
6. What is meant by "maladie de Roger"?
   ANS.: In 1861 the French pediatrician Henri Roger presented the first comprehensive de-
         scription of an *asymptomatic* VSD and described the murmur through the defect
         as loud and long, with its maximum intensity over the upper third of the medial
         precordial area (131). The expression is now used to refer to a small VSD with a
         loud murmur at the left lower sternal border. Roger, however, neither specified the
         size of the VSD nor placed the murmur at the lower sternal border.

The VSD Murmur Versus the MR Murmur

1. When does the effect of amyl nitrite on the VSD murmur differ from that on the MR murmur?

ANS.: Amyl nitrite causes all MR and uncomplicated VSD murmurs to become softer. However, amyl nitrite usually does not affect pulmonary artery pressure unless there is vasospastic constriction. In the presence of pulmonary artery constriction amyl nitrite may dilate the pulmonary arterioles and diminish pulmonary resistance *even more than systemic resistance*. The murmur, therefore, then becomes louder or stays the same. This may be used as a test for fixed pulmonary resistance with VSDs, because severe pulmonary hypertension fixed by hypertrophy or obliteration is not affected by amyl nitrite and the murmur becomes softer due to the fall in systemic resistance (129).

> *Note*: The combination of a VSD and MR is so rare that when it is found you should strongly suspect the presence of a corrected transposition in which the left AV valve (tricuspid valve) is incompetent (79).

2. When may a VSD murmur be loudest near the apex?

ANS.: When the ventricular septum ruptures because of infarction; it may do so in the muscle near the apex and mimic an MR murmur.

> *Note*: The murmur of a VSD due to a rupture is not loudest *exactly* at the apex; with careful attention it will be found to be louder slightly medial to the apex. The murmur of MR is usually also not loudest *exactly* at the apex, but with careful attention it will be found to be louder slightly lateral to the apex. If you compare the slightly lateral position with a slightly medial position to the maximum impulse, you will be able to distinguish a ruptured septum from MR. Furthermore, papillary muscle ruptures rarely have a grade 4/6 murmur, but about 50% of VSD murmurs have a murmur this loud. Also, a VSD due to a ruptured septum commonly has a presystolic murmur that is of medium to high frequency (41). If a congenital VSD is so large that it is functionally a single ventricle, a presystolic murmur is also often heard.

CONTINUOUS MURMURS

Definitions and Causes

1. What are the two definitions of a continuous murmur?

ANS.: a. The murmur never stops; that is, it is truly continuous throughout systole and diastole.

b. The murmur can be heard to go beyond the S_2 but stops before the next S_1; that is, it is not truly continuous but does envelop the second sound and go more than slightly beyond it (Fig. 19).

2. What is a systolic and diastolic murmur heard in the same area called if it is not continuous?

ANS.: A to-and-fro murmur. This implies that the systolic component is due to blood flowing in one direction and the diastolic murmur is due to flow in the opposite direction (e.g., an AS ejection murmur plus an AR murmur). (See Fig. 11 on page 301.) A continuous murmur, on the other hand, implies a murmur that is due to continuous flow in the same direction in both systole and diastole.

> *Note*: The systolic murmurs of a VSD or MR plus an AR diastolic murmur are also to-and-fro murmurs; that is, the forward and backward flow does not have to be through the same orifice.

3. When are continuous murmurs not due to regurgitation?

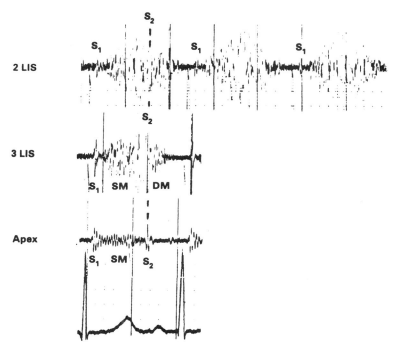

FIG. 19. Phonocardiograms from a patient with a PDA. The S₃ at the apex marks the beginning of diastole for the tracings of the continuous murmur, which envelops and obliterates the second sound at the left sternal border. This murmur did not sound truly continuous at the third left interspace (3 LIS) since it seemed to end in middiastole. The pulmonary artery systolic pressure was 35 mm Hg. The pulmonary flow was slightly more than twice the systemic flow.

    ANS.: Continuous murmurs may be caused by

        a. Partial obstruction to a vessel, as in bilateral peripheral pulmonary artery stenosis, or the collateral venous drainage caused by portal vein obstruction (heard in the epigastrium).

        b. Excessively rapid flow through tortuous vessels, as in

           1. Bronchial collateral circulation in cyanotic congenital heart disease with severe obstruction to pulmonary artery flow.

           2. An arteriovenous fistula, either pulmonary artery to pulmonary vein or internal mammary to adjacent vein.

           3. Large subcostal collaterals in coarctation of the aorta.

           4. Torrential venous flow as in

              (a) Total anomalous pulmonary venous drainage or connection into a left vertical vein (sometimes referred to as a left superior vena cava). See p. 275.

              (b) The venous hum in the neck or groin.

4. List the causes of continuous murmurs transmitted to the chest from the neck.

    ANS.: Those due to transmission from above the clavicle are

        a. The venous hum in children (see p. 272).

        b. An arteriovenous fistula in the neck, either congenital or acquired (usually by trauma).

     c. A partial subclavian artery obstruction due to atherosclerosis, with poor collateral circulation beyond the obstruction (113).

5. List the continuous murmurs involving the thoracic aorta besides PDA, coarctation collaterals, and the mammary souffle.

    ANS.: a. An aortic-pulmonary septal defect (see p. 272).

       b. An internal mammary-to-pulmonary vein fistula.

       c. A rupture of a sinus of Valsalva into the pulmonary artery, right atrium, or ventricle.

        Note: The continuous murmur of a ruptured sinus of Valsalva into the right heart is unlike a PDA murmur in that it does not peak before or after the S_2 and tends instead to be louder in systole or diastole, often creating the impression of a to-and-fro murmur.

6. List the intracardiac causes of continuous murmurs.

    ANS.: a. Flow through a small ASD in the presence of a high left atrial pressure due to MS. (An ASD with rheumatic MS is called Lutembacher syndrome.)

       b. Coronary artery to right heart fistula. (See p. 276.)

       c. A cor triatriatum.[1] A continuous murmur high in the left axilla has been noted in one such patient (54).

        Note: The descent of the base (mitral valve ring) during ventricular systole probably causes the systolic component of the murmur in cor triatriatum (i.e., from a "suction effect" by the decrease in pressure between the accessory chamber and the true left atrial chamber). This murmur is intermediate in frequency between that of an MS diastolic rumble and an aortic regurgitation high-frequency murmur (122).

7. Why should you search for a continuous murmur in the arms, legs, or abdomen in any patient in whom peripheral venous congestion (high venous pressure and peripheral edema) of obscure etiology is present?

    ANS.: A search must be made for an arteriovenous fistula, congenital or traumatic. If such a fistula is large (1 cm or more in diameter), signs and symptoms of failure may occur over a period of years.

       Note: This is a high-output type of failure without actual myocardial insufficiency. The arteriovenous shunt causes a low peripheral resistance for which the body tries to compensate by increasing blood volume and filling pressure. The sympathetic outflow that causes the high venous pressure may increase peripheral resistance. This in turn creates more shunt flow, causing a vicious cycle of more increase in blood volume and venous pressure until peripheral edema occurs.

8. What is the most common cause of a continuous murmur?

    ANS.: Persistent ductus arteriosus (usually called patent ductus arteriosus or PDA).

       Note: A ductus is patent or it is not a ductus. Therefore, it is more logical to use the term **persistent ductus arteriosus** than the term **patent ductus arteriosus**.

---

[1]Cor triatriatum is a congenital cardiac anomaly in which all the pulmonary veins join together to form a common chamber and empty into the left atrium through a small opening; that is, it is a kind of supravalvular mitral stenosis. The common chamber is usually situated inside the left atrium. Its major complication is secondary pulmonary hypertension.

Persistent Ductus Arteriosus Murmur

Shape and Duration

1. What are some of the other names for the continuous murmur of PDA when it is truly continuous?

   ANS.: Machinery murmur or Gibson murmur (37).

   > *Note*: A PDA murmur is continuous because there is a continuous aortic-pulmonary pressure gradient throughout both systole and diastole (if the pulmonary artery pressure is not far from normal).

2. When is the continuous murmur of PDA not "machinery" in quality or duration?

   ANS.: When it is not truly continuous; that is, when it begins slightly after the S_1 and crescendos to the S_2, ending after a short decrescendo in early or middiastole.

   > *Note*: a. About half of PDA murmurs in children are not truly continuous, and many are only pansystolic, exactly mimicking a VSD murmur. This is because with the aortic-pulmonary vasoconstriction secondary to the shunt, there is often moderate pulmonary hypertension that decreases the aortic-pulmonary artery gradient more in diastole than in systole. The low aortic pressure of infants and children, plus the reflex low diastolic pressure caused by the effect of a large volume of blood on the carotid sinus, tends to decrease the gradient further. When only a long systolic murmur is present, differentiation from a VSD is difficult. In any child with a VSD type of pansystolic murmur, a bounding pulse with a pulse pressure of more than 50 mm Hg should make you strongly suspect either a PDA or a PDA in addition to a VSD (105).
   >
   > b. Raising the aortic pressure with methoxamine or ephedrine is an excellent way of bringing out the continuous nature of the murmur. However, if norepinephrine is used, the murmurs may disappear altogether because the pulmonary artery pressure may increase more than the systemic pressure, presumably because the reactive pulmonary hypertensive arterioles are extremely sensitive to norepinephrine.
   >
   > c. The combination of clenched fists, overlapping fingers, rocker-bottom feet, and excessively wrinkled skin in infants with trisomy 16 to 18 suggests that both a PDA and a VSD are present.

3. Until what age is the aortic-pulmonary gradient usually small enough to prevent the diastolic component of the PDA murmur, so that only a VSD-like pansystolic murmur is heard?

   ANS.: Up to 1 year, the thick fetal pulmonary arterioles may not have involuted enough to keep the pulmonary artery pressure normal as it tries to accommodate the increased shunt flow. Despite this, about a third of newborns with PDA are said to have a continuous murmur (with a short diastolic component) for at least a few hours while the fetal ductus is still patent (it normally remains patent for about a week), and many typical PDA murmurs begin at age 6 weeks (11).

   > *Note*: A right-to-left shunt occurs in about 12% of newborns for a few hours, especially when they are crying (81).

4. Where in systole does the typical PDA murmur reach its maximum intensity?

   ANS.: It is crescendo to a peak at or slightly before the S_2; then it is decrescendo to beyond the S_2.

   > *Note*: a. The aortic-pulmonary gradient does not accurately reflect the shape of the murmur because the gradient is maximum in midsystole and the

murmur is maximum in late systole. A murmur shape is more related to the acceleration of flow than it is to gradient. The earlier the systolic peak, the greater the caliber of the ductus, as shown by the finding that when the shunt is large, the peak of the murmur occurs well before the A_2.

    b. If the PDA is in the low-pressure area distal to the site of an aortic coarctation, a continuous murmur may still be present, because despite the low pulse pressure, the mean pressure beyond the coarctation is almost the same as normal aortic mean pressure (23).

Loudness and Site

1. Where is a PDA murmur heard (a) loudest and (b) next loudest?
   ANS.: a. Loudest in the second left interspace.
       b. Next loudest in the first left interspace.
           Note: a. With a right-sided aortic arch, the PDA murmur may be best heard in the first or second *right* interspace.
               b. If the cause of the continuous murmur is not a PDA but some other cause in the chest or heart, the next loudest area is the third left interspace.
2. What can make a PDA murmur disappear transiently without any change in pulmonary artery pressure?
   ANS.: a. Some ducti are thought to kink or undergo spasm and so close off. One such ductus murmur paradoxically diminished with methoxamine (101). Another one intermittently disappeared with no constant maneuver; a slightly angulated course was found at surgery (113). In another case a valvelike structure was found inside the ductus (61).
           Note: a. Permanent closure of PDAs can occur with endarteritis due to infective endocarditis or with atheromatous thrombosis.
               b. A PDA murmur may be masked by an unimportant aortic stenosis and regurgitation.
       b. The most difficult differential diagnosis between a to-and-fro murmur and a continuous PDA murmur is when there is a small VSD with a crescendo murmur to the A_2, together with the decrescendo murmur of AR.

Other Auscultatory Signs of PDA

1. Explain the effect on the typical PDA murmur of (a) a vasopressor agent such as methoxamine and (b) a vasodilator such as amyl nitrite.
   ANS.: a. A vasopressor increases the murmur because it increases the aortic-pulmonary gradient.
       b. Amyl nitrite decreases the murmur because it decreases the gradient.
           Note: In the presence of hyperkinetic pulmonary hypertension, amyl nitrite may increase a PDA murmur because it may relax the hyperactive pulmonary arterioles more than it diminishes the peripheral system resistance.
2. List the auscultatory signs of a large PDA shunt flow besides the continuous murmur.
   ANS.: a. A paradoxically split S_2.
       b. A mitral diastolic murmur or even an opening snap due to an excess flow through the mitral valve.

c. Multiple systolic clicks or crackles (sometimes called "eddy sounds"), especially in the second half of systole and in early diastole.

> *Note*: Eddy sounds have been theorized to be a "head-on" collision of streams from the ductus and the pulmonary artery. They are usually heard only in large-flow ducti and may be present even if the diastolic component of the murmur is absent or very short (48).

PDA with High Pulmonary Artery Pressure

1. By inspection alone, how can you tell that a reversed shunt flow is through a PDA rather than at the atrial or ventricular level; that is, how can you differentiate between the Eisenmenger syndromes?

   ANS.: The feet may be more cyanotic and clubbed than the hands. This is known as **differential cyanosis and clubbing**. (See Fig. 17.)

   > *Note*: The differential cyanosis can be brought out by raising the pulmonary artery pressure still more with exercise.
   >
   > The ductus often joins the pulmonary artery to the aorta just beyond the left subclavian artery. Unsaturated pulmonary artery blood then passes beyond the left subclavian artery, and both hands are less clubbed and cyanotic than the feet. If, however, the ductus is at the junction of the aorta and the left subclavian artery, this artery may also receive unsaturated blood, and the left hand will be as cyanotic and clubbed as the feet.

2. Which component of the continuous murmur is the first to disappear as pulmonary artery pressure rises due to pulmonary hypertension?

   ANS.: The diastolic component disappears first because the diastolic gradient disappears first.

   > *Note*: There is a report of one adult patient whose systolic murmur disappeared with hyperkinetic pulmonary hypertension and a large left-to-right shunt. Only a pandiastolic murmur remained (84).

PDA Versus Aortic-Pulmonary Septal Defect Murmurs

1. What is meant by an aortic-pulmonary septal defect (sometimes called "aortic-pulmonary window")?

   ANS.: It is an opening between the ascending aorta and the pulmonary artery about 1 cm above the pulmonary valves.

2. What auscultatory clues are there to differentiate a PDA from an aortic-pulmonary septal defect murmur?

   ANS.: Although the site of maximum loudness may be at the second left interspace in both, the next loudest site in PDA is usually one interspace higher, whereas the aortic-pulmonary septal defect murmur is more likely to be second loudest one interspace lower.

   > *Note*: There is more likely to be a continuous murmur in PDA than in an aortic-pulmonary septal defect, because only about 15% of aortic-pulmonary septal defects are small enough to have pulmonary artery pressures that are sufficiently low to allow a continuous murmur (80).

The Venous Hum

1. Where is a venous hum best heard?

   ANS.: Just above the clavicle either medial to the sternocleidomastoid or between its insertions. It is best heard on the right side of the neck.

Note: A venous hum is more likely to be heard on the right side because the right jugular is larger than the left, since it carries about two-thirds of the intracranial venous drainage.

2. What does a venous hum sound like?

ANS.: Sometimes it is like a continuous roar; at other times it is like "the sound of the sea" heard by putting a seashell to the ear. Sometimes it is a whining sound. The diastolic component is often higher pitched and louder than the systolic. Probably the only quality that is *never* present is that of an actual hum.

3. What causes the venous hum?

ANS.: Two theories have been proposed.

a. Turbulence caused by a confluence of flow through the internal jugular and subclavian veins as they pour into the superior vena cava.

b. Anterior angulation of the internal jugular vein by the transverse process of the atlas (24). (This angulation and the murmur can be shown to increase by turning the head away from the side of the hum.)

4. How can you elicit a venous hum if you cannot hear it by merely placing the stethoscope on the neck?

ANS.: a. Ask the patient to sit up with his feet on the bed to bring maximum blood volume to the heart from both the lower body and head.

b. Apply the bell lightly to the right side of the neck, as closely as possible to the clavicle and anterior border of the sternocleidomastoid muscle or between its insertions. A small bell may be necessary to maintain a good air seal without excess pressure. Too much pressure eliminates the hum.

c. Turn the patient's head away. When maximum rotation is reached, raise the chin as high as possible (Fig. 20).

d. When a continuous roar or whine is heard, test for the presence of a hum by applying moderate pressure with the fingers a few inches above the stethoscope. A venous hum disappears with moderate pressure on the internal jugular vein.

5. What is the significance of a venous hum that can be heard without head turning?

ANS.: It suggests that the circulation time may be faster than normal.

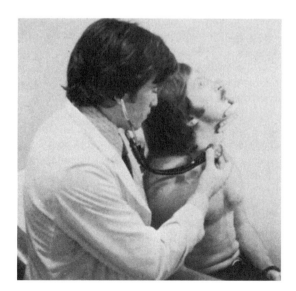

FIG. 20. A small bell is invaluable in enabling you to apply airtight light pressure anterior to the sternocleidomastoid muscle.

Note: a. An unelicited venous hum is commonly found in young children but only in about 10% of normal subjects over age 50. In about half of subjects over age 50, however, it can be elicited only by rotating and raising the head. The unelicited venous hum is of most help in confirming the presence of hyperthyroidism in the young and in suggesting the diagnosis of apathetic hyperthyroidism in the elderly, i.e., hyperthyroidism with no apparent symptoms or signs of thyrotoxicosis and often with atrial fibrillation (26). The nonelicited venous hum is also common in patients with severe uremia with a low hematocrit and also in pregnant women.

   b. If a venous hum is not only unelicited but actually difficult to obliterate, it is almost pathognomonic of a very rapid circulation time, as in thyrotoxicosis. A venous hum (continuous murmur) can also be heard over the femoral veins if the circulation is hyperkinetic (120).

   c. Although a venous hum should always be expected if you are diagnosing hyperthyroidism, the hum may disappear if heart failure slows venous flow.

   d. Although most thyroid bruits are actually venous hums, there are some in which you can obliterate the hum, and underneath a continuous murmur is located over the gland.

6. What are the methods of eliminating the venous hum besides applying pressure above the stethoscope?

   ANS.: Turn the patient's head toward the side of the hum or decrease venous return from the jugulars by placing the patient in a supine position.

   Note: a. When the diastolic component of a venous hum is high-pitched, it can be transmitted to the upper chest and may mimic AR. This hum is especially likely to be mistaken for AR because only the diastolic component of the hum may be transmitted downward. Such false AR can be found in approximately 10% of subjects with severe uremia and anemia who have a venous hum.

   b. Anemia alone may also cause a loud venous hum. One patient with a hematocrit of 30% had a venous hum that was heard by the patient himself as a loud roaring in both ears (40).

   c. A venous hum is common in the inguinal area in normal subjects in the supine position.

7. What besides the venous hum might cause a supraclavicular continuous murmur?

   ANS.: a. A traumatic or congenital arteriovenous fistula.

   b. Partial obstruction of any of the arteries arising from the aorta (aortic arch syndromes).

   Note: A continuous murmur due to aortic branch stenosis means that there is poor collateral circulation distal to the obstruction. (Good collateral circulation would raise the pressure enough distal to the obstruction to prevent a continuous gradient across the obstruction.)

8. When does a venous hum mimic a PDA?

   ANS.: If, as in some children, the total venous hum is transmitted downward to the upper chest.

   Note: a. The continuous murmur in some small tortuous PDAs may disappear in a sitting position. A venous hum responds in the opposite way to changes in posture (123).

    b. In patients with total anomalous pulmonary venous connection with a left vertical vein (which in turn drains into the innominate vein), the torrential flow may produce a continuous murmur like a venous hum that may be loudest slightly lower than the second left interspace (16). This may be due to partial obstruction of the vertical vein between the pulmonary artery and the left main bronchus (55). A continuous murmur of a venous hum may be audible in the first and second right interspace in these patients, probably due to an anomalous connection to the superior vena cava.

    c. The venous hum tends to increase with inspiration and in diastole, during which the pitch may be higher than in systole.

    d. The venous hum never radiates below the clavicle in adults.

Continuous Murmurs of Pulmonary Artery and Pulmonary Artery Branch Stenosis

1. What is necessary before a pulmonary artery stenosis can produce a continuous murmur? (This does not refer to pulmonary *valve* stenosis.)

    ANS.: The pulmonary artery stenosis must be multiple, causing pulmonary hypertension proximal to the obstruction. Experimentally, a continuous murmur can be produced by stenosis in a pulmonary artery only if the opposite artery is clamped (28).

        Note: a. You should suspect multiple pulmonary artery branch stenosis if you diagnose severe pulmonary hypertension with or without cyanosis and hear a continuous murmur over the posterior chest wall as well as anteriorly, especially if there is a normal main pulmonary artery on the x-ray (112).

           b. If there are severe multiple pulmonary artery stenoses, the continuous murmur may be due to enlarged, tortuous bronchial arteries supplying the lungs.

2. Where is a continuous murmur sometimes heard if a large pulmonary embolus causes partial obstruction of a left pulmonary artery?

    ANS.: Under the left scapula. It may increase with inspiration.

        Note: A thoracic aortic aneurysm can cause a continuous pulmonary arterial murmur by compressing a pulmonary artery so that there is a continuous gradient across the narrowed area.

Pulmonary Arteriovenous Fistulas

1. What is meant by a pulmonary arteriovenous fistula?

    ANS.: This is a right-to-left shunt from the pulmonary artery to a pulmonary vein, usually congenital.

2. What is the effect of respiration and body position on the continuous murmur of a pulmonary arteriovenous fistula?

    ANS.: Inspiration usually makes the murmur louder because it increases the pulmonary artery-to-pulmonary vein pressure gradient. Compression of the fistula caused by lying on the side of the malformation or by elevating the diaphragm by lying supine may attenuate or eliminate the murmur (42).

        Note: a. A continuous murmur is heard in only about two-thirds of patients with this fistula.

           b. Diagnostic clues by inspection alone are cyanosis and clubbing as well as telangiectasis on the skin or mucous membranes (Rendu-Osler-Weber disease).

Continuous Murmur of Bronchopulmonary Anastomoses

1. What should you suspect as a cause of a continuous murmur that is heard bilaterally in a patient with cyanosis and an x-ray that suggests no pulmonary artery at all?
   ANS.: Large bronchial arteries supplying the lungs in a patient with
   a. A persistent truncus arteriosus with small pulmonary arteries, or
   b. A solitary arterial trunk with pulmonary atresia.
2. What is suggested as a cause of a unilateral continuous murmur in a cyanotic patient with a PS murmur?
   ANS.: A tetralogy of Fallot with
   a. An absent pulmonary artery on one side. The continuous murmur may then be due to bronchial collateral circulation on that side.
   b. One pulmonary artery arising from the aorta.
   c. A PDA. However, a continuous murmur with uncomplicated tetralogy of Fallot is more likely to be due to the bronchial collateral circulation associated with pulmonary atresia because a PDA with an uncomplicated tetralogy of Fallot is very rare (14,87).
   Note: A continuous murmur in a cyanotic newborn may be due to mitral atresia with a forced left-to-right flow through a small ASD or stretched foramen ovale.

Continuous Murmurs of Coronary Artery or Aorta to Right Heart Fistulas

1. What, besides an aortic-pulmonary septal defect, can cause a continuous murmur that has either the maximum intensity or the second loudest area lower than the second left interspace?
   ANS.: a. A left or right coronary artery (usually dilated) that communicates with the coronary vein, right atrium, RV, or pulmonary artery.
   b. Rupture of a sinus of Valsalva into the right atrium or RV.
   Note: a. Both these lesions tend to produce diastolic accentuation of the murmur. But the murmur due to rupture of the sinus of Valsalva tends to be much louder than the coronary artery murmur and often has a cooing or musical quality. Look for a dicrotic pulse (see p. 40), which is very common in subjects with rupture of a sinus of Valsalva (79).
   b. The anomalous coronary artery to right heart fistula usually produces diastolic accentuation of the continuous murmur because there is more coronary flow in diastole than in systole.
   c. An anomalous left coronary artery originating from the pulmonary artery may occasionally produce in the adult a to-and-fro murmur, which is best heard at the fourth left interspace. If a vasopressor agent such as methoxamine causes the diastolic component to decrease, it suggests that most of the collaterals are passing through the ventricular septum and are squeezed off (132).
   d. A right coronary artery fistula to the LV may produce only a diastolic murmur that may be maximal at the apex or over the lower sternal border (59,117). It may, however, produce a to-and-fro murmur in which

the diastolic component is dominant and maximal in the epigastrium (82).

 e. If the continuous murmur is soft and is due to a left-coronary-artery-to-pulmonary-artery fistula, only the diastolic component may be heard at the third or fourth interspace, and that may mimic AR (50).

2. Which abnormal drainage areas of the coronary artery are suggested by a continuous murmur that is loudest at the (a) second or third right interspace, (b) second left interspace, (c) left lower sternal border, (d) upper sternum, and (e) lower sternum? (This question is for reference purposes and not for memorization.)

 ANS.: a. Right coronary artery to right atrium (43,63).

 b. Left coronary artery to pulmonary artery (63). Right coronary artery to pulmonary artery (47).

 c. Left coronary artery to pulmonary artery (63). Left coronary artery or circumflex artery to RV (72). Right coronary artery to pulmonary artery, or left coronary artery to left atrium (3).

 d. Right coronary artery to RV (63).

 e. Circumflex artery to coronary sinus (62). Left coronary artery to pulmonary artery or to apex of RV (63). Right coronary artery to coronary sinus or to right atrium (62,78). Left coronary artery to RV (78) (Fig. 21).

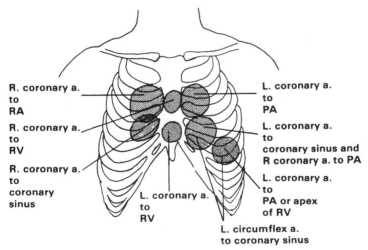

FIG. 21. Coronary artery fistules often give a clue to their site of drainage by the site of the loudest murmur.

 Note: Even if the murmur is loudest at the left lower sternal border, if it transmits well to the *right* lower sternal border or if only the diastolic component is louder to the right of the sternum, it should still suggest a shunt from the right coronary artery to the right atrium or ventricle (15,43).

3. Why may a rupture of a sinus of Valsalva into the RV produce diastolic accentuation of the continuous murmur?

 ANS.: The muscular walls encircling the orifice of the communication may relax in diastole, allowing more regurgitation (12).

Note: Because a continuous murmur that has a louder diastolic component than a systolic component is an important differentiation point from PDA, it is occasionally useful to use a maneuver that makes the diastolic component louder than the systolic if the murmur is not due to a PDA. Raising the systemic pressure by a post-Valsalva effect or isometric handgrip increases all diastolic components of a continuous murmur if the murmur is due to a sinus of Valsalva that has ruptured into the RV. If the diastolic components decrease with these maneuvers, suspect a coronary artery-to-right-heart fistula with collaterals passing through the ventricular septum.

4. Where is the continuous murmur loudest if a sinus of Valsalva ruptures into (a) the RV or (b) the right atrium?

   ANS.: a. If the sinus ruptures into the RV, the murmur is loudest at the third left or right interspace or at the left sternal border.

   b. If it ruptures into the right atrium, the murmur is loudest in the lower left or right sternal border or in the epigastrium (110).

   Note: If on turning the patient into the right lateral decubitus position the murmur is directed into the right chest, a communication with the right atrium is likely.

Continuous Murmurs of Coarctation

1. What causes the continuous murmur in coarctation?

   ANS.: Although the systolic and diastolic pressure gradient across a severe coarctation has been shown by intraaortic phonocardiography to produce a continuous murmur, collateral intercostal vessel flow is probably the most likely cause of a continuous murmur heard in coarctation. In mild or moderate coarctation, there is only a systolic murmur over the area of actual coarctation (just left of the vertebrae at midthorax level).

2. What is the clue for differentiating a PDA murmur from a coarctation murmur by auscultation of the posterior chest?

   ANS.: If the murmur is heard just as easily or even more easily over the posterior chest, it is much more likely to be due to coarctation (i.e., either to the collateral circulation on the chest wall or to the coarctation itself).

   Note: If a continuous murmur is heard only over the lower two or three ribs posteriorly, you should suspect an abdominal coarctation.

The Mammary Souffle

1. What is the cause of the mammary souffle?

   ANS.: It is a continuous arterial murmur due to a large flow into the breast during pregnancy and lactation, heard in a minority of pregnant women.

   Note: a. That the murmur arises in the superficial arteries of the breast is shown by the observation that firm pressure with the stethoscope or manual pressure lateral to the stethoscope can abolish the murmur. Its high pitch, systolic accentuation, and absence of any effect of a Valsalva maneuver suggests further that it is an arterial rather than a venous murmur. It is usually heard along the left sternal border, and it is rarely more than grade 4/6. It may disappear when the patient sits up.

b. There is a delay between the S_1 and the murmur, which often spills over the S_2 into early diastole. The delay is due to the time that must elapse before blood ejected from the LV arrives at the mammary arteries. Therefore, it must be distinguished from other causes of continuous murmurs. It may be systolic, to-and-fro, or continuous. It is more common on the left than on the right.

2. In which trimester of pregnancy does the mammary souffle begin, and how long does it last postpartum?

ANS.: Although it usually begins in the second or third trimester, it may not begin until the first postpartum week. It usually lasts from several weeks to 2 months postpartum.

REFERENCES

1. Agarwal AK. A new observation on capillary muscle dysfunction. *Chest* 1982;82:130.
2. Alexander MD, et al. Atrial septal aneurysm: A cause for midsystolic click. *Circulation* 1981;63:1186.
3. Arani DT, et al. Coronary artery fistulas emptying into left heart chambers. *Am Heart J* 1978;96:438.
4. Aravanis C. Silent mitral insufficiency. *Am Heart J* 1965;70:620.
5. Auger P, Wigle ED. Sudden, severe mitral insufficiency. *Can Med Assoc J* 1967;96:1493.
6. Barlow JB, et al. Late systolic murmurs and nonejection systolic clicks. *Br Heart J* 1968;30:203.
7. Beck W, et al. Hemodynamic effects of amyl nitrite and phenylephrine on the normal circulation. *Am J Cardiol* 1961;8:341.
8. Beck W, et al. The value of phonocardiography in the assessment of surgical closure of ventricular septal defect. *Am Heart J* 1964;67:742.
9. Bergland JM, et al. Pre-excitation as a cause of appearance and increased intensity of systolic murmurs. *Circulation* 1966;33:131.
10. Brown AK, Anderson V. Normal and prolapsed tricuspid valve leaflets. *Am J Cardiol* 1984;54:546.
11. Burnard ED. A murmur from the ductus arteriosus in the newborn baby. *Br Med J* 1958;1:806.
12. Buzzi A. Evaluation of a precordial continuous murmur. *Am J Cardiol* 1959;4:551.
13. Call T, et al. Cardiac defects in the Ehlers-Danlos syndrome. *Circulation* (Abstr) 1977;55(Suppl III):69.
14. Campbell M, Deuchar DC. Continuous murmurs in cyanotic congenital heart disease. *Br Heart J* 1961;12:173.
15. Carmichael DB, Davison DG. Congenital coronary arteriovenous fistula. *Am J Cardiol* 1961;8:846.
16. Carter REB, et al. Total anomalous pulmonary venous drainage. *Br Heart J* 1969;31:45.
17. Cha SD, et al. Intracardiac phonocardiography in tricuspid regurgitation. *Am J Cardiol* 1981;48:578.
18. Cheng TO. Characterization of late systolic murmur associated with coronary artery disease. *Circulation* (Abstr) 1971;43(Suppl II):31.
19. Cheng TO. Late systolic murmur in coronary artery disease. *Chest* 1972;61:346.
20. Cho K, et al. Tricuspid whoop: An autopsied case. *CV Sound Bull* 1974;4:655.
21. Chun PKC. Nonejection systolic click in mitral stenosis. *Am Heart J* 1981;3:463.
22. Chrysant SG, Frohlich ED. Autonomic sympathetic adjustments in patients with labile and fixed hypertension. *World Congress Cardiol* Tokyo, 1978:982.
23. Crevasse LE, Logue RB. Atypical patent ductus arteriosus. *Circulation* 1959;19:332.
24. Cutforth R, et al. The genesis of the cervical venous hum. *Am Heart J* 1970;80:488.
25. Dock W. Production of systolic clicks. *Arch Intern Med* 1973;132:114.
26. Dougherty MJ, Craige E. Apathetic hyperthyroidism presenting as tricuspid regurgitation. *Chest* 1973;63:767.
27. Ehlers KH, et al. Left ventricular abnormality with late mitral insufficiency. *Am J Cardiol* 1970;26:333.
28. Eldridge F, et al. Stenosis of a branch of the pulmonary artery. *Circulation* 1957;15:865.
29. Ewing DJ, et al. Static exercise in untreated systemic hypertension. *Br Heart J* 1973;35:413.
30. Farru O, et al. Auscultatory and phonocardiographic characteristics of supracristal ventricular defect. *Br Heart J* 1971;33:238.
31. Felner JM, et al. Systolic honks in young children. *Am J Cardiol* 1977;40:206.
32. Fox MB. Clicking pneumothorax. *Lancet* 1948;1:210.
33. Freedom RM, et al. The natural history of the so-called aneurysm of the membranous septum in childhood. *Circulation* 1974;40:375.
34. Friedman WF, et al. Multiple muscular ventricular septal defects. *Circulation* 1965;32:35.
35. Fujii J, et al. Echocardiographic and phonocardiographic study on the genesis of the musical murmur. *J Cardiol* 1976;6:385.
36. Fulkerson PK, et al. Calcification of the mitral annulus: Etiology, clinical associations, and therapy. *Am J Med* 1979;66:967.
37. Gibson GA. Clinical lectures on circulatory affections. *Edin Med J* 1900;8:1.

38. Gooch AS, et al. The use of hepatic pressure maneuver to identify the murmur of tricuspid regurgitation. *Clin Cardiol* 1983;6:277.
39. Hancock EW, Cohn K. The syndrome associated with the midsystolic click and late systolic murmur. *Am J Med* 1966;41:183.
40. Hardison JE, et al. Self-heard venous hums. *JAMA* 1981;1245:1146.
41. Haze K. et al. Interventricular septal perforation secondary to acute infarction. *CV Sound Bull* 1975;5:593.
42. Hazlett DR, Medina J. Postural effects on the bruit and right-to-left shunt of pulmonary arteriovenous fistula. *Chest* 1971;60:89.
43. Heidenreich RP, et al. A case of anomalous right coronary artery to right atrial fistula presenting as atypical coronary insufficiency. *Am J Cardiol* 1969;23:453.
44. Heikkila J. Mitral incompetence complicating acute myocardial infarction. *Br Heart J* 1967;29:162.
45. Hollman A, et al. Auscultatory and phonocardiographic findings in ventricular septal defects. *Circulation* 1963;28:94.
46. Honda M, et al. Observations of tapping sounds in pneumothorax. *J Cardiol* 1977;7:7.
47. Huang MTC, et al. Left and right coronary artery-pulmonary artery fistula. *N Y State J Med* 1979;79:1774.
48. Hubbard TF, Neis DD. The sounds at the base of the heart in patent ductus arteriosus. *Am Heart J* 1960;59:807.
49. Iemoto T, et al. An autopsied case of papillary muscle dysfunction with midsystolic click and late systolic honk. *CV Sound Bull* 1974;4:633.
50. Ishikawa T, et al. A case of coronary artery-to-pulmonary artery fistula. *J Cardiol* 1976;6:169.
51. Ishimitsu T, et al. Is this mitral valve prolapse? A case of mitral regurgitation with early systolic murmur due to early systolic prolapse of the posterior leaflet. *J Cardiol* 1989;19(Suppl XXI):97.
52. Isner JM, et al. Systolic click from a Swan-Ganz catheter. *Am J Cardiol* 1979;43:1046.
53. January LE, et al. Mitral insufficiency resulting from rupture of normal chordae tendineae. *Circulation* 1962;26:1329.
54. Jegier W, et al. Cor triatriatum: Surgical correction in early life. *Pediatrics* 1963;31:255.
55. Jensen JB. Total anomalous pulmonary venous return. *Am Heart J* 1971;82:387
56. Jeresaty RM. Mitral valve prolapse-click syndrome. *Progr Cardiovasc Dis* 1973;15:623.
57. Karliner JS, et al. Haemodynamic explanation of why the murmur of mitral regurgitation is independent of cycle length. *Br Heart J* 1973;35:397.
58. Kasai A, et al. Clinical evaluation of severe idiopathic tricuspid regurgitation. *J Cardiol* 1990;20:937.
59. Kawasaki S, et al. A phonocardiographic study of two cases of congenital coronary artery fistula. *CV Sound Bull* 1974;4:603.
60. Keenan TJ, Schwartz MJ. Tricuspid whoop. *Am Cardiol* 1973;31:642.
61. Keith TR, Sagarminaga J. Spontaneously disappearing murmur of patent ductus arteriosus. *Circulation* 1961;24:1235.
62. Kimbris D, et al. Coronary artery-coronary sinus fistula. *Am J Cardiol* 1970;26:532.
63. Koops B, et al. Congenital coronary artery anomalies. *JAMA* 1973;226:1425.
64. Kubota K, et al. Echocardiographic follow-up of mitral valve prolapse associated with atrial septal defect. *J Cardiol* 1979;9:123.
65. Liedtke AJ, Gault JH. Systolic click syndrome. *Circulation* 1973;58:453.
66. Limacher MC, et al. Tricuspid regurgitation during pregnancy: Two-dimensional and pulsed Doppler echocardiographic observations. *Am J Cardiol* 1985;55:1059.
67. Lindgren KM, Epstein SE. Idiopathic hypertrophic subaortic stenosis with and without mitral regurgitation. *Br Heart J* 1972;34:191.
68. Linsenmeyer GJ, et al. Adhesive pericarditis with unusual systolic click. *Am Heart J* 1984;108:1062.
69. Lipp H, et al. Intermittent pansystolic murmur after acute myocardial infarction. *Am J Cardiol* 1972;30:690.
70. Maisel AS. Hepatojugular reflux: Useful in the bedside diagnosis of tricuspid regurgitation? *Ann Intern Med* 1984;101:781.
71. Malcolm AD, et al. Clinical features in the presence of mitral leaflet prolapse. *Br Heart J* 1976;38:244.
72. Maranhao V, et al. Prolapse of the tricuspid leaflets in the murmur-click syndrome. *Cath Cardiovasc Diagn* 1975;1:81.
73. Markiewicz W, et al. Changing hemodynamics in patients with papillary muscle dysfunction. *Br Heart J* 1975;37:445.
74. Matsuhisa M, et al. Midsystolic click and late systolic murmur during inspiration in congenital absence of the pericardium. *J Cardiol* 1981;11:1009.
75. McDonald A, et al. Association of prolapse of posterior cusp of mitral valve and atrial septal defect. *Br Heart J* 1971;33:383.
76. Miki T, et al. Mitral valve prolapse in patients with myocarditis and collagen diseases. *J Cardiol* 1988;18(Suppl. XVIII):85.
77. Mittal AK, et al. Combined papillary muscle and left ventricular wall dysfunction as a cause of mitral regurgitation. *Circulation* 1971;44:174.
78. Morgan J, et al. Anomalies of the aorta and pulmonary arteries complicating ventricular septal defect. *Br Heart J* 1962;24:279.
79. Morgan J, et al. Ruptured aneurysms of the sinus of Valsalva. *Chest* 1972;61:640.

80. Morrow AG, et al. Congenital aortopulmonary septal defect. *Circulation* 1962;25:463.
81. Moss AJ, et al. Closure of the ductus arteriosus in the newborn infant. *Pediatrics* 1963;32:25.
82. Muraki H, Uozumi Z. A case of congenital fistula of right coronary artery to left ventricle. *CV Sound Bull* 1975; 5:159
83. Nakano T, et al. An autopsy case of tricuspid prolapse with special reference to the phonocardiographic and echocardiographic findings. *J Cardiol* 1979;9:133.
84. Nichimura M, et al. Loud holodiastolic murmur in patent ductus arteriosus. *J Cardiol* 1976;6:419.
85. Ochiai M. The relationship between mitral regurgitation and asynergy of the left ventricle in old myocardial infarction. *J Cardiol* 1989;19:775.
86. Oki T, et al. Mitral regurgitation in mitral valve prolapse. Its mechanisms and time course. *J Cardiol* 1987; 17:497.
87. Ongley PA, et al. Continuous murmurs in tetralogy of Fallot and pulmonary atresia. *Am J Cardiol* 1966;18:821.
88. Osterberger LE, et al. Functional mitral stenosis in patients with massive mitral annular calcification. *Circulation* 1981;64:472.
89. Phornphutkul C, et al. Cardiac manifestations of Marfan's syndrome in infancy and childhood. *Circulation* 1973;45:596.
90. Pombo E, et al. Aneurysm of the membranous septum. *Am Heart J* 1970;79:188.
91. Procacci PM, et al. Prevalence of clinical mitral valve prolapse in young women. *N Engl J Med* 1976;294:1086.
92. Ranganathan N, et al. Morphology of the human mitral valve. *Circulation* 1970;41:459.
93. Read RC, et al. Symptomatic valvular myxomatous transformation. *Circulation* 1965;32:897.
94. Rivero-Carvallo JM. Signo para el diagnostico de las insuficiencias tricuspidias. *Arch Inst Cardiol Mexico* 1946;16:531.
95. Rizzon P, et al. The praecordial honk. *Br Heart J* 1971;33:707.
96. Roberts WC. Anomalous left ventricular band. *Am J Cardiol* 1969;23:735.
97. Roberts WC, Perloff JK. Mitral valvular disease. *Ann Intern Med* 1972;77:939.
98. Robertson WS, Tavel ME. Mid-systolic sound associated with aortic insufficiency. *Chest* 1983;83:141.
99. Ronan JA Jr, et al. Effect of simple bedside maneuvers on the isolated systolic click. *Circulation* 1971;43(Suppl. II):105.
100. Sakakibara S, Konno S. Left ventricular-right atrial communication. *Ann Surg* 1963;158:93.
101. Sakamoto T, et al. Atypical response of intermittent continuous murmur of patent ductus arteriosus to vasoactive agents. *Jpn Heart J* 1967;8:318.
102. Salisbury PF, et al. Chordae tendineae tension. *Am J Physiol* 1963;205:385.
103. Sanders CA, et al. Severe mitral regurgitation secondary to ruptured chordae tendineae. *Circulation* 1965; 31:506.
104. Sanderson JN. Handy heart sound simulator. *Am J Cardiol* 1975;36:925.
105. Sasahara AA, et al. Ventricular septal defect with patent ductus arteriosus. *Circulation* 1960;22:254.
106. Scampardonis G, et al. Left ventricular abnormalities in prolapsed mitral leaflet syndrome. *Circulation* 1973; 48:287.
107. Schlesinger Z, et al. An unusual form of mitral valve insufficiency. *Chest* 1970;58:385.
108. Schreiber TL, et al. Effect of atrial septal defect repair on left ventricular geometry. *Circulation* 1980;61:888.
109. Schrire V, et al. Silent mitral incompetence. *Am Heart J* 1961;61:723.
110. Segal BL, et al. Rupture of a sinus of Valsalva aneurysm. *Am J Cardiol* 1963;12:544.
111. Shapiro HA, Weiss DR. Mitral insufficiency due to ruptured chordae tendineae. *N Engl J Med* 1959;261:272.
112. Shapiro W. Unusual experiences with precordial continuous murmurs. *Am J Cardiol* 1961;7:511.
113. Shapiro W, et al. Intermittent disappearance of the murmur of patent ductus. *Circulation* 1960;22:226.
114. Sheikh MU, Ali N. Systolic honk in heart failure: Its origin and mechanism of production. *Clin Cardiol* 1979; 2:52.
115. Sherman WT, et al. Competence of the tricuspid valve in pulmonary heart disease. *Circulation* 1965;31:517.
116. Shimada E, et al. Tricuspid valve prolapse associated with cor pulmonale. *J Cardiol* 1980;10:163.
117. Sonotani N, et al. A case of right coronary artery fistula to the left ventricle. *J Cardiol* 1976;6:573.
118. Steinfeld L, et al. The late systolic murmur of rheumatic regurgitation. *Circulation* 1971;44:106.
119. Steinfeld L, et al. Clinical diagnosis of isolated subpulmonic (supracristal) ventricular septal defect. *Am J Cardiol* 1972;30:19.
120. Strano A, et al. On the peripheral venous murmurs of the circulatory hyperkinetic syndrome. *Angiology* 1966; 17:213.
121. Takahashi T, et al. Echocardiographic features of small heart. *J Cardiol* 1985;15:867.
122. Tanaka M, et al. Acoustic characteristics and genesis of the heart murmur in cor triatriatum. *CV Sound Bull* 1974;4:457.
123. Thapar MK, et al. Changing murmur of patent ductus. *J Pediatr* 1978;92:939.
124. Upshaw CB. Precordial honk due to tricuspid regurgitation. *Am J Cardiol* 1975;35:85.
125. Venkataraman K, et al. Musical murmurs: An echophonocardiographic study. *Am J Cardiol* 1978;41:952.
126. Verani MS, et al. Mitral valve prolapse in coronary artery disease. *Am J Cardiol* 1976;37:1.
127. Vitums V, et al. Bedside maneuvers to augment the murmur of tricuspid regurgitation. *Med Ann DC* 1969; 38:533.

128. Vogelpoel L, et al. The atypical systolic murmur of minute ventricular septal defect. *Am Heart J* 1961;62:101.
129. Vogelpoel L, et al. Variations in the response of the systolic murmur to vasoactive drugs in ventricular septal defect. *Am Heart J* 1962;64:169.
130. Wann LS, et al. Prevalence of mitral prolapse by two-dimensional echocardiography. *Br Heart J* 1983;39:334.
131. Willius FA, Keys TE. *Cardiac Classics*. St. Louis: Mosby, 1941:623.
132. Yanagihara K, et al. Phonocardiographic features of anomalous left coronary artery. *J Cardiol* 1978;8:147.
133. Yoshida K, et al. Silent severe tricuspid regurgitation: A study by Doppler echocardiography. *J Cardiol* 1989; 19:187.

15

Diastolic Murmurs

DIASTOLIC ATRIOVENTRICULAR VALVE MURMURS

Mitral Stenosis Murmurs

Timing and Shape

1. When in the cycle does the diastolic murmur of mitral stenosis (MS) begin? How does it relate to the S_2?

ANS.: It begins just after the opening snap (OS). This means that there must be a pause due to isovolumic relaxation between the A_2 and the diastolic murmur. Because of the pause that usually occurs after the S_2, the MS murmur may be called an early delayed diastolic murmur (Fig. 1).

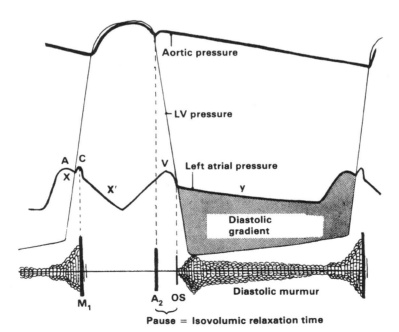

FIG. 1. There should be no mitral valve murmurs between the A_2 and the OS because this is isovolumic relaxation time. Note the slow Y descent of the left atrium due to the difficulty in emptying the left atrium through the stenotic valve. This accounts for the pressure gradient and murmur, both of which are decrescendo except for the very beginning and end.

Note: There often seems to be a slight additional pause between the OS and the diastolic murmur of MS when listening with the stethoscope. Although inflow into the left ventricle (LV) begins as soon as the mitral valve opens, the gradient and flow increase for a short period because the LV is still rapidly expanding. This increase in gradient often shows on a phonocardiogram as a short, early crescendo-decrescendo. We hear the OS and then the peak of the crescendo as if there were a pause between the OS and the beginning of the murmur (Fig. 2).

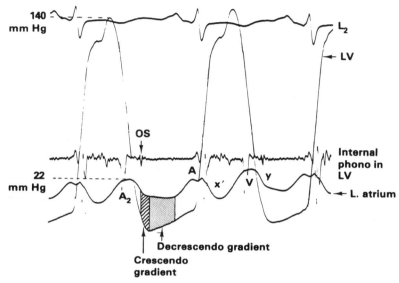

FIG. 2. Phonocardiogram and left atrial and left ventricle pressure tracings from a slightly hypertensive 50-year-old man with a mitral valve that was not calcified but that barely admitted the surgeon's finger. These tracings were taken with equisensitive micromanometers at the tips of the catheters to eliminate any time delays due to tubing. The diastolic murmur (not shown here) follows the gradient and therefore should have a short early crescendo before the decrescendo. This gives a rhythm of "one—two-du huuu" to the heart sounds, opening snap, and murmur. The distance between the "two" and the "du" is the time for isovolumic relaxation. The distance between the "du" and the "huuu" is the time to the peak of the early crescendo. The long 2OS interval of about 90 msec (0.09 sec) in this patient is probably due to his hypertension (see page 173 for explanation).

2. What is the typical shape of the diastolic murmur of MS on auscultation? Why?
   ANS.: After a very short crescendo, there is a decrescendo rumble that ends with a late crescendo up to the M_1. The decrescendo reflects the decrescendo gradient and flow between the left atrium and the LV. The late crescendo has a more complicated explanation (see the following section).

The Crescendo Murmur to the M_1 in Mitral Stenosis ("Presystolic Murmur")

1. What is the appearance of a murmur that is produced by atrial contraction forcing blood through a stenotic mitral valve?

ANS.: Although it should follow the curve of atrial pressure rise and fall (i.e., it should be crescendo-decrescendo), the actual shape is crescendo to the first sound. This murmur is often called "presystolic" (Fig. 3)

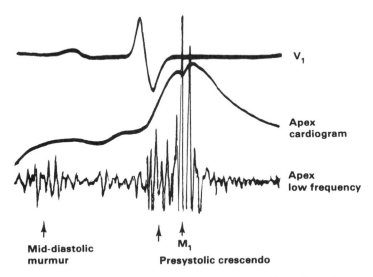

FIG. 3. The "presystolic" murmur in this 45-year-old woman with moderately severe MS begins with the onset of ventricular contraction, as shown by the simultaneous apex cardiogram tracing taken at very fast speed. However, blood is still flowing from the left atrium to the LV until mitral valve closure (M_1). Therefore, cardiologists prefer to consider this period as part of diastole.

2. What may we call the time between the onset of ventricular contraction and closure of the mitral valve or M_1?

  ANS.: The preisovolumic contraction period.

   Note: This period is prolonged in MS because both the high left atrial pressure and the stiffness of the mitral valve have to be overcome before the mitral valve can be closed. If systole is defined as beginning with ventricular contraction (physiologist's systole), then only the first part of the murmur in sinus rhythm is presystolic because it begins at the time of peak atrial contraction, before the ventricle contracts. Most of the murmur, however, is actually an early systolic murmur, because it occurs during the preisovolumic contraction period of LV contraction. This is apparent from the observation that most of the crescendo murmurs to the M_1 occur after the QRS. Also, if LV pressure or apex cardiograms are taken simultaneously with phonocardiograms, most of the murmur occurs with the onset of the LV pressure rise (Fig. 4).

However, because the auscultator's systole begins with the S_1, it is not necessary to change the traditional terminology of **presystolic murmur**. By a presystolic murmur, then, the auscultator means "immediately before the first heart sound."

Late diastolic mitral regurgitation (MR) has been proposed as the cause of the presystolic murmur. But this is impossible because left atrial pressure is higher than LV pressure during much of the preisovolumic LV contraction (52,82).

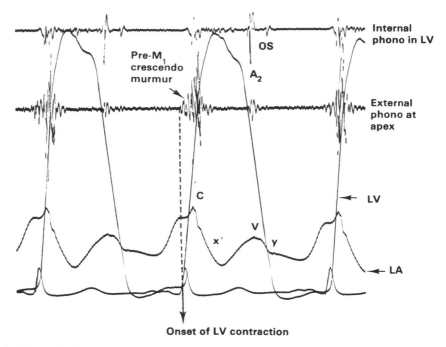

Onset of LV contraction

FIG. 4. These simultaneous phonocardiograms and left atrial and left ventricle pressure tracings were taken with catheter-tip micromanometer pressure transducers to eliminate any time delays due to tubing. Note that the "presystolic" crescendo of the MS murmur occurs during ventricular systole. This is from a 43-year-old man, mildly symptomatic, with severe MS but with only a small amount of calcium in his mitral valve. His left atrial A wave was 32 mm Hg, but his cardiac index was 2.7, which is low-normal. He had a grade 3/6 diastolic rumble at the apex, of which only the presystolic component is seen well in these phonocardiograms.

3. If blood is entering the LV during early (preisovolumic) ventricular contraction, how can a murmur become gradually louder (crescendo) when the pressure gradient as well as the volume of the flow across the orifice is being rapidly reduced?

ANS.: As the mitral orifice is reduced by LV contraction, the velocity of flow increases as long as the pressure is higher in the left atrium than in the LV (15). Several studies have shown that even the slightest closing motion of a stenotic mitral valve during diastole can produce a diastolic murmur (29,84).

Because the intensity of a sound is proportional to the fourth power of its velocity, a small change in blood velocity may cause marked changes in the intensity of a murmur. The increase in the loudness of a murmur as the mitral valve is closed by ventricular contraction can be compared with the effect of very rapid narrowing of the nozzle of a hose, whereas the decreasing gradient is analogous to turning the tap off. In effect, while the tap is being turned off, the velocity of flow is increasing.

Note: a. Angiograms or echocardiograms of the LV, together with simultaneous phonocardiograms, show that the valve is moving into a closed position at the time of the presystolic murmur (85).

b. Doppler studies in MS have shown a steady increase in velocity of flow during the QRS complex, reaching a peak 80 to 100 msec after the onset of the QRS (16).

4. Is atrial contraction required to produce the presystolic crescendo murmur?

ANS.: No. In atrial fibrillation the late crescendo occurs at the end of the short diastoles because only during short diastoles is the left atrial pressure high enough to maintain high-velocity flow during preisovolumic ventricular contraction (15). It requires a gradient of more than 10 mm Hg at the onset of LV contraction to create a crescendo murmur to the M_1 (15) (Fig. 5).

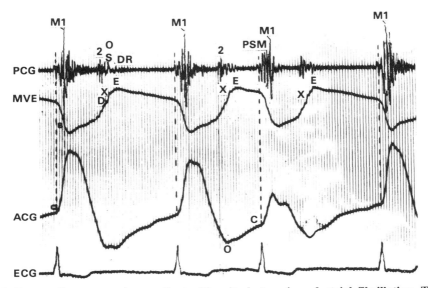

FIG. 5. Presystolic murmur in a patient with mitral stenosis and atrial fibrillation. The best presystolic crescendo to the M_1, occurring at the end of a short diastole, begins with the start of mitral valve closure on the mitral valve "gated" echocardiogram (MVE) and with the start of LV contraction, point C of the apex cardiogram (ACG). The presystolic murmur occurs during preisovolumic LV contraction. (From P. Toutouzas et al. Mechanism of diastolic rumble and presystolic murmur in mitral stenosis. *Br Heart J* 1974;36:1096.)

This also explains why atrial contraction helps to produce the pre-M_1 crescendo. Atrial contraction can elevate left atrial pressure sufficiently to create the necessary increased velocity of forward flow as the mitral valve orifice is being reduced by ventricular contraction.

5. What does the presence of a crescendo murmur to the M_1 tell you about the mitral valve in MS?

ANS.: The valve must be sufficiently flexible to change the size of the orifice; that is, it must not be rigidly calcified (although it may be too fibrosed or calcified for a valvotomy) (50).

Note: Important MR complicating MS can eliminate this pre-M_1 accentuation even in sinus rhythm (90). The loss of presystolic accentuation here may be due to a poorly contracting left atrium secondary to both the dilatation and the greater rheumatic damage of the atrium associated with the combined lesion.

Pitch and Quality

1. Is the MS diastolic murmur high or low in pitch? Why?

   ANS.: Low, because a murmur that is produced more by flow than by gradient produces low frequencies. The gradient across the mitral valve in diastole is relatively low as gradients go, no matter how severe the stenosis is; that is, in the usual case of severe MS, the maximum diastolic gradient is about 30 mm Hg at the beginning of diastole and about 10 mm Hg at the end.

   Note: a. Some of the descriptions of the MS diastolic murmur that suggest the low frequencies include the following: rumbling (like distant thunder or like a ball rolling down a bowling alley) and "blubbering." (Austin Flint used this word in 1884.)

   b. The early rumble followed by a late crescendo to a loud M_1 may be likened to the growl and bark of a dog. The growl is the rumble and the presystolic crescendo murmur is the bark.

2. Under what circumstances are high frequencies present in a mitral diastolic murmur?

   ANS.: High frequencies are present if the velocity of flow across the orifice is increased due to a good circulation time, a strong LV expansion, a strong atrial contraction, MR, or a tadpole-shaped orifice in which commissural fusion and valvular thickening are more marked anterolaterally than posteromedially (46).

   Note: The crescendo to the M_1 is usually rich in high frequencies (54). Therefore, if a wide, rough S_1 is confused with a presystolic crescendo, firm pressure with the diaphragm brings out the high-pitched crescendo components leading to the M_1. A rough S_1, on the other hand, separates into split sound components (Fig. 6).

Factors Increasing MS Murmur Loudness

1. Besides pushing the stethoscope farther from the heart, why does the MS murmur become softer on inspiration?

   ANS.: Blood is sequestered in the lungs and therefore withheld from the left side of the heart during inspiration. (It is useful to think of the lungs as a sponge that expels its blood into the left atrium during the squeezing effect of expiration and fills with blood from the RV during inspiration.)

2. What factors besides a high left atrial pressure can increase the flow across a moderately to severely obstructed mitral valve?

   ANS.: The powerful force of a healthy LV can pull blood into the LV. Concomitant MR also increases the loudness of the murmur and makes the MS murmur louder, because MR not only makes the LV larger and brings the apex closer to the stethoscope but also elevates the V wave during systole. Therefore, there is more pressure forcing blood through the mitral valve in diastole.

   Note: A grade 4/6 mitral diastolic murmur means that there is at least moderate stenosis (in the absence of MR). If, however, it radiates to the base (very unusual), it almost always signifies severe MS. (It also denies systemic levels of pulmonary hypertension [91].)

3. How can you bring out a mitral diastolic murmur that is almost inaudible?

   ANS.: a. Bring the LV closer to the stethoscope by turning the patient into the left lateral decubitus position and listen during end-expiration over the site where your fin-

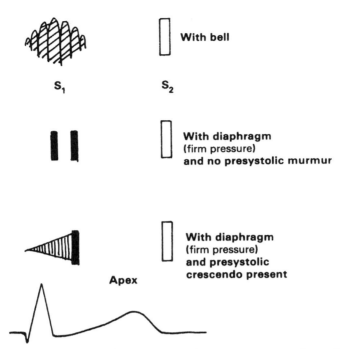

FIG. 6. A wide, rough first sound due to many low-frequency components can be differentiated from a presystolic murmur of MS plus M₁ by eliminating the low frequencies as much as possible with firm pressure.

ger feels the apex beat. The left lateral decubitus position also has been shown to increase the pressure gradient across the mitral valve and thus increases the flow in about one-third of patients with MS (1).

b. Use very light pressure with the largest bell available that allows a good air seal.

c. Increase the flow across the mitral valve by

1. Having the patient cough a few times, or listening after a Valsalva strain during the release phase. In the post-Valsalva release phase, the obstructed vena caval venous flow floods the lungs and pours into the left atrium a few seconds later. There is a more pronounced post-Valsalva rise of pressure in the left atrium in MS than in the normal heart (6).

2. Listening after digitalis has slowed the rate and increased the volume of diastolic flow into the LV. (Digitalis may also increase the force of LV expansion or "suction.")

3. Listening when the patient is squatting or during a handgrip maneuver. Cardiac output is increased for a few beats after squatting. During handgrip the mitral diastolic gradient has been shown to increase as a result of both the increase in cardiac output and the increase in heart rate (24).

4. Asking the patient to exercise. (Merely turning the patient into the left lateral decubitus position may be sufficient, and you should listen immediately, before the effect of this exertion is lost.) The maximum effective duration for

the supine straight leg-raising exercise beyond which there is probably not much increase in cardiac output is, at the most, 3 minutes; that is, physiologists consider 3 minutes of moderate exercise sufficient to reach a steady state. The more vigorous the exercise, the longer it takes to reach a steady state.

5. Administering amyl nitrite. See p. 250 for an explanation of how amyl nitrite increases venous return and cardiac output.

Factors Softening the MS Murmur

1. What can make MS diastolic murmurs soft besides mild MS, obesity, emphysema, or low flow?

    ANS.: a. A large right ventricle (RV) pushing the LV posteriorly. The RV is an anterior chamber, and if it enlarges, as it often does in MS, it pushes the LV away from the anterior chest wall.

    b. A coincidental atrial septal defect (ASD).

2. What, besides the mitral obstruction itself, can cause a low flow in MS?

    ANS.: a. Severe pulmonary hypertension. This causes an additional obstruction to flow for which RV hypertrophy and a rise in RV pressure do not compensate completely.

    b. Other valves causing obstruction (i.e., tricuspid or aortic stenosis).

    c. A very dilated left atrium due to severe rheumatic damage can lower the left atrial pressure even with severe MS and decrease the flow and therefore loudness of the murmur.

    d. A cardiomyopathy, usually on either a rheumatic or coronary basis. The flow can be reduced by the decreased diastolic "suction" of a poorly functioning ventricle.

    e. Atrial fibrillation. Atrial fibrillation often causes too fast a ventricular rate for good diastolic flow through the mitral obstruction, but even when the heart rates are slow, the loss of atrial contraction reduces flow. It has been shown that a well-placed atrial contraction can increase cardiac output by about 25% in significant MS (40).

    Note: In atrial fibrillation, the murmur of MS may disappear at the end of a long diastole for two opposite reasons.

    a. There may be such mild MS that the gradient disappears by the end of diastole.

    b. There may be such low flow that although the gradient is still high at the end of a long diastole, the flow is too low to permit a murmur to be heard at the end of a long diastole.

3. What is peculiar about the site of some soft MS murmurs that may make them difficult to hear?

    ANS.: They may occasionally be so localized that the murmur may disappear a few millimeters away from the exact apex area. You should palpate the apex beat with the patient in the left lateral decubitus position and place the stethoscope bell exactly at the area of the apex beat.

4. What anatomic factors have been thought to correlate with completely silent MS (i.e., no apical diastolic rumble at any time, even when the patient is in sinus rhythm and not in failure)?

ANS.: Any one or a combination of the following.
   a. An almost completely immobile mitral valve, usually with adhesions, thickening, and shortening of the chordae, which causes a second area of stenosis below the valve (88).
   b. A posteromedially deviated mitral valve orifice (88).
   c. A large left atrial thrombus deviating the stream away from the apex (70,88).
   d. A large ASD (Lutembacher syndrome).
      Note: If there is a large ASD, left atrial blood crosses the ASD rather than the obstructed mitral valve, thus diminishing the MS murmur.

Etiology and Differential Diagnosis

1. What is the usual etiology of MS?
   ANS.: Rheumatic fever, which causes a chronic process of valvular fibrosis, fusion, and calcification, together with shortened thickened chordae.
      Note: The normal valve orifice measures 4 to 6 cm^2. It must be reduced to about 2.5 cm^2 to elevate left atrial pressure significantly. Critical stenosis occurs at 1 cm^2.
2. What are some unusual causes of MS?
   ANS.: a. A left atrial myxoma.
      Note: Left atrial myxoma may produce a grade 4/6 diastolic murmur that may vary in loudness and position in the cycle from beat to beat and from one position of the chest to another.
   b. Congenital MS. Ninety percent of such patients die by age 2 if not treated surgically. Even the exceptional patients who live until adolescence are in heart failure from infancy (79).
      Note: The leaflets in one form of congenital MS, known as "parachute" mitral valve (a single papillary muscle sending chordae to fused, thickened, and fibrosed leaflets), may function normally or even be purely regurgitant.
   c. A calcified bacterial vegetation, as large as 2 cm in diameter, obstructed the mitral valve in a patient who had only MR prior to the infective endocarditis (3).
      Note: Verrucous endocarditis (Libman-Sacks valvulitis of disseminated lupus) does not usually cause enough mitral obstruction to produce even a diastolic murmur (48).
   d. Mitral ring constriction due to localized constrictive pericarditis of the atrioventricular ring (very rare).
3. What may imitate the MS diastolic murmur despite no significant diastolic gradient across the mitral valve?
   ANS.: a. A diastolic flow murmur due to excessive flow across the mitral valve, as in severe MR or ventricular septal defect (VSD).
   b. Hypertrophic cardiomyopathy with or without outflow obstruction (75,83). The reason is unknown. A small cavity usually is present and the ventricle is severely noncompliant. The murmur is characteristically short.
   c. A diastolic murmur across a porcine valve may be due to deflection of the blood flow through the valve toward the septum or posterior ventricular wall rather than toward the apex. It can be heard in about half the patients with normally

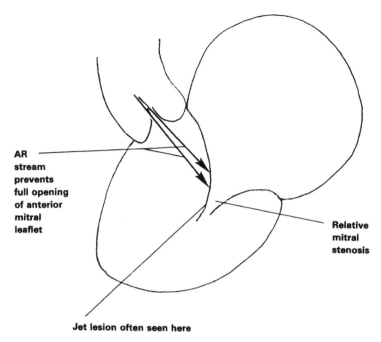

AR
stream
prevents
full opening
of anterior
mitral
leaflet

Relative
mitral
stenosis

Jet lesion often seen here

FIG. 7. The aortic regurgitant stream holds the anterior leaflet up in a semiclosed position. This accounts for the mitral diastolic rumble mimicking mitral stenosis and for the attenuated opening snap in patients with both mitral stenosis and aortic regurgitation.

functioning porcine valves (55). Fluttering of the respective ventricular walls can be seen on echocardiography (32).

Note: a. The finding of a low-frequency diastolic rumble across a St. Jude Medical or Byork-Shiley prosthesis in the mitral position, although occasionally a normal finding, should prompt careful evaluation, including fluoroscopy, to ensure that the function of the valve is in fact normal.

b. A mitral diastolic rumble may not be due to true MS if an S_3 precedes a short murmur. Only rarely does a true S_3 precede any MS murmur, in which case there is usually a good presystolic crescendo.

c. The Austin Flint murmur.

d. A mitral diastolic murmur is occasionally heard in coarctation of the aorta; the explanation is unknown. It may be due to coincidental fibroelastosis involving the valve. It persists after successful excision of the aortic obstruction.

The Austin Flint Murmur Versus the MS Murmur

1. What is the Austin Flint murmur?

ANS.: It is an apical diastolic rumble similar to the murmur of organic MS but is due to an aortic regurgitation (AR) stream that prevents the mitral valve from opening fully (Fig. 7).

Note: Right-sided Austin Flint murmurs due to pulmonary regurgitation, secondary to pulmonary hypertension, have been recorded (37). They have inspiratory and presystolic accentuation (44).

2. What is the most plausible theory explaining the mechanical cause of the Austin Flint murmur?

ANS.: The AR stream may impinge on the undersurface of the anterior leaflet of the mitral valve and push it up, creating a relative MS. Support for this theory is found in the following facts.

    a. A yellow plaque (jet lesion) has been seen on the septal surface of the anterior mitral leaflet of some patients with the Austin Flint murmur. This may be a jet lesion (20,61,87).

    b. When an Austin Flint murmur is present, the amplitude of opening of the mitral anterior leaflet is reduced on echocardiograms.

        Note: Echocardiograms often show fluttering of the anterior mitral leaflet in patients with Austin Flint murmurs. This was once thought to be the cause of the murmur, but some patients with the vibrating leaflets have no Austin Flint murmur, and some with the Austin Flint murmur have no leaflet vibrations.

3. What suggests that the apical diastolic murmur in severe AR is at least sometimes due to transmission of the low-frequency components of the AR murmur to the apex?

ANS.: a. It sometimes starts with the S_2 (i.e., before the mitral valve has had a chance to open). Also, it occasionally persists when Doppler flow studies showed that mitral inflow had ceased at the end of diastole when left ventricular pressure had exceeded left atrial pressure.

    b. If the AR is severe, its murmur is rich in low frequencies, which can be transmitted downstream to the apex. (The low-frequency components of murmurs tend to be best transmitted downstream [8].)

        Note: Austin Flint's explanation for the apical diastolic rumble in AR was that the increased ventricular volume due to double filling (from both the normal mitral flow and AR flow) floats the mitral valves upward into the nearly closed position, producing a relative MS (25). However, this theory requires the LV pressure to become higher than the left atrial pressure, in which case the valves would close completely, as in sudden, severe AR (see p. 303). The Austin Flint murmur would then disappear. Austin Flint's theory also requires that the LV be empty in early diastole, an impossible concept.

4. Why did Austin Flint describe the position of this murmur as presystolic?

ANS.: He described it as a "blubbering presystolic murmur" because the timing and quality sounded to him exactly the same as the murmur of MS. Since he thought that the atrium contracted just after the early filling phase, he considered almost all of diastole to be "presystolic" except for the very early filling phase. He recommended that all MS diastolic murmurs also be called presystolic (26).

        Note: a. In one study, a definite presystolic accentuation of the Flint murmur was not demonstrable in any patient in an entire series of 17 patients (61). In another study, a presystolic component was completely absent in two of 15 patients with an Austin Flint murmur (87). The pre-M_1 accentuation of the Austin Flint murmur, even when present, is often a subtle finding and does not have the marked crescendo to the S_1 heard in patients with MS (87) (Fig. 8).

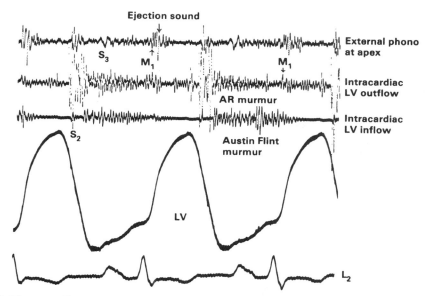

FIG. 8. Phonocardiograms and LV pressure tracing from a 45-year-old man with marked orthopnea who had an Austin Flint murmur due to severe AR, resulting from a previous infective endocarditis. Note that the diastolic rumble at the apex begins even before the S_3 was recorded externally. Note also the absence of a presystolic crescendo and the soft M_1.

   b. In severe AR, there is often a reversal of the pressure gradient across the mitral valve in late diastole (28). Because angiograms in such patients have shown late diastolic MR, the presystolic component of the Austin Flint murmur in severe AR has been said to be due to this late diastolic MR (52). Intracardiac phonocardiograms, however, have shown that although a reversed gradient can produce a recordable presystolic murmur in the left atrium, this murmur cannot be recorded on either a chest surface or LV inflow tract phonocardiograms (Fig. 9).

5. How can you differentiate an Austin Flint murmur from the murmur of MS by auscultation?

   ANS.: a. If there is no loud S_1 or OS, the chances that MS is present are diminished. But remember that AR can attenuate or eliminate an OS.

   b. If an S_3 is heard, it is more likely to be an Austin Flint murmur. But an S_3 occasionally can introduce an MS murmur.

   c. If there is no obvious presystolic crescendo to the S_1 despite short diastoles, it is more likely to be an Austin Flint murmur.

   d. Amyl nitrite produces a louder MS murmur after about 20 sec, whereas an Austin Flint murmur immediately becomes softer or even disappears. This is because amyl nitrite lowers peripheral resistance, thus increasing the peripheral runoff and decreasing the amount of AR. (In the presence of severe congestive failure, amyl nitrite may have no effect [74].)

6. When can the detection of an Austin Flint murmur be clinically useful?

   ANS.: It may be the only auscultatory clue to the presence of at least a moderate degree of AR if there is only a soft AR murmur (61). It also means a high LV end-diastolic pressure (62).

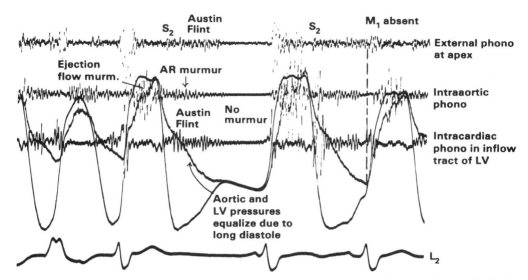

FIG. 9. Phonocardiograms and aortic and LV pressure tracings from a 51-year-old man who had severe AR with dyspnea on exertion and paroxysmal nocturnal dyspnea following infective endocarditis 2 months prior to this tracing. He had a grade 3/6 aortic ejection murmur due to excessive forward flow, a grade 3/6 aortic diastolic blowing murmur at the left sternal border, and a grade 3/6 diastolic rumble (Austin Flint murmur) at the apex. Note the sudden pause (due to sinus suppression secondary to a premature ventricular contraction with retrograde conduction) that allowed the LV pressure to rise as high as aortic pressure. The Austin Flint murmur stopped, even though the LV pressure must have exceeded left atrial pressure; that is, late MR is not the cause of any part of the Austin Flint murmur. Note also how the amount of AR is limited by the rapid rise of pressure in the LV. This is why, with sudden, severe AR, the diastolic murmur may be short.

MITRAL DIASTOLIC FLOW MURMURS (INFLOW MURMURS)

1. What is meant by a mitral diastolic inflow murmur?
   ANS.: The murmur is a low-pitched rumble, heard over the apex area, that is produced by a relative MS (i.e., by an excessive flow through a normal mitral valve).
2. List some common causes of excessive flow through a mitral valve that can produce a diastolic flow murmur besides severe MR and hyperkinetic states such as thyrotoxicosis.
   ANS.: a. A very slow ventricular rate with a healthy heart, for example, congenital complete atrioventricular (AV) block (2,63).
      Note: In complete AV block or when the PR interval is long, a diastolic flow murmur that coincides with the forward flow through the AV valves after atrial contraction can occur; that is, atrial contraction causes a semiclosure movement to follow the initial maximum opening effect, and if this leaflet apposition occurs at the same time as the early rapid filling phase, a flow murmur may be produced as blood is forced in through the almost-closed leaflets.
      b. A left-to-right shunt (e.g., a VSD or persistent ductus arteriosus with the shunt having a ratio of at least 2:1).
      Note: The advantage of hearing a flow murmur in a VSD with findings of pulmonary hypertension is that it indicates that the condition is operable;

that is, the pulmonary hypertension is not fixed (no pulmonary vascular disease) but is caused instead by an excessive flow into the pulmonary arterioles (hyperkinetic vasospastic pulmonary hypertension).

3. How does a mitral diastolic flow murmur differ from the murmur of MS, besides being short?

   ANS.: A flow murmur usually starts with an S_3 and has no presystolic component. See Fig. 8, p. 249.

   Note: An S_3 plus an S_4 close together can mimic a middiastolic flow murmur (81).

4. Why does the diastolic flow murmur not start exactly with the onset of opening of the mitral valve?

   ANS.: The mitral valve at its immediate opening probably makes too large an orifice for a murmur to be produced. Echocardiograms have shown that immediately after the initial opening movement of the mitral valve, the valve moves rapidly into a semi-closed position, probably as a result of eddy currents. At the time of the S_3, the mitral cusps are moving up and rapidly become more opposed to one another; a murmur then occurs while rapid flow is still continuing for a short time. The murmur is thus probably due to the increasing velocity of flow as a result of a dynamically narrowing mitral orifice, much like the effect of narrowing the nozzle of a hose.

   Note: A Carey Coombs murmur is the diastolic inflow murmur usually ushered in by an S_3 and is heard in subjects with cardiomegaly and MR due to acute rheumatic fever (13,14). Many writers tend to ignore the MR and imply that the inflow murmur is a special type of mitral murmur caused by the valvulitis itself, rather than a flow murmur heard commonly in any patient with substantial MR and torrential flow through the valve. Carey Coombs thought that it was due to dilatation of the LV.

TRICUSPID DIASTOLIC FLOW MURMURS

1. What is the site of the tricuspid inflow murmur?

   ANS.: Anywhere over the RV area. This includes all the lower right and left parasternal area as well as the epigastrium. When the RV is very large, the entire left lower chest area can also become the RV area.

2. What are the common causes of increased flow through the tricuspid valve?

   ANS.: Shunt flows (ASD and anomalous pulmonary venous connection with the right atrium) and tricuspid regurgitation (TR).

   Note: A tricuspid inflow murmur in a primum type of atrial septal defect is louder and longer, and it more often radiates to the apical area than in the usual secundum ASD.

3. How can a tricuspid inflow murmur be exaggerated besides by exercise or deep inspiration?

   ANS.: a. By holding the legs up or bending the knees toward the chest with the subject supine.

   b. By panting, rapid respirations.

   c. By amyl nitrite inhalation, which opens up arteriovenous communications and constricts veins by means of sympathetic reflexes.

4. How does an ASD tricuspid diastolic flow murmur differ in timing from a VSD mitral diastolic flow murmur?

ANS.: In an ASD the murmur starts earlier, at about the time of the opening of the tricuspid valve, and is not preceded by an S₃ (58). It may occasionally be presystolic
as well (23). In a VSD it is almost always initiated by an S_3 (Fig. 10).

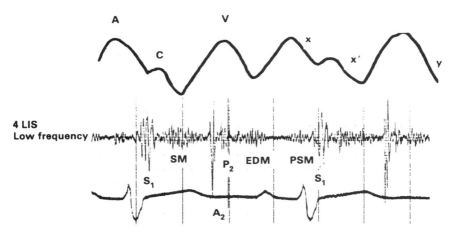

**FIG. 10. Phonocardiogram and jugular pulse tracing from a teenaged girl with an ostium pri-
mum ASD. The presystolic murmur (PSM) is unusual in ASDs, but, when present, is crescendo-
decrescendo and not crescendo to the first sound, as in MS. Note that the Y descent in the jugular tracing is almost equal to the combination of X + X' descents. This is due to the high V wave,
which results from the addition to the right atrium of blood from some additional source (i.e., not
only from the venae cavae but here also from the left atrium and even from the LV because of
MR, which is expected with primum defects).**

Note: If an ASD has an anomalous pulmonary venous connection with the right
atrium, then even when pulmonary hypertension is high enough to
markedly decrease the shunt through the ASD, a tricuspid flow murmur
may persist, probably because the pulmonary venous pressure remains
higher than the right atrial pressure and maintains an increased flow into
the right atrium (64).

5. With what is a tricuspid inflow murmur confused?

ANS.: The murmur of tricuspid stenosis (TS). In the presence of a normal sinus rhythm,
however, the TS murmur is almost always only presystolic and has many high frequencies in it.

TRICUSPID STENOSIS DIASTOLIC MURMURS

1. Where is the TS murmur heard on the chest wall?

ANS.: In the same place as the tricuspid inflow murmur (i.e., the RV area).

2. How does the TS murmur differ from the MS murmur?

ANS.: a. In sinus rhythm it is a presystolic murmur but has no presystolic crescendo to
the S₁; that is, it is nearly always a short crescendo-decrescendo murmur, and it
sounds like an S₄ murmur. Only if atrial fibrillation is present is there a delayed
early diastolic murmur (21).

Note: In MS a presystolic murmur may also be crescendo-decrescendo if there is a long PR interval and low flow due to heart failure.

b. It always increases with inspiration, often markedly, whereas the MS murmur characteristically decreases with inspiration.

c. The MS murmur is louder in the left lateral decubitus position. The TS murmur is accentuated in the right lateral decubitus position (49).

d. The MS murmur is usually predominantly low-pitched and rumbling; the TS presystolic murmur is often scratchy.

e. Rheumatic TS is probably never present without MS, even though on rare occasions the TS may be the dominant lesion (56). Therefore, if no MS can be diagnosed, a presystolic murmur at the left sternal border should make you suspect either a right atrial myxoma, an ASD, or carcinoid stiffening of the tricuspid valve.

f. One study has shown that presystolic crescendo-decrescendo murmurs with high-pitched components can be recorded in about one-fifth of normal subjects as well as in some patients with ASD, hypertensive obstructive cardiomyopathy (HOCM), or a variety of other conditions (42). Another study showed that such murmurs were present in patients with ischemic heart disease; they were heard best at the left lower sternal border (69).

3. Why does the TS murmur become louder on inspiration?

ANS.: Interestingly, it does not appear to be due to an increase in right atrial pressure alone, because right atrial pressure has been shown to rise relatively little during inspiration with TS. Inspiration increases inflow into the right heart, and because RV inflow is restricted by the TS, the volume in the RV is not increased as much as it is in the right atrium, where venous inflow is unrestricted (92). The mean right atrial pressure tends to remain unchanged with inspiration, whereas RV pressure falls and the relatively higher pressure in the right atrium increases the gradient across the tricuspid valve (21).

Note: The TS murmur increases both during moving inspiration and during inspiratory apnea. (An inadvertent Valsalva maneuver during the apnea makes the TS murmur softer.)

4. What should you consider besides rheumatic TS if either a middiastolic inflow murmur or a presystolic murmur increases with inspiration?

ANS.: Ebstein's anomaly (which often has both TS and TR), an ASD with large flow, or a right atrial myxoma.

Note: a. Some patients with a right atrial myxoma and a middiastolic inflow murmur also have a murmur between the M_1 and the second component of a widely split S_1 (3,45). The second component is probably the tricuspid component of the S_1. The short murmur may be due to TR with upward movement of the tumor through the tricuspid valve before the valve closes.

b. Constrictive pericarditis can occasionally cause a localized constriction around the tricuspid annulus and can produce the gradient and murmur of TS (72).

c. Occasionally, the TR in the Ebstein's anomaly is so severe that the ECG shows RVH and the RV becomes palpable despite the downward displacement of the tricuspid valve into the RV.

DIASTOLIC SEMILUNAR VALVE MURMURS

Aortic Regurgitation Murmurs

Causes of Aortic Regurgitation

1. What are the most common causes of severe AR (a) in the child and (b) in the adult?
   ANS.: a. In the young child, a VSD with aortic valve prolapse may be the most common cause of severe AR.

   b. Although in the adult, rheumatic heart disease, endocarditis, or paraprosthetic valve leaks are probably equally common as causes of severe AR, one study showed that the most common cause was idiopathic myxomatous degeneration of the aortic valve, similar to that seen in mitral valve prolapse, which gradually accumulates varying amounts of calcium (67).

   Note: The most common cause of mild AR in the adult is severe hypertension, usually with a bicuspid valve. In one series of severely hypertensive patients, 60% had AR (53). In another series of hypertensive patients, 6% had AR, all trivial. Those with AR had diastolic blood pressures of at least 110 mm Hg (65). Usually, when the diastolic pressure is reduced below 115 mm Hg, the AR disappears. The aortic annulus is not significantly dilated at systolic pressures below 170, or diastolic pressures below 105. The cause of the reversible AR has been thought to be high pressure above a bicuspid or fenestrated aortic valve. Fenestrations are common in both the aortic and pulmonary valves. In one autopsy study, 82% of all semilunar valves had fenestrations (30). However, bicuspid valves do not tolerate very high pressures above them either.

2. What should make you suspect, by auscultation, that a bicuspid aortic valve is the cause of the AR?
   ANS.: In the presence of mild AR, an ejection click followed by an early ejection murmur that is loudest in the second right interspace, ending with a loud A_2.

   Note: The following theory may explain the incompetence of a bicuspid aortic valve. If the valve edges were straight between their attachments, the valves would be obstructive as they opened. Obstruction is avoided if at least one of the leaflets has a voluminous or redundant (and pleated) free-edge length that is greater than the straight-line distance between its attachments to the aortic wall. This redundant valvular tissue may allow free forward flow in systole but may prolapse downward during diastole, producing at least mild regurgitation, especially if only one leaflet has the extra diameter (19).

3. List some rare causes of AR (a) with arthritis and (b) without arthritis.
   ANS.: a. With arthritis
   1. Ankylosing spondylitis. The cusps are shortened and thickened by fibrous tissue, and occasionally this produces AR a few years before the symptomatic spondylitis, although x-ray evidence of spondylitis may be seen and tissue typing with the antigen HLA-B27 may be positive (22). However, the incidence rises with the duration of the arthritis (5).
   2. Reiter syndrome. AR may be found from 1 to 20 years after diagnosis, and it occurs in about 5% of patients with this syndrome.

3. Rheumatoid or psoriatic arthritis (57).
4. Disseminated lupus erythematosus.
5. The arthritis associated with ulcerative colitis.
   b. Without arthritis
1. Syphilis (luetic aortitis).
2. Osteogenesis imperfecta. The AR here is due to dilatation of the aortic root (17).
3. Marfan syndrome. The AR is due to dilatation of the aortic root and myxomatous degeneration of the cusps (69).
   Note: Although both males and females with Marfan syndrome may have MR, only males (usually under age 40) develop AR. When a patient has only some but not all of the features of Marfan syndrome (forme fruste), cystic medial necrosis of the aorta with or without a dissecting aneurysm is usually an associated lesion (66). Although myxomatous transformation of the aortic valve is characteristic of Marfan syndrome, it can occur without this syndrome, and when it does, it can result in rupture of an aortic cusp (60).
4. Dissecting aneurysm of the ascending aorta.
5. Supravalvular AS. The AR here is due either to fusion of a cusp with the supravalvular membrane or to the valve leaflets adhering to the aortic wall (80).
6. Uremia. If the early diastolic murmur is localized to the apex and disappears or decreases with sitting, an atypical friction rub and not AR may be the cause of the murmur (4). AR correlates not with the level of uremia, but with the presence of at least two of the three conditions commonly seen in uremia: severe anemia, volume overload, and diastolic pressure of 120 mm Hg or more. It is not always due to the effect of hypertension on a bicuspid or rheumatic valve because it can occur when the blood pressure has been made normal by dialysis and when the valve is found to be normal at autopsy.
7. Aortic arch syndrome, or Takayasu disease (pulseless disease). The AR here is due to dilatation of the aortic ring.
8. Rupture of a sinus of Valsalva.
9. Giant cell arteritis (41).
10. Aortic-annular ectasia.

Timing and Shape

1. When in the cycle does the AR murmur begin, and what is its shape?
   ANS.: It begins with the aortic component of the second sound (A_2). In general, it is decrescendo.
   Note: There is often a very early and very short crescendo-decrescendo to the murmur. This crescendo-decrescendo is due to the shape of the aortoventricular gradient and flow, which increases in early diastole as ventricular pressure drops precipitously below aortic pressure to nearly zero, while aortic pressure falls slowly. A good dicrotic wave to the aortic pressure curve may also be partly responsible for this crescendo-decrescendo. Because the presence of a good dicrotic wave in AR suggests mild or, at the most, moderate AR, a marked crescendo-decrescendo effect in the early part of the murmur suggests that the AR is not severe.

The dicrotic wave is thought to be caused by a "rebound" effect of the aortic leaflets immediately after their abrupt closure in early diastole. If true, then a good dicrotic wave would be expected only when the valve is least insufficient (Fig. 11).

The auscultatory effect of the short and early crescendo-decrescendo is that the murmur appears to start after a short silent period following the A_2. The background rhythm is 1 to 2-HAaaaaaaa-1 to 2-HAaaaaaaa.

A pandiastolic murmur suggests that the AR is at least moderate in severity, provided that the heart rate is not so fast that even a short diastolic murmur would be pandiastolic.

Systolic and diastolic murmurs

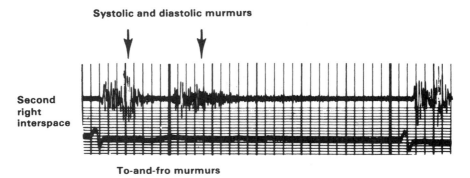

Second right interspace

To-and-fro murmurs

FIG. 11. **This murmur was due to mild syphilitic AR. It was loudest at the second and third right interspaces. Note the slight early crescendo-decrescendo. A systolic murmur due to blood going in one direction together with a diastolic murmur due to blood going in the opposite direction is called a to-and-fro murmur.**

Quality and Loudness

1. What is the dominant frequency or pitch of the usual AR murmur? Why?

   ANS.: The dominant frequency is high. If the AR is mild, then the murmur is due more to a large gradient than to flow; that is, there is a small but high-velocity regurgitant jet, and the murmur, therefore, is purely high-pitched. If the AR is moderate, the murmur is due to a greater flow, and it has mixed frequencies but still is dominantly high. If AR is severe, the murmur may be very rough due to an excess of low and medium frequencies.

   Note: The more low frequencies there are, the more severe the AR, but the reverse is not necessarily true (i.e., a pure high-frequency murmur may be present with moderately severe AR); presumably, the low-frequency components are transmitted to areas not accessible to the stethoscope. However, a grade 1 AR murmur is rarely if ever due to severe AR.

2. How can you best imitate by voice the sound of a typical, mild AR murmur (i.e., a purely high-pitched murmur)?

   ANS.: In Mexico this has been called an "aspirative" AR murmur and is imitated by noisily breathing *in* through the mouth. If you breathe *out* quickly, with the mouth open or whisper "ah," you can easily imitate the classic AR murmur.

   Note: Because it sounds so much like a breath sound, the patient should hold his breath on expiration to allow you to perceive this murmur better.

3. How can you increase the loudness of the very soft AR murmur?
   ANS.: a. You can get the stethoscope closer to the heart by having the patient sit up and
      lean forward. Then press hard with the diaphragm during held expiration.
      b. You can increase peripheral resistance as follows.
         1. Ask the patient to squat, and auscultate the chest immediately. The increase
            in venous return for a few beats also helps increase the murmur.
            Note: a. Squatting is effective in bringing out a grade 1/6 murmur but has
               little effect on the murmur of moderate to marked AR.
               b. Kinking of the lower body arteries is probably unimportant in the
                  effect of squatting on blood pressure because drawing the knees up
                  to the chest in the supine position has little effect on blood pres-
                  sure. Squatting may be a form of isometric exercise.
         2. Have the patient do isometric exercise by means of handgrip. The elevation
            of systolic blood pressure after 3 minutes of 33% maximum handgrip pres-
            sure is greater in patients with AR than in normal subjects (38).
         3. Administer a vasopressor drug.
            Note: a. AR with a soft murmur is probably trivial if the diastolic blood
               pressure is more than 70 mm Hg and the pulse pressure is less than
               40 mm Hg (11).
               b. AR severity is clinically underestimated in the presence of signifi-
                  cant MS, which prevents the left ventricular volume and pulse pres-
                  sure from reflecting the severity of the AR (35).
               c. More than 50% of patients with mild or moderate AR by pulsed
                  Doppler have no AR murmur (68).
               d. Combine squatting with handgrip or the "squat and squeeze ma-
                  neuver" for maximum effect on the murmur loudness.

Musical AR Murmurs

1. What is the significance of a musical AR murmur?
   ANS.: Musical aortic diastolic murmurs often occur in patients with a perforated leaflet
      as in infective endocarditis, everted leaflets (often luetic), or rupture of an aortic
      sinus of Valsalva. Ruptures of leaflets are usually secondary to myxomatous trans-
      formation or infective endocarditis.
2. What is the timing and shape of musical AR murmurs?
   ANS.: a. The same as that of the actual AR murmurs; that is, pandiastolic decrescendo
         after the usual initial short crescendo, or
      b. The musical parts may occur only in early diastole and are then followed by the
         usual high-frequency decrescendo murmur for the rest of diastole, or
      c. There may be a mid- or late-diastolic crescendo-decrescendo musical compo-
         nent.
         Note: The dove-coo musical murmur has a peculiar shape (see Fig. 12), sug-
            gesting it is made by vibrations of the aorta itself. The regurgitant stream
            acts on the aortic valve, which probably acts like a reed that in turn
            causes the aorta to vibrate. The shape of the murmur may be due to the
            effect of the mitral valve, which, when open, allows the aortic posterior
            wall freedom to resonate. In the semiclosed position, the mitral valve
            pulls on the aorta and keeps it more rigid, thus muting the vibrations
            (47).

L. lower sternal border   High frequency

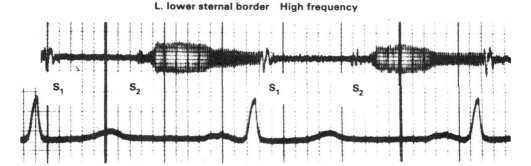

S_1 S_2 S_1 S_2

FIG. 12. Luetic AR was suspected as the cause of this aortic diastolic murmur. Note the regular vibrations seen in all phonocardiograms of musical murmurs.

Site

1. Where, as a rule, is the AR murmur best heard?

    ANS.: Over the midsternum or just to the left of the sternum at the level of the third or fourth intercostal space.

    Note: a. The AR murmur is best heard at the second or third interspace to the right of the sternum in the presence of marked poststenotic dilatation of the aorta (when AS is also present) or when marked atherosclerotic tortuosity pushes the ascending aorta anteriorly and to the right. However, it is best heard in the *fourth* right interspace only if it is due to nonrheumatic conditions that cause the regurgitant stream to flow in peculiar directions (i.e., when it is secondary to infective endocarditis, an aortic aneurysm, a prolapsed aortic valve, or rupture of a sinus of Valsalva).

    b. The murmur may be even louder in the high mid-left thorax, at the apex, or in the midaxillary line, than in the sternal edge. This has been called the Cole-Cecil murmur (12). The cause for these unusual radiations is unknown. Occasionally, the murmur may be heard *only* in the axillary area or at the apex. This may have been one of the reasons that "silent" AR was reported in 16 patients with significant AR on cineangiography (68).

Sudden, Severe Aortic Regurgitation

1. What are the most likely causes of sudden, severe AR?

    ANS.: Infective endocarditis or rupture of an aneurysm of the sinus of Valsalva.

    Note: a. At the apex there is often a soft or absent S_1 and a loud S_3 (89). The soft or absent S_1 is due to the rapid and marked rise of LV pressure in diastole. It is so marked that it rises above the left atrial pressure in middiastole, at which time it closes the mitral valve prematurely. The loud S_3 may be a middiastolic S_1, which occurs at the moment that LV pressure becomes higher than left atrial pressure. It may be the result of tensing of the chordae rendineae and papillary muscles by mitral valve closure (89).

b. The tachycardia of sudden, severe AR often causes diastole to be equal to or even shorter than systole, so that it is difficult to tell systole from diastole by auscultation. This occurs because ejection is prolonged by the severe LV volume overload, and the diastolic period may be further shortened by tachycardia. Carotid or apical palpation during auscultation is mandatory to avoid confusing systole with diastole.

2. Why may an AR murmur not be pandiastolic in sudden, severe AR even with diastoles that are shorter than normal?

ANS.: In sudden, severe AR, the LV does not expand as well as it does in chronic AR; that is, it is less distensible because of the inability of the pericardium to stretch acutely. Indeed, the LV pressure in diastole may rise so high and so fast that it may even reach aortic diastolic pressure in middiastole. The equalization of aortic and ventricular pressures limits the amount and duration of AR that can occur. (See Fig. 9, p. 295.) The AR murmur not only may be short (not pandiastolic) but may be surprisingly soft.

Differential Diagnosis

1. What are the common imitators of an AR murmur?

ANS.: a. A pulmonary regurgitation murmur caused by high pressure in the pulmonary artery (Graham Steell murmur).
   b. The high-frequency components of MS murmurs transmitted to the left sternal border.

2. What are the rare imitators of an AR murmur?

ANS.: a. The diastolic component of a soft, continuous murmur due to a coronary-to-pulmonary artery fistula (43) or a right-coronary-to-LV fistula if the systolic component is inaudible (33).
   b. Inflation of an aortic balloon pump during diastole produces a short, slightly delayed diastolic murmur with a blowing, spurting, or blubbering quality (10).
   c. A flail posterior mitral leaflet during the rapid movement from its prolapsed position in the left atrium to its open position in the LV, pushing blood from the left atrium to the LV (31).
   d. The soft, AR-like diastolic murmur heard at the second or third left interspace in some patients with moderate obstruction (not more than 50% occluded) of the anterior descending coronary artery (9).

THE MURMUR OF ANTERIOR DESCENDING CORONARY ARTERY STENOSIS

1. What are the characteristics of the diastolic murmur of coronary artery stenosis?

ANS.: It is
   a. High-pitched (71) and crescendo-decrescendo, corresponding to the pattern of diastolic coronary flow, which is maximum in the first quarter of diastole.
   b. Most easily audible when the patient is sitting up.

Note: This murmur has been observed to disappear after infarction and after aortocoronary bypass surgery (9).

The diastolic murmur of coronary artery stenosis suggests that the obstruction is not major; that is, it allows enough flow to produce the turbulence necessary to cause a diastolic murmur. It is not surprising that an obstruction of not more than 50% has been found in those cases that have been investigated.

PULMONARY REGURGITATION MURMURS

Murmurs with High Pressure in the Pulmonary Artery (Graham Steell Murmur)

1. Does the pulmonary artery pressure have to be very high to produce a pulmonary regurgitation (PR) murmur?

    ANS.: It is usually very high (i.e., at nearly systemic levels). Pulmonary regurgitation murmurs are rarely present with pulmonary artery pressures of below 80 mm Hg systolic unless the main pulmonary artery is markedly dilated.

    Note: a. A Graham-Steell murmur is a PR murmur that is secondary to pulmonary hypertension, regardless of whether the hypertension is primary or secondary.

    b. A PR murmur with a VSD may occur even with normal pulmonary vascular resistance if the pulmonary pressure is over 80 mm Hg.

2. How does the Graham Steell murmur differ from the AR murmur?

    ANS.: It may not differ; that is, both are dominantly high-pitched, may be from grade 1 to 6, may have an early crescendo-decrescendo, and (when soft) may even become louder on expiration (73). The Graham Steell murmur, however, usually increases with inspiration when it is loud (Fig. 13).

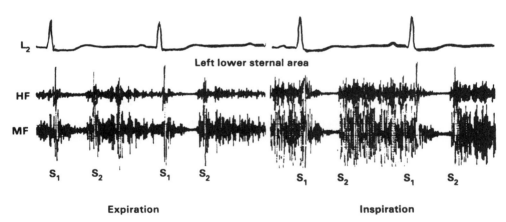

FIG. 13. These phonocardiograms are from a patient with a PDA whose pulmonary artery pressure was 145 mm Hg and whose aortic pressure was about the same. This loud diastolic murmur (Graham Steell murmur) increased markedly on inspiration. A soft Graham Steell murmur may not increase with inspiration.

Note: a. A Graham Steell murmur that is soft may decrease with inspiration despite the increase in pulmonary artery flow because the soft PR murmur is usually best heard in the second left interspace where the effect of inspiration pushing the stethoscope away from the heart is most marked. Also, inspiration may not increase flow to the lungs in patients with severe pulmonary hypertension if concomitant TR is present.

b. Isometric handgrip and squatting will selectively increase the murmur of AR.

3. How can a Valsalva strain help in differentiating a PR from an AR murmur?

ANS.: Immediately on release of the Valsalva strain, the PR murmur resumes its pre-Valsalva loudness. The AR murmur returns to its normal intensity only after four or five beats.

Note: a. In patients with a dilated pulmonary artery there may be an early short diastolic decrescendo scratch without AR or PR. Such scratches may result from an extracardiac effect of adhesions between the pulmonary artery and the surrounding lung.

b. The Graham Steell murmur was once erroneously thought to be common in patients with MS because the murmur of AR was misinterpreted as being due to PR.

PR Murmurs with Normal Pressure in the Pulmonary Artery (Primary Pulmonary Regurgitation)

1. What are the two most likely causes of primary PR murmurs, besides congenital absence of the pulmonary artery?

ANS.: a. Idiopathic dilatation of the pulmonary artery. (In some series, about a third of patients with idiopathic dilatation have PR.)

b. Surgery for pulmonary stenosis. Pulmonary valvotomy invariably leaves some degree of PR.

Note: a. A patient with tetralogy of Fallot with PR almost invariably has no pulmonary valve, and the pulmonary obstruction is due to a constricted valve ring.

b. The occasional PR in patients with an ASD might really be another instance of coincidental idiopathic dilatation of the pulmonary artery. In one series of patients with uncomplicated ASDs, a small number had an early basal diastolic murmur that was recorded externally and only in the outflow tract of the RV by internal phonocardiography (23). In another series of patients with uncomplicated ASDs who were over age 20, 40% had a grade 2/6, medium-frequency, diastolic decrescendo murmur that increased on inspiration, was of maximum loudness at the second left interspace, and radiated to the lower right sternal border (51).

c. A diastolic murmur at the left lower sternal border that begins with the P_2 in some ASD patients with normal pulmonary artery pressure has been shown to sometimes be the diastolic component of a continuous murmur at the ASD caused by a high left atrial pressure due to MR, plus a small to moderate-sized ASD (76).

d. Multivalvular or single valve stenosis and/or regurgitation can be caused by ergot alkaloids taken chronically for migraine. The valves are thickened and retracted but not calcified.

2. How do the shape, length, and pitch of a primary PR murmur differ from those of the Graham Steell murmur?

ANS.: a. With high pressures in the pulmonary artery, the shape, length, and pitch of the PR murmur are the same as those of AR. With *normal* pressures in the pulmonary artery, there is sometimes a slight delay after the P_2 before any murmur is heard. However, even if it starts with the P_2, the murmur tends to be short and rough, due to dominant medium and low frequencies.

b. When the PR is mild, the murmur may have characteristics that are between those of the Graham Steell murmur and the primary PR murmur; that is, it may start earlier, last longer, and have higher frequencies than the more severe primary PR murmur (59).

c. One intracardiac phonocardiogram study showed no pause between the P_2 and the murmur (27). But in another such study, the PR murmur was markedly delayed (7).

d. Immediately after the regurgitant pulmonary valve closes, the pressure falls rapidly, the gradient between the pulmonary artery and RV increases rapidly, and the murmur loudness increases (crescendo) until the RV pressure reaches its nadir. Then the gradient rapidly tapers off and the murmur decreases in loudness (decrescendo). Thus, the regurgitant PR murmur of a patient with normal PA pressure is a short crescendo-decrescendo medium-frequency murmur because the gradient is not high as in pulmonary hypertension high-frequency PR murmurs (Fig. 14).

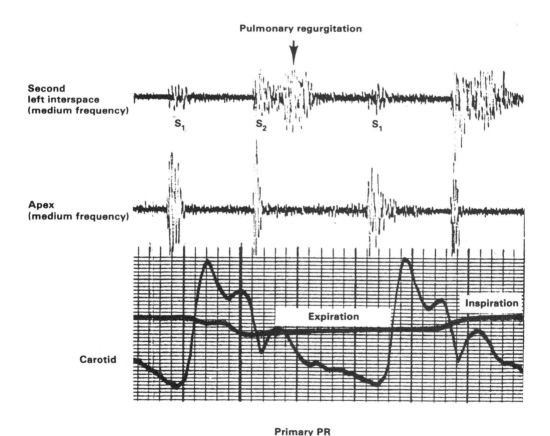

FIG. 14. This murmur of primary PR in a teenaged boy was early diastolic and had many low and medium frequencies in it. It did not increase with inspiration at the second left interspace because too much air was interposed between heart and stethoscope in that area. The murmur was softer at the left lower sternal border, where, however, it did become louder with inspiration.

3. Why is the primary PR murmur short?

ANS.: Diastolic pressure in the pulmonary artery falls rapidly because it begins with a normal pressure at the pulmonary incisura and has diastolic runoff in two directions, so that pulmonary artery and RV pressure rapidly equalize.

Note: Pulmonary regurgitation was found to be due to distortion rather than dilatation of the pulmonary valve annulus (86).

PERICARDIAL FRICTION RUBS

Pericarditis

1. What is the mechanism that causes friction rubs?

ANS.: It is usually assumed that the rub sounds are caused by the two roughened pericardial membranes (the visceral and parietal pericardia) sliding over one another. When the overlying pleura is also involved, perhaps the noises are caused by the pleura rubbing against the outer layer of pericardium. The rub then would be a pleuropericardial friction rub.

Note: The three most common causes of generalized pericarditis are viral pericarditis, disseminated lupus, and uremia. The most common cause of a localized pericarditis is acute myocardial infarction. If there has been neither infarction nor trauma to the heart (including radiation to the chest), then consider a metastatic tumor involving the heart.

Recognizing a Pericardial Friction Rub

1. What adjectives and analogies have been used to describe the quality of friction rubs?

ANS.: They usually are crunching, scraping, creaking, grating, crackling, or scratching. They often sound like squeaky shoes or like two pieces of sandpaper rubbed against one another. Occasionally, however, they sound no different from any other mixed-frequency murmur. They often sound surprisingly superficial (i.e., closer to the ears than the usual murmur, as if they were half-way up the stethoscope tubing).

2. When are the three components heard in most friction rubs?

ANS.: One is heard in systole and two are heard in diastole. One of the diastolic rubs occurs in early diastole, near the end of early rapid expansion of the ventricle, at the time when an S_3 would occur. The other occurs at the end of diastole, when atrial contraction produces sudden ventricular expansion. This is when an S_4 would occur.

Note: The systolic rub may replace the first or second heart sound or occur only in midsystole. There is, therefore, the possibility that three rubs may occur in systole.

3. If one major rub replaces the first heart sound (the most common occurrence) and two rubs occur in diastole, what is the cadence of a friction rub that is heard as a background rhythm?

ANS.: The cadence is the same as that of a quadruple rhythm due to a double gallop (i.e., "ch-DUP-sh-sh—ch-DUP-sh-sh," where the "DUP" is the S_2).

Note: Because the systolic rub may replace both the S_1 and the S_2, it is common to hear the rhythm as "CH-sh-sh—CH-sh-sh." When one of the diastolic rubs is absent, it is usually the S_3; that is, an S_4 rub is the last to disappear, probably because the heart is maximally distended at the end of diastole, tending to bring the inflamed pericardial surfaces into contact.

4. Is the friction rub usually louder during inspiration or expiration? Why?

ANS.: In about a third of patients, it increases during inspiration (18,77). This may be due to several possible causes.

    a. The downward pull of the diaphragm on the pericardium may draw the pericardium more tautly over the heart. The diaphragm is attached to the pericardium, and it is conceivable that a small amount of fluid between the visceral and parietal pericardium could be squeezed out by the tightening of the two layers with inspiration.

    b. It may be a pleuropericardial rub. Even when there is pericardial effusion, there may still be a pericardial rub, and this may be accounted for either by the squeezing out of a small amount of fluid by inspiration or by the expanded lung pressing on the pericardium during inspiration if it is a pleuropericardial rub.

5. Of the three major rub components, which one is almost always present? Which is the next most common component?

ANS.: The systolic component is almost always present. The atrial systolic component is next in frequency of occurrence, but rarely does an atrial systolic rub occur alone as the only rub sound. It almost always occurs together with at least a systolic rub. It is not surprising, then, that a systolic rub alone (rare) is more likely to occur in atrial fibrillation than in sinus rhythm (39).

    Note: When only a systolic rub is present, it can best be differentiated from a murmur by searching the chest for a site where it increases on inspiration—a rare phenomenon with murmurs. There is almost always one place on the chest where you can elicit an inspiratory increase. Placing the patient with the face and chest down and resting on knees and elbows can not only bring out a questionable rub but may exaggerate the effect of respiration.

6. Where are most friction rubs best heard?

ANS.: Near the left sternal border, at about the third or fourth left interspace.

7. When is the friction rub transient?

ANS.: During the course of acute myocardial infarction, when it may last only a few hours. However, in the postmyocardial infarction syndrome (Dressler syndrome), it may last for weeks.

8. What can imitate a friction rub?

ANS.: A noisy left-sided pneumothorax. A shallow pneumothorax at the left lung apex (occasionally seen only on a film taken on full expiration) can apparently cause air pockets on the medial aspect of the lung. The contraction of the LV against these bubbles of air may produce sounds at the apex that are synchronous with systole and diastole (74). They have been described as grinding, clicking, and crunching, and may be heard at a distance from the patient. They do not occur with a right-sided pneumothorax and seem to occur almost entirely in young males.

    Note: a. A mixture of fluid and air in the pericardium, as when a few milliliters of air are introduced into the pericardium to replace the fluid withdrawn, produces a metallic tinkle that is synchronous with systole. A large amount of injected air can produce a churning, splashing sound (millwheel murmur) (78).

    b. Temporary transvenous pacemakers have been associated with friction rubs thought to be caused by contact of the pacing wire with the inner surface of the myocardium; that is, they may be endocardial friction rubs, although occasionally they are a sign of perforation (36).

c. Mediastinal emphysema can produce crackles, bubbles, and churning sounds with each cardiac contraction (Hamman sign). They may be very soft or may be loud enough to be heard at a distance. The Hamman crunch may also be caused by a dilated lower esophagus, or gastric dilatation, and by bullous emphysema involving the lingula. Immediately postoperatively the crunching Hamman sign may be heard over the cardiac apex in the left lateral decubitus position.

REFERENCES

1. Anan R. et al. Mechanism of increment of the diastolic rumble in mitral stenosis in left lateral position. *Circulation* (Abstr) 1991;84:165.
2. Ayers CR, et al. Congenital complete heart block in children. *Am Heart J* 1966;72:381.
3. Barlow J, et al. A case of right atrial myxoma. *Br Heart J* 1962;24:120.
4. Barratt LJ, et al. The diastolic murmur of renal failure. *N Engl J Med* 1976;295:121.
5. Benisch BM. Mitral stenosis and insufficiency. *Am Heart J* 1971;82:39.
6. Bjork VO, Malmstrom G. Simultaneous left and right atrial pressure curves during Valsalva's experiment. *Am Heart J* 1955;50:742.
7. Brayshaw JR, Perloff JK. Congenital pulmonary insufficiency. *Am J Cardiol* 1962;10:282.
8. Bruns DL. A general theory of the cause of murmurs. *Am J Med* 1959;27:360. (Classic article.)
9. Burg JR, et al. Disappearance of coronary artery stenosis murmur. *Chest* 1973;63:440.
10. Clements SD Jr, et al. Phonocardiographic study of sounds produced by a circulatory assist device. *Arch Intern Med* 1977;137:1619.
11. Cohn LH, et al. Preoperative assessment of aortic regurgitation. *Circulation* 1966;31(Suppl):76.
12. Cole R, Cecil AB. The axillary diastolic murmur in aortic insufficiency. *Bull Johns Hopkins Hosp* 1908;19:353.
13. Coombs CF. Rheumatic myocarditis. *Quart J Med* 1908;2:26.
14. Coombs CF. *Rheumatic Heart Disease.* Bristol, England: Wright, 1924:203.
15. Criley JM, Hermer AJ. The crescendo presystolic murmur of mitral stenosis. *N Engl J Med* 1971;285:1284.
16. Criley JM, et al. Presystolic murmur in atrial fibrillation. *Circulation* 1977;56:133.
17. Criscitiello MG, et al. Cardiovascular abnormalities in osteogenesis imperfecta. *Circulation* 1965;31:255.
18. Dressler W. Effect of respiration on the pericardial friction rub. *Am J Cardiol* 1961;7:130.
19. Edwards JE. The congenital bicuspid aortic valve. *Circulation* 1961;23:485.
20. Edwards JE, Burchell HB. Endocardial and intimal lesions. *Circulation* 1958;18:946.
21. El-Sherif N. Rheumatic tricuspid stenosis. *Br Heart J* 1971;33:16.
22. Eversmeyer WH, et al. Aortic insufficiency with mild ankylosing spondylitis. *JAMA* 1978;240:2652.
23. Feruglio GA, Sreenivasan A. Intracardiac phonocardiogram in thirty cases of atrial septal defect. *Circulation* 1959;20:1087.
24. Fisher ML, et al. Hemodynamic response to isometric exercise. *Br Heart J* 1973;35:422.
25. Flint A. On cardiac murmurs. *Am J Med Sci* 1862;44:29.
26. Flint A. *Diseases of the Heart,* 2nd ed. New York: Macmillan, 1870:206.
27. Fontana ME, Wooley CF. The murmur of pulmonic regurgitation in tetralogy of Fallot. *Circulation* 1978;57:986.
28. Fortuin NJ, Craige E. On the mechanism of the Austin Flint murmur. *Circulation* 1972;45:558.
29. Fortuin NJ, Craige E. Echocardiographic studies of the genesis of mitral diastolic murmurs. *Br Heart J* 1973;35:75.
30. Foxe AN. Fenestrations of the semilunar valves. *Am J Pathol* 1929;5:179.
31. Fuchs RM, Achuff SC. Auscultatory findings of mitral prolapse. *Am Heart J* 1981;101:351.
32. Futamata H, et al. The diastolic rumble and fluttering of the ventricular wall after atrioventricular valve replacement. *J Cardiol* 1981;11:371.
33. Galioto FM Jr, et al. Right coronary artery to left ventricular fistula. *Am Heart J* 1971;82:93.
34. Gamble WH, Reddy PS. Preservation of the third heart sound in mitral stenosis. *N Engl J Med* 1983;309:498.
35. Gash AK, et al. Left ventricular function in combined mitral stenosis and aortic regurgitation. *Circulation* (Abstr) 1983;68(Suppl III):237.
36. Glassman RD, et al. Pacemaker-induced endocardial friction rubs. *Am J Cardiol* 1977;40:811.
37. Green EW, et al. Right-sided Austin Flint murmur. *Am J Cardiol* 1973;32:370.
38. Gumbiner CH, Gutgesell HP. Response to isometric exercise in children and young adults with aortic regurgitation. *Am Heart J* 1983;106:540.
39. Harvey WP. Auscultatory findings in disease of the pericardium. *Am J Cardiol* 1961;7:15.

40. Heidenreich FP, et al. Left-atrial transport in mitral stenosis. *Circulation* 1969;40:545.
41. How J, Strachan RW. Aortic regurgitation as a manifestation of giant cell arteritis. *Br Heart J* 1978; 40:1052.
42. Ide Y, et al. A study of atrial presystolic murmurs. *J Cardiol* 1978;8:505.
43. Ishikawa T, et al. A case of coronary-pulmonary artery fistula. *J Cardiol* 1976;6:169.
44. Kambe T, et al. Clinical study on the right-sided Austin Flint murmur. *Am Heart J* 1979;98:701.
45. Kaufmann G, et al. Heart sounds in atrial tumors. *Am J Cardiol* 1961;8:350.
46. Kawano K. Two-dimensional and Doppler echocardiographic studies of the genesis of a high-pitched diastolic rumble in mitral stenosis. *J Cardiol* 1989;19:155.
47. Kohno K, et al. Aortic regurgitation with dove-coo murmur with special reference to the mechanism of its generation using dual echocardiography. *Jpn Heart J* 1981;22:861.
48. Kong TO, et al. Clinical diagnosis of cardiac involvement in systemic lupus erythematosus. *Circulation* 1962; 26:7.
49. Laake H. Rheumatic tricuspid stenosis. *Acta Med Scand* 1958;161:109.
50. Lakier JB, et al. Primary degeneration: The most common etiology of isolated aortic regurgitation. *Circulation* 1983;68(Suppl III):297.
51. Liberthson RR, et al. Pulmonary regurgitation in large atrial shunts without pulmonary hypertension. *Circulation* 1976;54:966.
52. Lochaya S, et al. Late diastolic mitral regurgitation. *Am Heart J* 1967;74:161.
53. Luisada AA, Argano B. The phonocardiogram in systemic hypertension. *Chest* 1970;58:598.
54. Luisada AA, diBartole G. High-frequency phonocardiography. *Am J Cardiol* 1961;8:51.
55. Mirro MJ, et al Auscultatory and phonocardiographic features of normally functioning porcine mitral valve. *Circulation* 1977;55,56(Suppl III):69.
56. Morgan JR, et al. Isolated tricuspid stenosis. *Circulation* 1971;44:729.
57. Muna WF, et al. Psoriatic arthritis and aortic regurgitation. *JAMA* 1980;244:363.
58. Nadas AS, Ellison RC. Phonocardiographic analysis of diastolic flow murmurs in secundum atrial septal defect and ventricular septal defect. *Br Heart J* 1967;29:684.
59. Nemickas R, et al. Isolated congenital pulmonic insufficiency. *Am J Cardiol* 1964;14:456.
60. O'Brien KP, et al. Spontaneous aortic cusp rupture. *Circulation* 1968;37:273.
61. O'Brien KP, Cohen LS. Hemodynamic and phonocardiographic correlates of the Austin Flint murmur. *Am Heart J* 1969;77:603.
62. Parker E, et al. The Austin Flint murmur and the A wave of the apex cardiogram in aortic regurgitation. *Circulation* 1971;43:349.
63. Paul MH, et al. Congenital complete atrioventricular block. *Circulation* 1958;18:183.
64. Perloff JK. Auscultatory and phonocardiographic manifestations of pulmonary hypertension. *Progr Cardiovasc Dis* 1967;9:303.
65. Puchner TC, et al. Aortic valve insufficiency in arterial hypertension. *Am J Cardiol* 1960;5:758.
66. Read RC, et al. Symptomatic valvular myxomatous transformation. *Circulation* 1965;32:897.
67. Rosenthal T, Kariv I. A pathognomonic murmur of atypical patent ductus. *Chest* 1969;56:350.
68. Sadanandan S, et al. Diagnostic accuracy of auscultation in aortic regurgitation. *J Am Coll Cardiol* (Abstr) 1988; 11:175A.
69. Sagara T, et al. The clinical significance of the presystolic murmur in ischemic heart disease. *CV Sound Bull* 1974;4:471.
70. Saksena FB, et al. Massive left atrial thrombus. *Cardiology* 1976;61:298.
71. Sangster JF, Oakley CM. Diastolic murmur of coronary artery stenosis. *Br Heart J* 1973;35:840.
72. Schire V, et al. Unusual diastolic murmurs in constrictive pericarditis and endocarditis. *Am Heart J* 1968;76:4.
73. Schwab RH, Killough JH. The phonocardiographic differentiation of pulmonic and aortic insufficiency. *Circulation* 1965;32:352.
74. Semple T, Lancaster WM. Noisy pneumothorax. *Br Med J* 1961;1:1342.
75. Shabetai R, Davidson S. Asymmetrical hypertrophic cardiomyopathy. *Circulation* 1972;54:37.
76. Somerville J, Resnekov L. The origin of an immediate diastolic murmur in atrial ventricular defects. *Circulation* 1965;32:797.
77. Spodick DH. Pericardial friction. *N Engl J Med* 1968;278:1204.
78. Spodick DH. Acoustic phenomena in pericardial disease. *Am Heart J* 1971;81:114.
79. Starkey GWB. Surgical experience in the treatment of congenital mitral stenosis and insufficiency. *J Thorac Cardiovasc Surg* 1959;38:336.
80. Starr A, et al. The supravalvular aortic stenosis. *J Thorac Cardiovasc Surg* 1961;41:134.
81. Taquini AC, et al. Phonocardiographic studies of early rheumatic mitral disease. *Am Heart J* 1940;20:295.
82. Thompson ME, et al. Sound, pressure and motion correlates in mitral stenosis. *Am J Med* 1970;49:436.
83. Tominaga T, et al. Apical mid-diastolic rumble in hypertrophic cardiomyopathy: A pulsed Doppler echocardiographic study. *J Cardiol* 1985;15:1071.
84. Toutouzas P, et al. Double diastolic murmur in mitral stenosis. *Br Heart J* 1980;43:92.
85. Toutouzas P, et al. Mechanism of diastolic rumble and presystolic murmur in mitral stenosis. *Br Heart J* 1974; 36:1096.

86. Tsuneyoshi H, et al. Pulmonic regurgitation with special reference to the shape of the pulmonic valve ring. *J Cardiol* 1985;15:1145.
87. Ueda H, et al. The Austin Flint murmur. *Jpn Heart J* 1965;6:294.
88. Ueda H, et al. "Silent" mitral stenosis. *Jpn Heart J* 1965;6:206.
89. Wigle ED, Labrosse CJ. Sudden, severe aortic insufficiency. *Circulation* 1965;32:708.
90. Wood P. An appreciation of mitral stenosis. *Br Med J* 1954;1:1051. (Classic article.)
91. Wood P. An appreciation of mitral stenosis. *Br Med J* 1954;1:1113. (Classic article.)
92. Wooley CF, et al. Intracardiac sound and pressure events in man. *Am J Med* 1967;42:248.
93. Wunsch CM, Tavel ME. Patent ductus and pulmonary valve insufficiency. *Chest* 1970;57:572.

16

Abdominal Murmurs

1. List the common causes of abdominal murmurs, besides renal artery stenosis.
    ANS.: a. Normal arterial and venous flow murmurs, usually heard only in young people.
        b. Hepatic malignancies, alcoholic hepatitis, and portal-systemic vein anastomoses in portal hypertension (4).
        c. Splenic artery aneurysms or stenosis.
        d. Aortic atheromatous obstruction.
        e. Superior mesenteric or iliac artery stenosis (4).

NORMAL ABDOMINAL MURMURS

1. How common are abdominal murmurs in normal subjects?
    ANS.: They occur in almost half of subjects under age 25 but in only about 5% of those over age 50. (Thus, an abdominal murmur in an older adult should probably be considered abnormal [2].)
        Note: Normal murmurs are heard in the epigastrium or over the inferior vena cava, where a venous hum is heard in about 5% of normal subjects (2). In very thin patients, these murmurs may radiate to the left lower sternal border of the chest and may be confused with a cardiac murmur.
2. How can amyl nitrite inhalation indicate the degree of stenosis producing the arterial murmur?
    ANS.: With moderate stenosis, the arterial murmur is intensified by increasing the flow through the stenotic area. With severe stenosis, on the other hand, the murmur may soften, because amyl nitrite can dilate collateral vessels to the area beyond the obstruction, and the blood escapes via these collaterals (3).

RENAL ARTERY STENOSIS MURMURS

1. What is the pitch and timing of the stenosing renal vascular murmur?
    ANS.: It is high-pitched, sometimes to-and-fro with systolic accentuation, sometimes only a short systolic murmur, and sometimes continuous.
        Note: a. With the palm of your hand, press the diaphragm chestpiece firmly over various parts of the upper abdomen, with the patient in expiratory apnea.
            b. The best sites for hearing renal vascular murmurs are beneath the costal margin anteriorly, lateral to the aorta and lumbar spine, or just above the umbilicus, usually to the left of the midline.

313

c. In a hypertensive patient a murmur over a femoral artery due to atherosclerosis suggests the presence of renal artery stenosis.

MISCELLANEOUS ABDOMINAL MURMURS

1. What does a venous hum over the abdominal wall suggest?

   ANS.: If it is not the normal venous hum in a young person, it suggests portal hypertension and an anastomosis between the portal and systemic veins.

   > *Note*: A continuous murmur means either an arteriovenous fistula of the portal system or renal artery stenosis. If the venous hum over the xiphoid region or umbilical area is heard over the chest, you should suspect hepatic cirrhosis with portal-systemic anastomosis (Cruveilheir-Baumgarten syndrome). Systolic accentuation occurs with inspiration or sitting up. Firm pressure at the site of a thrill may cause the murmur to disappear.

2. What should a systolic murmur in the left hypochondrium suggest?

   ANS.: a. An aneurysmal or tortuous and calcified splenic artery, a huge spleen, a traumatized spleen, or compression of the splenic artery by carcinoma of the pancreas.

   b. Renal artery stenosis.

   > *Note*: a. A friction rub over the splenic area suggests splenic infarction.
   >
   > b. An epigastric murmur is more likely to be due to celiac artery compression than to renal artery stenosis (1).

3. After what kind of surgery should a patient who develops congestive heart failure postoperatively have the abdomen explored for a continuous murmur?

   ANS.: After lumbar disc surgery because a fistula may have occurred between the aorta (or iliac artery) and the inferior vena cava.

REFERENCES

1. McLoughlin MJ, et al. Abdominal bruits. *JAMA* 1975;232:1238.
2. Rivin AU. Abdominal vascular sounds. *JAMA* 1972;221:699.
3. Ueda H, et al. Quantitative assessment of obstruction of the aorta and its branches in "aortitis syndrome." *Jpn Heart J* 1966;7:3.
4. Zoneraich S, Zoneraich O. Diagnostic significance of abdominal arterial murmurs in liver and pancreatic disease. *Angiology* 1971;22:197.

17

Prosthetic Valve Sounds

PROSTHETIC VALVE ABNORMALITIES

Aortic Prosthetic Valve Abnormalities

1. What can make the OC of a ball valve softer than normal?
   ANS.: The OC may be muffled (less than 50% of the loudness of the OC on a phonocardiogram) if
      a. There is a clot on the cage that cushions the impact of the ball as it strikes the cage, or
      b. There is a cardiomyopathy, with resultant poor myocardial contractility (1).
2. How can you tell that a metallic (titanium or "stellite") ball is malfunctioning due to clot formation?
   ANS.: A normal metallic ball valve produces multiple systolic clicks (like the rapid firing of a machine gun) due to fluttering of the ball. When these clicks disappear, metallic ball valve malfunction is probable.
3. What usually causes an aortic prosthetic valve to become regurgitant?
   ANS.: A paravalvular (suture line) leak.
       Note: a. Small aortic paravalvular leaks occur in at least 15% of such valves (5).
            b. When *severe* aortic regurgitation occurs with a prosthetic aortic valve, preoperatively there usually has been a heavily calcified valve that has involved the valve ring and does not hold sutures well.
            c. When an aortic prosthesis becomes detached and has a rocking motion as it hangs by only a hinge of sutures (usually at the site of the former posterior noncoronary cusp), the detached prosthesis may push up the anterior mitral leaflet during diastole, resulting in a relative stenosis. This can cause a middiastolic murmur (5). The abnormal rocking motion can usually be detected by fluoroscopy.
4. What is the major difference between the OC and CC of a disc valve and those of a ball valve?
   ANS.: The OC of a disc valve is normally softer than the CC and therefore sounds like an abnormal ball valve.

Mitral Prosthetic Valve Abnormalities

1. How does the murmur of a paravalvular, prosthetic, mitral valve leak differ from that of native valve regurgitation?

ANS.: a. A systolic apical murmur due to a paravalvular leak often is not audible even when severe (7).

b. It may be audible only in unexpected places, such as the posterior chest wall.

Note: The development of unexplained heart failure in a patient with a prosthetic mitral valve should always raise the suspicion of silent, severe mitral regurgitation due to a paravalvular leak.

PORCINE HETEROGRAFTS

1. Which valve is taken from the pig's heart to be used for mitral valve replacement? Why?

ANS.: The aortic valve. An aortic valve does not require chordae tendineae or papillary muscles.

Note: a. Only about two-thirds of normally functioning porcine heterografts in the mitral position have an OS. About one-half have a "mitral" diastolic rumble (3).

b. Ejection murmurs can be heard in about two-thirds of patients with a porcine mitral bioprosthesis because of the turbulent flow past the stent, which projects into the outflow tract enough to produce some obstruction (8).

c. When a bioprosthetic valve in the aortic position becomes fibrotic or calcified, the pitch of the A_2 increases (6).

TILTING DISC VALVES

1. What is characteristic of the opening and closing sounds of tilting disc valves?

ANS.: Although the Lillehai-Kaster valve can open silently, the Bjork-Shiley and St. Jude valves usually produce multiple clicks often followed by a middiastolic rumble.

Note: The multiple opening clicks of a mitral disc valve often sound like an early diastolic crackle (2).

REFERENCES

1. Delman AJ. Aortic ball variance. *Am Heart J* 1972;83:291.
2. Kupari M, et al. Auscultatory characteristics of normal functioning Lillehai-Kaster, Bjork-Shiley, and St. Jude heart valve prostheses. *Br Heart J* 1986;55:364.
3. Schluger J, et al. Auscultatory and phonocardiographic sign of ball variance in a mitral prosthetic valve. *Am Heart J* 1971;81:809.
4. Shah PM, et al. Spread of the mitral sound over the chest: A study of five subjects with the Starr-Edwards valve. *Circulation* 1963;28:1102.
5. Smith ND, et al. Auscultation of the normally functioning prosthetic valve. *Ann Intern Med* 1981;95:5.
6. Stein PD, et al. Frequency spectra of the first heart sound and the aortic component of the second heart sound in patients with degenerated porcine bioprosthetic valves. *Am J Cardiol* 1984;53:557.
7. Sutton GC, et al. Major detachment of aortic prosthetic valves. *Br Heart J* 1970;32:337.
8. Yoshida K, et al. Left ventricular outflow obstruction by the mitral porcine bioprosthesis. *Circulation* (Abstr) 1979;74:298.

18

Systolic Time Intervals

DEFINITIONS AND METHODS OF MEASUREMENT

1. What are the systolic time intervals (STIs)?

    ANS.: They are the left ventricular (LV) ejection time (ET) and the preejection period (PEP).

    > *Note*: Measuring and interpreting STIs is probably the most simple and accurate noninvasive method of evaluating myocardial function because they reveal not only the degree of ejection but also the heart's ability to undergo isovolumic contraction.

2. What is meant by the *LVET*? How is it measured?

    ANS.: It is the time between the opening and closing of the aortic valves. It can be measured directly from an echocardiographic study of aortic valve motion. It can also be measured indirectly as the interval between the upstroke and the dicrotic notch of an external carotid pulse tracing (Fig. 1).

3. What is meant by the *PEP*?

    ANS.: It is the time between the beginning of electrical activation of the heart (the onset of the Q or R wave of the QRS) and the opening of the aortic valve (indirectly measured by the onset of the rise in carotid pressure on the tracing or opening of the aortic valve on an M-mode echocardiogram). Changes in isovolumic contraction time are reflected in changes in PEP.

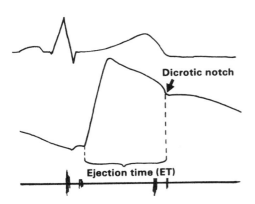

FIG. 1. The ET is measured from the upstroke of the carotid to the dicrotic notch. A slight hump is often seen preceding the first sharp upstroke. This probably represents isovolumic contraction time and should not be included in the ET. The ET is often called the LVET, but the LV seems redundant, because we assume that we are dealing with left-sided events unless told otherwise.

317

PHYSIOLOGIC CHANGES

1. How are the STIs affected by (a) heart rate, (b) sex, (c) age, and (d) active occupation?
   ANS.: a. The faster the heart rate, the shorter the STIs (both PEP and ET are short-ened).
   b. Women have slightly longer STIs than men, due mainly to a prolongation of the ET. This difference begins at puberty (23).
   c. Children have slightly shorter STIs than adults. Older subjects have slightly longer PEPs and ETs. (The ET increases by about 2 msec [0.002 sec] per decade, so that by age 80, it is about 10 to 20 msec [0.01 to 0.02 sec] longer than normal by the usual regression equation that corrects for heart rate.)
   d. Active people have been found to have shorter PEPs than those who are seden-tary (67).
   Note: To correct the STIs for heart rate and sex, three methods are used.
   a. Read the upper and lower limits of normal for rate and sex from graphs made from established linear regression equations. The graphs use one standard deviation (SD) as the limits (Figs. 2–5) .

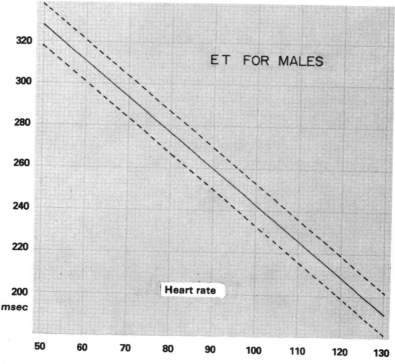

FIG. 2.   This graph can be used for male adults. Older and female subjects have slightly longer ejection times. Children have shorter ejection times.

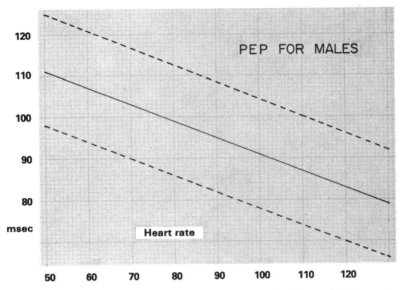

FIG. 3. This graph shows that, for a heart rate of 90, the preejection period for male subjects should not be much longer than 105 msec. This reflects isovolumic contraction.

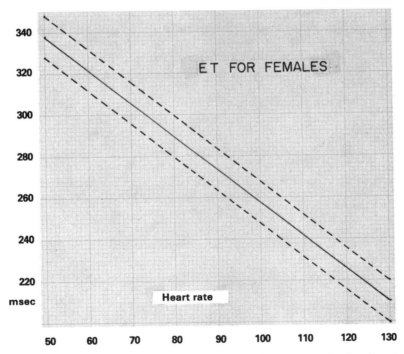

FIG. 4. This graph shows that, if the heart rate is 90, the upper normal ejection time for female subjects is 280 msec (longer than for male subjects). A linear relation exists between heart rate and ejection time for heart rates between 50 and 120.

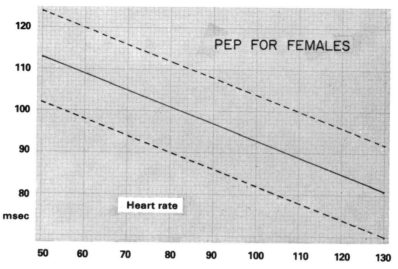

FIG. 5. This graph shows that, if the heart rate is 90, the preejection period for female subjects can be as long as 110 msec, which is longer than for male subjects.

b. Use a single number calculated from the regression equation. This is the STI index. It offers a convenient expression for studying serial changes and for comparing patients (33,63).

The ET index for males is the ET plus 1.7 times the heart rate. The normal index is 413 ± 10 msec. For females, use 1.6, and the normal index is 418 ± 11 msec. The PEP index for males and females is the PEP plus 0.4 times the heart rate. The normal PEP index for males is 131 ± 10; for females it is 133 ± 10.

c. Use the ratio of PEP/ET to ignore heart rate and sex. PEP/ET ratios are unrelated to age or heart rates from age 1 month to 15 years, when the mean is 0.31 (SD = 0.05). For adults the mean is 0.34 (SD = 0.04). Adolescents have a PEP/ET ratio between that of children and adults because although both PEP and ET increase with age, the PEP lengthens slightly more than does the ET (12,68). The upper normal for adults should therefore be considered to be 0.42 (i.e., 2 SDs).

Note: In the normal adult a linear relation may be accepted between the ET and heart rate for heart rates of between 50 and 120 mm (66).

2. How does a change in volume of the LV affect the STI?

ANS.: Although the increased Starling effect of increased volume tends to shorten the PEP, the volume effect lengthens the ET (42). Conversely, the decreased Starling effect of a decreased volume, such as occurs with diuretics, raising the chest, or standing, lengthens the PEP and shortens the ET. If the chest is raised to 45 degrees, the PEP/ET is 28 ± 0.03 (39). If the chest is raised to 60 degrees, there is almost a 25% decrease in return of blood to the heart and lungs.

FACTORS AFFECTING STIs

Myocardial Damage

1. How does total time for contraction of a piece of muscle from a subject in heart failure compare with normal muscle?

    ANS.: Surprisingly, the total time for contraction is *unchanged*; that is, if it takes 300 msec (0.30 sec) for total contraction time before failure, it will take about 300 msec for total contraction after heart failure (49).

2. How has it been shown that the entire LV takes the same amount of time for total contraction after heart failure as before failure?

    ANS.: The QS_2 (PEP $\pm$ ET) is the same in patients with and without failure.

3. Does the heart in failure take a longer or shorter time to raise pressure to open the aortic valve; that is, how is isovolumic contraction time affected?

    ANS.: Isovolumic contraction time is prolonged (which is the same as saying that the PEP is prolonged).

    Note: If the PEP is prolonged in heart failure, and the total contraction time is unchanged, the ET must shorten.

4. What is Hegglin syndrome? Significance?

    ANS.: It means the Q-T is prolonged and the Q-2 is shortened. Normally, Q-T is less than Q-2 by 26 $\pm$ 13 msec. Patients with Hegglin syndrome have various degrees of depressed myocardial function.

Hypertension

See references 15, 27, 48, 56.

Coronary Artery Disease

1. Coronary disease at rest. See references 10, 12.
2. Exercise. See references 3, 7, 8, 10, 33, 41, 54, 69.
3. Effect of acute myocardial infarction on STIs. See references 34, 44, 59.
4. Effect of prognosis on STIs. See reference 22.
5. Effect of ejection fraction on STIs. See references 46, 50.

Valvular Heart Disease

1. Aortic stenosis and regurgitation. See references 4, 6, 26, 34, 37, 51, 52, 66.
2. Mitral stenosis and regurgitation. See references 7, 19, 31, 43, 53, 60.

Constriction and Tamponade

See references 2, 13, 21, 28, 29, 30.

Conduction Defects and Arrhythmias

1. Bundle branch block. See references 5, 6, 11, 24, 40, 65, 70.
2. Atrial fibrillation. See references 6, 47, 57.
3. Premature beats 66.

Drugs and Hormones

1. Amyl nitrite effect. See reference 45.
2. Propranolol effect. See references 17, 18, 35, 36, 65.
3. Digitalis effect. See references 25, 63, 62.
4. Adriamycin. See reference 14.
5. Hypothyroidism. See references 9, 16, 25.
6. Hyperthyroidism. See references 1, 11, 25, 36, 40, 56, 64.
7. Diabetes. See reference 55.

Shunts

ASD and VSD. See references 38, 53, 61.

Anemia

See reference 58.

REFERENCES

1. Amidi M, et al. Effect of the thyroid state on myocardial contractility. *Circulation* 1968;38:229.
2. Armstrong TS, et al. Systolic time intervals in constrictive pericarditis. *Am Heart J* 1973;85:6.
3. Aronow WS, et al. External isovolumic contraction times and left ventricular ejection time/external isovolumic contraction time ratios at rest and after exercise in coronary heart disease. *Circulation* 1971;43:59.
4. Bache RJ, et al. Left ventricular ejection times in aortic stenosis. *Circulation* 1973;47:527.
5. Baragan J, et al. Chronic left complete bundle branch block. *Br Heart J* 1968;30:196.
6. Bonner AJ Jr, Tavel ME. Systolic time intervals. *Arch Intern Med* 1973;132:816.
7. Boudoulas H, et al. Abbreviation of systolic time intervals in acute mitral regurgitation. *Am J Cardiol* 1979; 44:595.
8. Boudoulas H, et al. Effect of propranolol on post-exercise left ventricular ejection time index. *Am J Cardiol* 1981;48:357.
9. Bough EW, et al. Myocardial function in hypothyroidism. *Arch Intern Med* 1978;138:1476.
10. Bowlby JR. Effects of exercise on left ventricular ejection time in patients with hypertension or angina pectoris. *Am Heart J* 1979;97:348.
11. Braunwald E, Morrow AG. Sequence of ventricular contraction in human bundle branch block. *Am J Med* 1957; 23:205.
12. Buyukozturk K, et al. Systolic time intervals. *Am J Cardiol* 1971;28:183.
13. Carter WH, et al. Respiratory variation of left ventricular ejection time in pericardial effusion. *Am J Cardiol* 1972;29:427.
14. Chaudron J-M, et al. Adriamycin cardiotoxicity and systolic time intervals. *World Congress Cardiol Tokyo* 1978;367.
15. Cousineau D, et al. Circulating catecholamines and systolic time intervals. *Am Heart J* 1978;96:227.
16. Crowley WF, et al. Noninvasive evaluation of cardiac function in hypothyroidism. *N Engl J Med* 1977;296:1.
17. Frankl WS, et al. The effect of propranolol on left ventricular function in angina pectoris as measured by systolic time intervals. *Res Commun Chem Pathol Pharmacol* 1972;4:77.
18. Frishman W, et al. Noninvasive assessment of clinical response to oral propranolol. *Am J Cardiol* 1975;35:635.
19. Fujiki A, et al. Noninvasive assessment of left ventricular performance and grade of regurgitation in mitral insufficiency. *J Cardiol* 1980;10:521.
20. Garrard CL Jr, et al. The relationship of alterations in systolic time intervals to ejection fraction. *Circulation* 1970;42:455.
21. Ghose SK, et al. Differential diagnosis between constrictive pericarditis and cardiomyopathy. *Br Heart J* 1976; 38:47.
22. Gillilan RE, et al. The prognostic value of systolic time intervals in angina pectoris. *Circulation* 1979;60:268.
23. Golde D, Burstin L. Systolic phases of the cardiac cycle in children. *Circulation* 1970;42:1029.
24. Haft JI, et al. Left bundle branch block. *Circulation* 1971;42:279.
25. Hillis WS, et al. Systolic time intervals in thyroid disease. *Clin Endocrinol* 1975;4:617.
26. Ibrahim M, et al. Systolic time intervals in valvular aortic stenosis and idiopathic hypertrophic subaortic stenosis. *Br Heart J* 1973;35:276.
27. Inoue K, et al. Left ventricular function in essential hypertension. *Am J Cardiol* 1973;32:264.

28. Ito M, et al. Echocardiography, phonocardiography and carotid artery pulse wave in patients with pericardial effusion. *Jpn J Clin Cardiol* 1976;5:15.
29. Jain AC, et al. Left ventricular function after cigarette smoking by chronic smokers. *Am J Cardiol* 1977;39:27.
30. Khullar S, Lewis RP. Usefulness of systolic time intervals in constrictive pericarditis and restrictive cardiomyopathy. *Br Heart J* 1976;38:43.
31. Kligfield P, et al. Effect of additional lesions on left ventricular ejection time in aortic stenosis. *Br Heart J* 1977; 39:1259.
32. Kligfield P, Okin P. Effect of ventricular function on left ventricular ejection time in aortic stenosis. *Br Heart J* 1979;42:438.
33. Lewis RP, et al. Enhanced diagnostic power of exercise testing for myocardial ischemia by addition of post-exercise ejection time. *Am J Cardiol* 1977;39:767.
34. Lewis RP, et al. A critical review of the systolic time intervals. *Circulation* 1977;56:146.
35. Lopez-Arostegul F, et al. Effect of beta blockade on response of systolic time intervals to exercise. *Circulation* 1971;43,44 (Suppl II):196.
36. Mazzaferri EL, et al. Propranolol as a primary therapy for thyrotoxicosis. *Arch Intern Med* 1976;136:50.
37. Nandi PS, Spodick DH. Determination of systolic intervals utilizing the carotid first derivative. *Am Heart J* 1973;80:495.
38. Nesje OA. Systolic time intervals in isolated ventricular septal defect in the adult. *Circulation* 1980;62:609.
39. Northover BJ. Left ventricular systolic time intervals in patients with acute infarction. *Br Heart J* 1980;43:506.
40. Parisi AF, et al. The short cardiac pre-ejection period. *Circulation* 1974;49:900.
41. Pouget JM, et al. Abnormal responses of the systolic time intervals to exercise. *Circulation* 1971;43:289.
42. Rubler S, et al. Systolic time intervals in pregnancy and the postpartum period. *Am Heart J* 1973;86:182.
43. Sakamoto T, et al. Systolic time intervals in left ventricular function of mitral stenosis. *CV Sound Bull* 1973; 3:253.
44. Samson R. Changes in systolic time intervals in acute infarction. *Br Heart J* 1970;32:839.
45. Sawayama T, et al. Influence of amyl nitrite inhalation on systolic time intervals in normal subjects and in patients with ischemic heart disease. *Circulation* 1969;40:327.
46. Sawayama T, et al. Polygraphic studies on the effect of nitroglycerin in patients with ischaemic heart disease. *Br Heart J* 1973;35:1234.
47. Sawayama T, et al. Noninvasive evaluation of diastolic filling patterns in patients with atrial fibrillation. *Am J Cardiol* 1980;45:1005.
48. Shaver JA, et al. The effect of steady-state increases in arterial pressure on ejection time. *J Clin Invest* 1968; 47:217.
49. Spann JF, et al. Contractile state of cardiac muscle. *Circ Res* 1967;21:341.
50. Stack RS, et al. Left ventricular performance in coronary artery disease evaluated with systolic time intervals. *Am J Cardiol* 1976;37:331.
51. Stefadouros MA, et al. Internally recorded systolic time intervals in hypertrophic subaortic stenosis. *Am J Cardiol* 1977;40:700.
52. Stefadouros MA, et al. Post-extrasystolic changes in systolic time intervals in the assessment of hypertrophic cardiomyopathy. *Br Heart J* 1982;47:261.
53. Sutton R, et al. Noninvasive assessment of left ventricular function in chronic heart disease. *Am Heart J* 1977; 93:289.
54. Sugimoto T, Inasaka T. The measurement of systolic time intervals in left ventricular performance. *CV Sound Bull* 1975;3:241.
55. Sykes CA, et al. Changes in systolic time intervals during treatment of diabetes. *Br Heart J* 1977;39:255.
56. Tarazi RC, et al. Left atrial abnormality and preejection period in hypertension. *Dis Chest* 1969;55:214.
57. Tavel ME, et al. Ejection time in atrial fibrillation. *Circulation* 1972;46:744.
58. Val-Mejias J, et al. Left ventricular performance during and after sickle cell crisis. *Am Heart J* 1979;97:585.
59. Waagstein F, et al. Apex cardiogram and systolic time intervals in acute myocardial infarction. *Br Heart J* 1974; 36:1109.
60. Wanderman KL, et al. Left ventricular performance in mitral regurgitation assessed with systolic time intervals. *Am J Cardiol* 1976;38:831.
61. Wanderman KL, et al. Left ventricular performance in patients with atrial septal defect. *Am J Cardiol* 1978; 41:487.
62. Weissler AM, et al. Prognostic significance of systolic time intervals after infarction. *Am J Cardiol* 1981;48:995.
63. Weissler AM, Schoenfeld CD. Effect of digitalis on systolic time intervals. *Am J Med Sci* 1970;259:4.
64. Welch TG, Lewis RP. Hyperadrenergic state in coronary artery disease. *Clin Res* 1974;22:155.
65. Wennemark JR, et al. Cardiodynamic effect of experimental bundle branch block. *Circ Res* 1962;10:280.
66. White WC, Zimmerman TJ. Prolonged left ventricular ejection time in the postpremature beat. *Circulation* 1975; 52:306.
67. Whitsett TL, Naughton J. The effect of exercise on systolic time intervals. *Am J Cardiol* 1971;27:252.
68. Willems JL, et al. The left ventricular ejection time in elderly subjects. *Circulation* 1970;42:37.
69. Winter WG, et al. The effect of exercise on intrinsic myocardial performance. *Circulation* 1973;48:50.
70. Wong B, et al. Effect of intermittent left bundle branch block on left ventricular performance in the normal heart. *Am J Cardiol* 1977;39:459.

Subject Index

A

Abdominal aneurysm
  double murmur, 234
  pistol shot sound, 234
Abdominal compression test, 73–76
Abdominal jugular test, 74
Abdominal murmur, 313–314
Acquired facies, 19–21
Adams Stokes attack. *See* Stokes-Adams attack
Amyl nitrite
  action of, 250–251
  administration of, 250–251
  in PS, 231
  in VSD, 266–267
Amyloid heart disease
  cardiomyopathy and S_3, 189
  square root sign, 89
Amyloidosis, 18
Anacrotic notch, 33
Anacrotic pulse, 33
Anacrotic shoulder, 31, 33
Anemia, and AR, 300
Aneroid manometer, 46–47
Aneurysm
  abdominal
    double murmur, 234
    pistol shot sound, 234
  and atrial septal click, 259
  dissecting
    and AR, 300
    double murmur in, 234
    septal and click, 259
Angioid streaks, 24
Angle of Louis, 69
Ankylosing spondylitis
  AR in, 299
Annulus
  calcified mitral, 240, 241
  distortion and PR, 308
Anomalous left coronary artery, and MR, 240
Anomalous pulmonary vein, and jugular waves, 86
Anomalous pulmonary vein connection
  and fixed split, 162

and murmurs, 268
Anti-Hegglin syndrome, 143
Anulo-aortic ectasia, 143, 300
Aortic aneurysm, palpation for, 114
Aortic-annular ectasia, 143, 300
Aortic arch syndromes, and venous hum, 274
Aortic area, 221
Aortic dissection, 12–13
Aortic-pulmonary septal defect, 269, 272
Aortic regurgitation. *See* Murmurs;
      Regurgitation, aortic
Aortic root sound theory, 128
Aortic sclerosis
  murmur of, 219–220
  and septal angulation, 220
Aortic stenosis. *See* Stenosis, aortic
Aortic valve. *See* Murmurs, diastolic;
      Murmurs, systolic; Regurgitation,
      aortic; Valves, aortic
A_2P_2
  vs. A_2OS, 176–179
  vs. tricuspid OS, 180
Apex beat, 94–99
  in AS, 34
  in ASD, 100–101
  "A" wave of, 111–113, 116
  in cardiac enlargement
    false displacement of, 102
    in left lateral decubitus position, 99–101
    in sitting position, 97–98
  in endocardial cushion defect, 101
  left *vs.* right ventricular, 99
  in LV hypertrophy, 101
  in mitral stenosis, 102
  normal, 110
  normal site of, 96–97
    determination of, 97–98
  palpation of, 95–96, 97
    chest position for, 95–96
  vs. PMI, 95
  in PS, 101
  as sign in cardiac enlargement, 99–101
  sustained, 110–111

Apex cardiogram, 115–116
  and palpable A wave, 196
  and S$_3$, 183, 184
AR. *See* Regurgitation, aortic
Arcus, corneal, 22
Argyll Robertson pupil, 21
Arm, palpation, 30
Arrhythmias
  etiology, 13
  and jugular waves, 91–92
Arteriosclerosis
  rate of rise, 33
  retinal signs, 23
Arteriovenous fistula
  bounding pulses in, 36
  continuous murmur, 268, 274
AS. *See* Stenosis, aortic
Ascites, in congestive heart failure, 25
ASD. *See* Atrial septal defect
ASH. *See* Asymmetric septal hypertrophy
Asthma, blood pressure in, 60
Asymmetric septal hypertrophy, 223
Atrial clicks, 195, 207
Atrial fibrillation
  and clicks, 195
  and jugular waves, 91–92
  and S$_1$ loudness, 140
  on split S$_2$, 160
Atrial flutter. *See* Atrial fibrillation
Atrial gallop. *See* Heart sound, fourth (S$_4$)
Atrial hump, 111, 116
Atrial kick, 112, 113–114, 199. *See also* Apex
      beat
Atrial myxoma, 5
  left
      and loud S$_1$, 191
      murmurs in, 291
      S$_4$ in, 199
      tumor plop *vs.* S$_3$ in, 191
      and widely split S$_2$, 155
  right
      murmurs in, 298
      vs. TS, 298
Atrial regurgitation
  bounding pulses in, 36
  pulses in, 37
Atrial septal defect
  apex beat in, 100–101
  chest movement in, 104
  and cleft mitral valve, 240
  and continuous murmur, 215–216
  and Down syndrome, 20
  and Ellis-van Creveld syndrome, 27

  and endocardial cushion defect, 257
  extremity abnormalities with, 26
  and Holt-Oram syndrome, 27
  and jugular waves, 86, 87
  and Lutembacher syndrome, 215
  and Marfan syndrome, 27
  and mitral valve prolapse, 257
  and MR, 257
  murmurs, 215–216
  and OS, 179
  and P$_2$ at apex, 149
  persistent left superior vena cava in, 68
  and P$_2$ loudness *vs.* A$_2$, 150–151
  and pulmonary flow murmur, 236
  with pulmonary hypertension
      in RV enlargement, 105
  and pulmonary regurgitation, 306
  and S$_3$, 188
  and S$_4$, 204
  and split S$_2$
      after long pause, 160
      after surgery, 155
      and Eisenmenger syndrome, 165
      fixed, 155, 157–158
      narrow, 160
      vs. pulmonary hypertension, 162
      with pulmonary stenosis, 161
      on standing, 160, 161
      and Valsalva maneuver, 161
      wide, 154
  tricuspid flow murmur, 296
  and tuft erythema, 18
Atrial septum, 259
Atrial sounds, 195
Atrioventricle, 67, 112
Atrioventricular block
  complete
      inaudible S$_4$ in, 195
      mitral flow murmur in, 295
      split S$_4$ in, 198
Atrioventricular valve regurgitation
  and Down syndrome, 20
Auscultatory gap, 48
Auscultogram, 123–126
AV block. *See* Atrioventricular block
A wave, 111–112, 116. *See also* Apex
      cardiogram; Jugular waves and contours
  palpable, 196

B

Barlow syndrome. *See* Valves, mitral, prolapse
      of

Beriberi, 18
Bernoulli effect, 223
Bicuspid aortic valve
    in AR, 299
    and ejection sound, 299
Billowing mitral valve syndrome. *See* Valves,
        mitral, prolapse of
Bisferiens pulse, 38–40
Bjork-Shiley valve, 292, 316
Blood pressure, 42–51
    in AS, 42–43
    accuracy of, 49–51
    in AR, 43
    arm differences in, 43
    in asthma, 60
    calcified brachial arteries effect on, 51
    and chestpiece pressure, 50
    in children, 42
    circadian rhythm and, 50
    cuff size and, 47
    deflation and inflation rates for, 48–49
    diastolic pressure recording, 46
    disappearance point in, 46
    by Doppler, 49
    in embolism, 60
    and exercise, 49
    false-negative, 60–62
    false-positive, 60–62
    in infants, 42, 49
    in legs, 54–62
        in AR, 56
        vs. arms, 54
        auscultation, 54–55
        in coarctation, 56–58
        by Doppler, 55
        Hill sign in, 56
        in infants, 55–56
    marked inspiratory fall, 59–61
    mechanism, 60
    muffling point in, 46
    by palpation alone, 44
    reproducibility of, 49–50
    respiration effect on, 58–59
    in shock, 49
    systolic pressure recording errors, 46–49
    without cuff, 43–44
Blue sclerae, 24
Brachial arteries, medial sclerosis of, 51
Bradycardia, and opening snap, 174
Bradydactyly, congenital syndromes in, 27
Brockenbrough effect, 35, 36
Bronchial collateral flow. *See*
        Bronchopulmonary anastomosis

Bronchopulmonary anastomosis
    with congenital cyanosis, 268
    continuous murmur, 268
    murmur, 276
Bruit *vs.* murmur, 233
Bypass surgery murmur, 234–235

C

Cannon waves. *See* A wave, palpable; Jugular
        waves and contours
Capillary pulsation, 62
Carcinoid heart disease
    history in, 5
    and TR, 261
Cardiac dilatation, identification of, 99–101
        by apex beat, 98–99
        in left lateral decubitus position, 99–101
        by percussion, 99
Cardiac enlargement
    identification of, 99–100
Cardiac malpositions, 102
Cardiac rhabdomyomas, 19
Cardiac size
    determination of, 99
    x-ray evaluation of, 107–109
Cardiac tumors, history in, 5
Cardiomegaly, apex beat in, 97
Cardiomyopathy
    amyloid, 189
    hypertrophic subaortic (HSS or HOCM)
        and asymmetric septal hypertrophy, 223
        and Bernoulli effect, 223
        ejection murmur in, 222–227
            and maneuvers, 225–226
            vs. MR, 226–227
            vs. valvular AS, 224–225, 226
        ejection sound in, 131–132
        and fluttering leaflet, 224
        and inflow gradients, 223
        and MR, 223. 226–227
        with right ventricle obstruction, 223
        S_2 split in, 166
        S_3 split in, 189
        and systolic anterior motion, 223
Cardiorespiratory murmurs, 261
Cardiothoracic (C/T) ratios, 107
Carey Coombs murmur, 296
Carotid artery, murmur, 233
Carotid-cavernous sinus arteriovenous fistula,
        and exophthalmos, 23
Carotid pulse, in AS, 34
Carotid shudder, 39

Carvallo sign, 259
Chest
    examination of, 27–28
        for ventricular hypertrophy, 94–99
Chest pain, etiology, 11–13
Chest wall, aortic and arterial pulsations,
        114–115
Cheynes-Stokes respiration, 28
Chondroectodermal dysplasia, 27
Chordae
    anatomy of, 243
    rupture of, 200, 243–246
        murmur characteristics, 243–244
Chordal snap theory, 257
Chronic obstructive pulmonary disease, split S_2
        in, 169
Click late-systolic syndrome. See Valves,
        mitral, prolapse of
Clicks
    and absence of pericardium, 258
    in aneurysm of septum, 263–264
    in AR, 259
    atrial, 195
    from balloon catheter, 258
    ejection. See Heart sounds, first (S_1)
    non-ejection, 251–253
    and pericardial adhesions, 258
    in VSD with aneurysm, 263–264
Closing snap, 178
Clubbing, 16–17
Coarctation of aorta, 25
    abdominal, 278
    bounding pulses in, 36
    leg pulses in, 56–58
        radial-femoral lag, 56–58
    murmurs in, 233–234
        continuous, 268
        subcostal, 234
    palpation for, 114–115
    vs. PS and bicuspid valve, 228
    symptoms, 6, 14
    and Turner syndrome, 21
Cole-Cecil murmur, 303
Complete AV block. See Atrioventricular block
Concentric hypertrophy. See Ventricular
        hypertrophy
Congenital facies, 19–21
Congenital heart disease, history in, 6
Congestive heart failure
    abdominal compression in, 73–74
    blood pressure in, 61
    and crackles, 117–118
    and exophthalmos, 23

and jugular waves, 86
Constriction, blood pressure in, 60
Constrictive pericarditis
    and jugular waves, 86, 88–90
    lateral retraction in, 104
    and loud S_1, 191
    and pericardial knock, 192–193
    RV enlargement in, 104, 105
    and S_4, 197
    square root sign, 89
Contraction ring theory, 257–258
COPD. See Chronic obstructive pulmonary
        disease
Corneal arcus, 22
Coronary artery
    bypass murmur, 234–235
    fistula, 276
        vs. AR murmur, 304
        to left ventricle, 276
        to right heart, 276–278
    and to-and-fro murmur, 276–277
Coronary artery stenosis, murmurs, 304
Cor pulmonale, history in, 4
Corrected transposition. See Transposition,
        corrected
Cor triatriatum, 269
Crackles, 28, auscultation for, 117–118
Cubitus valgus, 25
C wave. See Jugular waves and contours
Cyanosis
    central vs. peripheral, 16
    with continuous murmurs, 275
    differential, 17
    with PS murmurs, 230–231

D
DaCosta syndrome, 18
de Musset sign, 20
Dextrocardia, and right ventricular impulse,
        101
Dextroversion, 102
    and right ventricular impulse, 101
Diagramming murmurs, 126–127
Diastolic pressure. See Blood pressure
Dicrotic, wave and pulse, 40
    and AR murmur, 300–301
    cause of, 300–301
    in ruptured sinus of Valsalva, 276
Dilatation, vs. enlargement and hypertrophy,
        109
Discrete subvalvular AS, 227
Dissecting aneurysm

and AR, 300
   double murmur in, 234
   septal and click, 259
Diuretics
   effect on S$_3$, 187
Dizziness, etiology, 10–11
Double gallop, 202
Dove-coo musical murmur, 302
Down syndrome, 22
   facies, 20
Dressler syndrome, 309
Dyspnea, etiology, 7

E

Earlobe crease, 20
Ebstein's anomaly
   loud S$_1$ in, 138
   and opening snap, 179
   sail sound in, 138
   and TR *vs.* MR, 240
   and TS, 298
Eccentric hypertrophy. *See* Ventricular
   hypertrophy
Eddy sounds, 272
Eddy *vs.* vortex theory, 209
Edema, 24–25
   in bedridden patients, 24
   etiology, 9
   grading, 24
Ehler-Danlos syndrome, and mitral valve
   prolapse, 256
Eisenmenger syndrome
   definition, 165
   S$_2$ split in, 165
Ejection sound or click, 127
Ejection time. *See* Systolic time intervals
Electrical alternans, 53
Elfin facies, 227
Ellis-van Creveld syndrome, 27
Embryocardia, 152
Emphysema, mediastinal, 310. *See also*
   Chronic obstructive pulmonary disease
Endocardial cushion defect
   apex beat in, 101
   MR in, 240
Endocarditis
   and AR, 299
   infective and MS, 291
   verrucous, 291
Enlargement, *vs.* dilatation and hypertrophy,
   109
Erb point, 228

Ewart's sign, 28
Exophthalmos, 22–23
Extremities, examination of, 25–27
Eyes, examination of, 21–24

F

Facies, 19–21, 227
False tendon murmur, 217–218
Fenestrated valves, 299
"Fingerized thumb," 26
Fistulas. *See* Arteriovenous fistula; Coronary
   artery, fistula ; Murmurs, continuous;
   Pulmonary arteriovenous fistula
Floppy valve syndrome, 246
Flow murmurs. *See* Murmurs
Frequency, defined, 119
Friction rubs, 308–310
   components, 308
   and pacemakers, 309–310
   pleuropericardial, 308–310
   respiratory effect, 309
   site of, 309
   splenic, 314

G

Gallavardin phenomenon, 220
Gallop rhythm. *See also* Heart sounds, fourth
   (S$_4$); Heart sounds, third (S$_3$)
   augmented, 186
   double, 202
   and quadruple rhythm, 202
   summation, 186
   train-wheel, 202
Gibson murmur, 270
Gradient
   impulse, 213
   and pitch of murmur, 248
Grading sounds and murmurs, 127–128
Graham Steell murmur, 265, 305–306

H

Handgrip
   and AR loudness, 302
   and congestive heart failure, 250
   hemodynamic effects of, 202
   and HSS or HOCM, 225
   and mitral stenosis murmur, 289
Heart size. *See* Apex beat; Cardiac dilatation;
   Cardiac size

Heart sounds
  ejection
    aortic
      in AS, 127, 131–132, 135
      and bicuspid valve, 131
      in discrete subvalvular AS, 228
      in HSS or HOCM, 131–132
      in hypertension, 131
      in tetralogy of Fallot, 135
    in mitral valve prolapse, 135
    in persistent truncus arteriosus, 135
    pulmonary, 132–135
      in ASD, 137
      hypertension, 127, 136
      in idiopathic dilatation, 136–137
      in poststenotic dilatation, 134–135
      and posture, 134
      and Q-click interval, 135
      before QRS, 133
      respiration effect on, 134
      site of, 134
      in stenosis, 132–135
  first (S_1)
    in AS, 140
    changing
      in atrial fibrillation, 140
      in AV dissociation, 139
      in second degree AV block, 139–140
    in Ebstein's anomaly, 138
    factors controlling loudness, 137–141
    in LBBB, 140
    in mitral stenosis, 130
    in MR, 141
    and M sound, 128
    in myocardial infarction, 137–138
    nonejection clicks or sounds, 135
    and papillary muscle MR, 242–243
    physiology of, 127–130
    and PR interval, 138–139
    quality of
      and closing snap, 141
      in MS, 141
      in porcine valve, 141
      vs. S_2, 153
    splitting of
      in ASD, 130
      in bundle branch block, 130
      components in, 127, 128
      in infarction, 131
      in MS, 130
      origins of, 127, 129–130
    ventricular pressure rise in, 137–138
  fourth (S_4), 195–207
    after long diastoles, 202
    in angina, 200
    in AV block, 198
    and bell pressure, 201
    in constrictive pericarditis, 197
    and excess catecholamines, 200
    and held respiration, 201
    and hypertrophic cardiomyopathy, 199
    inaudible, 195
    increasing loudness of, 201
    mechanism for, 197
    in mild AS or hypertension, 204
    and MS, 196
    murmur, 297
    in myocardial infarction, 200
    and pacemaker click, 206–207
    pathological, 198–200
    physiological, 197–198
    and PS_4 and S_4S_1 intervals, 205–206
    rhythm, 197–200
    right-sided, 204–205
    vs. S_3, 202
    vs. split S_1, 203–204
    synonyms for, 195
    in volume overload, 200
    and A wave, 196
  second (S_2)
    and impedance, 144
    loudness of, 147–153
      in AR, 151
      and arterial recoil velocity, 147
      P_2 in ASD and MS, 150–151
      P_2 in pulmonary hypertension, 150–151
      vs. S_1, 153
      A_2 *vs.* P_2, 147
    mechanism of production, 143
    pulmonary component (P_2)
      and hangout interval, 144
      and impedance, 144
      in PS, 152
      split, 145–146
    single, in tetralogy of Fallot, 149
  vs. S_1 loudness and quality, 153
  soft
    causes of, 151–152
  split
    after age 50, 147
    bell *vs.* diaphragm in, 147
    eliciting, 147
    expiratory, 167
    fixed, 157–162
    and held respiration, 146, 155
    movement physiology in, 145–147

in MR, 155
narrow, 153–154
nonparadoxical, reversed, 168–169
in obesity, 149
paradoxical, 165–167
persistent expiratory, 154
A_2P_2 sequence, 144–147
QS_2 and Hegglin syndrome, 143
reduplicated, 145
reversed, 162–163, 166–167
in right chest, 149
in tamponade, 155
in transposition, 149
in truncus arteriosus, 145
vocal imitations of, 154
in VSD, 149
wide, 153–156
third (S_3)
and amyloid infiltrate, 189
and aneurysm, 185
and apex cardiogram, 183
and AR, 189
audibility of, 187
and augmented gallop, 186
with diastolic dysfunction, 189
in dogs, 183
and filling rates, 189
and gallop, 186
with heterograft valves, 183
with homograft valves, 183
in hypertrophic cardiomyopathy, 189
loudness of, 185
in mitral stenosis, 193
and mitral valve apparatus, 183
murmur after, 190
vs. opening snap, 191–192
pathological, 189
physiological, 185–186
vs. pathological, 189–190
production of, 183–185
with prosthetic ball valve, 183
respiration effects on, 187
right ventricular, 190–191
and sarcoid infiltrate, 189
standing in, 187, 190
and summation gallop, 186
timing of, 182–183
Hegglin syndrome, 143, 321
Hemic murmur, 215
Hepatojugular reflux, 73–76
terminology, 73
HOCM. *See* Hypertrophic obstructive
cardiomyopathy

Hollen-Horst bodies, 23
Holosystolic, definition, 238
Holt-Oram syndrome, 27
Honk, systolic, 253
HSS. *See* Hypertrophic subaortic stenosis
Hurler syndrome, 22
Hypertelorism, 21–22
Hypertension
and aortic sclerosis, 220
and AR, 299
"A" wave in, 112
and ejection sound, 131
etiology, 13–14
pulmonary
apex beat in, 100–101
classification, 164
and continuous murmur, 275
and diastolic flow murmur, 295–296
in Eisenmenger syndrome, 164–165
ejection sound in, 136
and jugular waves, 86–88
in MS, 176, 290
primary
and fixed split, 162
and Graham Steell murmur, 265
split S_2 width, 154
and vibratory S_1, 136
RVH, left parasternal impulse in, 104–105
and S_3, 188
and S_4, 204
and TR, 261
tricuspid whoop or honk, 253
retinal signs, 23
and S_4, 204
and split S_2, 162
and S_4S_1 and QM_1 intervals, 205–206
and tambour S_2, 150
Hyperthyroidism
arterial and continuous murmurs, 234
and atrial click, 207
and venous hum, 274
Hypertrophic obstructive cardiomyopathy
apex beat in, 97–98
"A" wave in, 112–113
bisferiens pulse, 39
brisk pulse, 34–35
midsystolic dip in, 117
Hypertrophic subaortic stenosis
"A" wave in, 112
brisk pulse, 34, 35
midsystolic dip in, 117
Hypertrophy, *vs.* dilatation and enlargement,
109

Hystidiastolic, definition, 181

I

Idiopathic dilatation of pulmonary artery. *See* Pulmonary artery, idiopathic dilatation of
Impedance and hangout interval, 144–145
Impulse gradient, 213
Inching, 153
Incisura, 40, 144
Incompetence *vs.* regurgitation, 240. *See also* Murmurs, diastolic; Murmurs, systolic
Infarction. *See* Myocardial infarction
Infective endocarditis
  eye signs, 21
  history in, 5
  skin signs secondary to, 17
Infiltrative cardiomyopathy, history in, 5
Insufficiency *vs.* regurgitation, 240. *See also* Murmurs, diastolic; Murmurs, systolic
Intercostal murmurs, 234
Intercostal pulsations, 234
Internal mammary murmurs, 269
Intestinal carcinoid disease, cutaneous manifestations of, 18
Iridodonesis, 23
Ischemic heart disease, history in, 3–4

J

Jaccoud's arthritis, 26
Janeway lesions, 17
Jugular veins
  pressure in. *See* Venous pressure
  valves in, 67–68
Jugular waves and contours, 76–92
  abnormal, 82–83
  in adult *vs.* child, 81
  in arrhythmias, 91–92
  "A" wave and X' descent, 76–77
    Cannon, 13, 83, 84
    giant, 82–83
    in HSS or HOCM, 83
    vs. carotid, 81–82
  C wave
    cause of, 78, 80
    and X' descent, 77–78
  H wave, 92
  normal, 76–79
    timing, 81
  recognition, 80–81
  V wave and Y descent, 79–80

abnormalities, 85–88
  after surgery, 86
  in anomalous pulmonary vein, 86
  in ASD, 86, 87
  in atrial fibrillation and flutter, 91–92
  in congestive heart failure, 86
  in constrictive pericarditis, 86, 88–90
  in MR, 86
  in pulmonary hypertension, 86–88
  in tamponade, 88–90
  in TR, 85, 87, 88
  in VSD, 86
  X descent, 76–78, 88
    abnormalities, 83–85
  X prime (X')
    in absent pericardium, 84
    after surgery, 84
    vs. descent, 76–78
    and Mackenzie, 78
    normal, 76–78
    and stiff right atrium, 84
    in tamponade, 88
    in TR, 84

K

Kartagener syndrome, 102
Kortokoff sounds, 44–46, 53–54
  causes and phases of, 44
  loudness of, 44–46, 50–51
  pitch of, 45
Kussmaul sign, 76

L

LA enlargement, left parasternal movement in, 106
LBBB. *See* Left bundle branch block
Left bundle branch block
  and S_1 loudness in, 140
  and split S_2, 162, 166
Left parasternal movement, left-sided causes of, 105–107
Left ventricle
  enlargement, left parasternal movement in, 105–106
  stiffness of, 112
Left ventricular failure
  dyspnea in, 8
  history in, 2
Left ventricular hypertrophy, 94
  apex beat in, 97–98, 101
  and displaced left ventricular impulse, 101

left ventricular impulse in, 110
Left ventricular impulse
    displaced, cause, 101–102
    in LVH, 110
Levoversion, 102
Lillehai-Kaster valve, 316
"Liver palms," 18
Livido reticularis, 18
Lupus erythematosus, AR in, 300
Lutembacher syndrome
    and continuous murmur, 215, 269
    and silent MS, 291
LV. See Left ventricle
LVH. See Left ventricular hypertrophy

M

Machinery murmur, 270
Maladie de Roger, 266
Malar flush, 21
Mammary souffle, 278–279
Manometer
    jugular, 69–70
    mercury vs. aneroid, 46–47
    pulsation, 68
Marfan syndrome
    and AR, 300
    hand and wrist signs of, 26–27
    iridodonesis in, 23
    and mitral valve prolapse, 240, 256
    and MR, 240
"Masking" of sounds, 120
Mercury manometer, 46–47
Methoxamine, 254
Mill-wheel murmur, 309
Mitral annular or ring calcium. See Annulus;
        Valves, mitral
Mitral atresia murmur, 276
Mitral opening snap. See Opening snap
Mitral regurgitation. See Murmurs, systolic;
        Regurgitation, mitral
Mitral stenosis. See Stenosis, mitral
Mitral valve. See Valves, mitral
Mitral valve prolapse. See Valves, mitral,
        prolapse of
Mönckeberg arteriosclerosis, 51
MR. See Regurgitation, mitral
MS. See Stenosis, mitral
"M" sound. See Heart sounds, first (S₁)
Müller maneuver, in HSS or HOCM, 226
Multiple lentigines, 19

Murmurs
    arterial. See Vascular murmurs
    carotid, 233
    continuous
        in anomalous pulmonary venous
            connection, 275
        in aortic pulmonary septal defect, 269
        in bronchopulmonary anastomoses, 276
        in coarctation, 233
        and collateral circulation, 275
        coronary artery to right heart, 269
        definition, 238, 267
        in hyperthyroidism, 234
        internal mammary, 269
        mammary souffle, 278–279
        in mitral atresia, 276
        in newborn, 276
        in PDA, 270–272
            amyl nitrate effect on, 271
            with coarctation, 271
            and diastolic flow murmur, 271
            and eddy sounds, 271
            intermittent, 271
            loudness and site, 271
            in newborn, 270
            pansystolic vs. VSD, 270
            S₂ reversal in, 271
            vs. to-and-fro murmur, 271
            and vasopressor agent effect, 271
            vs. venous hum, 274–275
        and pulmonary arteriovenous fistula, 276
        in pulmonary artery stenosis, 275
        in pulmonary atresia, 276
        and pulmonary embolus, 276
        renal, 313–314
        and sinus of Valsalva rupture, 269
        in tetralogy of Fallot, 276
        in truncus arteriosus, persistent, 276
        vascular. See Vascular murmurs
        venous hum, 272–275
            abdominal, 314
            in anemia, 274
            in aortic arch syndrome, 274
            vs. AR, 274
            vs. arteriovenous fistula, 274
            causes of, 273
            character of, 273
            eliciting, 273
            in neck, 272–275
            vs. PDA, 274
            unelicited, 274
    diastolic

Murmurs, diastolic (*contd.*)
  aortic
    vs. balloon pump, 304
    Cole-Cecil, 303
    Doppler *vs.* auscultation, 302
    dove-coo murmur, 302
    loudest site, 303
    vs. MS murmur, 304
    musical, 302
    severity, 302
    in sudden severe AR, 293
    syphilitic, 300
    timing and shape, 300–301
  Austin Flint, 292–294
    and jet lesion, 293
    vs. MS murmur, 294
    presystolic murmur in, 293–294
  mitral
    flow, 291–292
      in AV block, 295
      Cary Coombs, 296
      in MR, 249
      vs. MS, 296
      in PDA, 271
      in VSD, 265
    stenosis, 283–292
      and atrial fibrillation, 290
      vs. Austin Flint, 294
      growl and bark in, 288
      localization of, 291
      loudness maneuvers, 288–290
      pitch, 288
      post-Valsalva effect on, 289
      presystolic, 284–287
      and S_3, 292
      severity and loudness, 288
  presystolic
    in ASD, 204
    and Austin Flint, 293–294
    crescendo, 287
    in MS, 284–287
    in normal subjects, 298
    in TS, 298
  pulmonary, Graham Steell, 265
  tricuspid
    flow
      in ASD, 158
      vs. TS, 298
    stenosis
      in constriction, 298
      in Ebstein's anomaly, 298
      vs. MS, 298
      vs. right atrial myxoma, 298
      site of, 297

systolic
  ejection
    aortic
      and aging effect, 222
      and amyl nitrite, 226
      and gradient estimation, 213
      and heart failure effect, 222
      vs. HSS or HOCM, 222–227. *See also* Cardiomyopathy, hypertrophic subaortic (HSS or HOCM)
      imitation of with fingernail, 220
      loudness and site, 220–222
      and MS effect, 222
      musical, 222
      vs. PS murmur, 232
      respiration effect on, 232
      and sclerosis, 219–220
      and severity of, 213
      upward radiation of, 221–222
    definition, 211–212
    eddy or vortex theory, 209
    flow
      in anemia, 215
      aortic *vs.* pulmonary, 215
      in ASD, 215–216
      benign, 215
      functional, 215
      hemic, 215
      innocent, 214
      in pregnancy, 215
      and relative stenosis, 215
      in soundproof rooms, 214
      in the young, 214
    frequency and gradient, 209
    and Gallavardin phenomenon, 220
    gradient *vs.* loudness, 213
    humming, 217–218
    impulse gradient, 213
    and long diastole, 210, 211
    physical causes of, 208–209
    and premature ventricular contractions, 210
    pulmonary stenosis
      vs. AS, 228
      vs. coarctation, 228
      degree estimation, 229–230
      respiration effect on, 232
      sinus arrhythmia effect on, 232
      standing effect on, 232
      with tetralogy of Fallot, 230–231
      valvular *vs.* infundibular, 228
      with VSD, 230–231
    supraclavicular, 233
  musical, 253

regurgitant
    characteristics of all, 238
    drugs and maneuvers in, 249–251
    vs. incompetence or insufficiency, 240
    long diastoles on, 238–240
    mitral
        vs. AS with amyl nitrite, 250–251
        and annulus sphincter, 240
        in anomalous left coronary artery, 240
        in ASD, 240
        vs. cardiorespiratory murmur, 261
        and corrected transposition, 240
        and diastolic flow murmur, 249
        drugs and maneuvers on, 249–251
        duration, 247
        vs. Ebstein's anomaly, 240
        in endocardial cushion defect, 240
        and HSS or HOCM, 241–242
        and ischemia, 247
        and long diastoles, 238–240
        loudest site of, 267
        loudness and radiation, 246–247
        and Marfan syndrome, 240, 256
        and papillary muscle dysfunction, 238
        pitch, 247
        and prosthetic valves, 247
        quantifying degree of, 248–249
        respiration effect on, 248
        rheumatic *vs.* papillary muscle,
            245–246
        and ruptured chordae, 243–244
        vs. septal rupture, 267
        shape, 247
        silent severe, 247
        standing effect on, 251
        vs. TR, 261
        and widely split S$_2$, 247
    mitral prolapse
        after long diastoles, 239
        drugs and maneuvers in, 253–255
        murmurs, 251–259
        vs. papillary muscle dysfunction, 241–242
        standing effect on, 251
        vasopressors and, 254–255
    pansystolic *vs.* holosystolic, 238
    in PDA, effect of long diastole on, 239
    pitch, gradient, 248
    tricuspid
        acute severe, 259
        from carcinoid disease, 261
        and Carvallo sign, 259
        and COPD, 261
        in Ebstein's anomaly, 240
        loudness and shape of, 259–260

and pregnancy, 261
    from prolapse, 261
    from pulmonary hypertension, 261
    from RV infarction, 261
    site of, 259
    VSD
        amyl nitrite effect on, 260
        with AR, ASD, and PDA, 266
        with diastolic flow murmur, 265
        if supracristal, 266
        long diastole effect on, 239
        loudness factors on, 264–265
        with LV to right atrium shunt, 266
        vs. MR, 267
        muscular, 262
        vs. or with PS, 266
        vs. papillary rupture, 267
        with pulmonary hypertension,
            263–264
        vs. ruptured chordae, 243
        shapes of, 261–262
        Swiss cheese defect, 266
        to-and-fro murmur, 267
        whoops and honks in, 253
MVP. *See* Valves, mitral, prolapse of
Myocardial infarction
    and friction rubs, 309
    and reversed split, 166
    of right ventricle, and TR, 261
    and S$_1$, 137
    and split S$_1$, 131
    square root sign, 90
    and S$_4$S$_1$ interval, 206
Myocarditis
    history in, 5
    and reversed split, 166
Myxedema
    facies, 20
Myxoma, atrial. *See* Atrial myxoma
Myxomatous degeneration, mitral, 240

N

Neck webbing, 21
Neurofibromatosis, 19
New York Heart Association functional
    classification, 14
Nonejection clicks or sounds, 135, 251–259
Noon syndrome, 22

O

Obesity, and site of split S$_2$, 149
Opening click, in ball and disc valves, 315

Opening snap, 171–180
  in Ebstein's anomaly, 139
  mitral
    and bioprosthetic valve, 175
    and commissurotomy, 176
    differential diagnosis, 179
    loudness of, 175–176
      with low frequencies, 176
    mechanisms and timing, 171–172
    in MR, VSD, and prolapse, 171
    in PDA, 271
    respiration effect on, 177
    vs. reversed split, 177
    on right chest, 176
    snare drum vs. triple second sound, 178
    and S₂OS interval, 173–175
      with AR, 174
      with atrial fibrillation, 174
      with bradycardia, 174
      with hypertension, 174
      vs. A₂P₂, 176–179
      vs. S₃, 192
      standing effect, 178
      vs. tumor plop, 179
  tricuspid, 179
    in ASD, 179
    in Ebstein's anomaly, 179
    vs. mitral OS, 179
    vs. A₂P₂, 180
    respiration effect on, 179–180
    in TS absence, 179
Orthopnea, etiology, 7
Osler's nodes, 17

P
Pacemaker
  click, 206–207
  and endocardial rubs, 309–310
  murmurs from, 261
Palmary erythema, 18
Palpitations, etiology, 13
Pansystolic, definition, 238
Papillary muscle dysfunction murmurs. See
      Murmurs, systolic, regurgitant
Papilledema, and hypoxic cor pulmonale with
      hyperpnea, 21
Parachute valve, 291
Paradoxical splitting. See Heart sounds, second
      (S₂)
Paroxysmal nocturnal dyspnea, etiology, 8
Patent ductus. See Persistent ductus arteriosus
Patient history, 1–14

PDA. See Persistent ductus arteriosus
Pectus excavatum, 27–28
  and displaced left ventricular impulse, 102
Percussion, for cardiac size, 99
Percussion wave, 32
Pericardial knock, vs. S₃, 192–193
Pericardiectomy, and atrial click, 207
Pericarditis
  and atrial click, 207
  constrictive
    and loud S₁, 191
    and pericardial knock, 192–193
    and S₄, 197
  symptoms, 5
Pericardium
  and clicks, 258
  congenital absence of, and displaced left
      ventricular impulse, 102
  widely split S₂ in, 154
Persistent ductus arteriosus, 17
  bounding pulses in, 36
  closure, spontaneous, 271
  with coarctation, 271
  continuous murmurs, 269
  and Eisenmenger syndrome, 165
    and differential cyanosis, 272
    and murmur change, 272
    split S₂ in, 165
  flow murmurs, 271
  kinked or with spasm, 271
  LV volume in, 37
  murmurs. See Murmurs, systolic, regurgitant
  opening snap in, 271
  vs. patent ductus term, 269
  and S₃, 188
  split S₂ in, 162
  with VSD, 266
Persistent truncus arteriosus
  and continuous murmurs, 276
  split S₂ on right, 149
  S₂ split in, 145
Phenylephrine, 250, 254
Pheochromocytoma, 19
  and QS₂, 143
Physical examination, 16–19
Pistol shot sounds, sound and aneurysm, 234
Pitch, defined, 119
PMI. See Point of maximum impulse
Pneumothorax, and midsystolic clicks, 258
Pneumothorax rubs, 309
Point of maximum impulse, 95
Polydactyly, congenital syndromes in, 27
Popliteal arteries, palpation, 41–42
Porcine valve, 316

S_1 in, 141
S_2 in, with degeneration, 152
Positive abdominal compression test, 74
Postextrasystolic potentiation
and ejection murmur, 211
and S_1 loudness, 140, 141
Poststenotic dilatation
of aorta and split S_2, 163
of pulmonary artery
and ejection click, 135
and P_2, 152
PR. See Regurgitation, pulmonary
Precordium, examination of, for ventricular
hypertrophy, 109–114
Preejection period. See Systolic time intervals
Pregnancy
and mammary souffle, 278–279
murmurs in, 215
and TR, 261
Preisovolumic contraction period, 285
Premature ventricular contractions
and ejection murmur, 210, 218
and systolic regurgitant murmur, 238–239
Presyncope. See also Syncope
etiology, 10–11
Presystolic gallop. See Heart sounds, fourth
(S_4)
Prolapsed mitral valve. See Valves, mitral,
prolapse of
Prosthetic valves, 316
aortic
and cage clot or detachment, 315
OC vs. CC, 315
mitral
murmurs, 247
opening clicks, 315
porcine, murmurs in, 316
porcine, 316
tilting disc, 316
Protodiastole, 181
Protodiastolic gallop sound. See Heart sound,
fourth (S_3)
PS. See Stenosis, pulmonary
Pseudohypertension, 51
Psoriatic arthritis, and AR, 300
Pulmonary area, 148
A_2 vs. P_2 in, 228
Pulmonary arterial stenosis
of multiple branches, 235–236
murmurs in, 235–236
S_2 split in, 154
and supravalvular AS, 227
Pulmonary arteriovenous fistula, 275–276

Pulmonary artery
atresia, 276
idiopathic dilatation of
and ejection murmur, 213
and P_2 characteristics, 152
S_2 split in, 154, 157
palpation of, 106
pressure, normal, 144
Pulmonary atresia
continuous murmur in, 276
Pulmonary ejection murmurs. See Murmurs,
ejection
Pulmonary embolism
blood pressure in, 61
and continuous murmurs, 276
and fixed split, 157
massive, S_2 in, 152
and S_3, 191
Pulmonary hypertension. See Hypertension,
pulmonary
Pulmonary regurgitation. See Regurgitation,
pulmonary
Pulmonary stenosis. See Stenosis, pulmonary
Pulmonary valve. See Valves, pulmonary
Pulmonary valve stenosis, facies, 21
Pulse
bounding, 36, 37
brisk
with increased pulse pressures, 36–39
with normal pulse pressures, 34–35
carotid vs. jugular, 72–73
collapsing, 37
Corrigan, 37
femoral, 57
jugular, 69
leg, 41–42, 54–62
normal rates of rise, 31
palpation, 30, 41
radial, 57
slow rates of rise, 32–33
water-hammer, 37
Pulsus alternans, 51–53
and cuff deflation, 48–49
Pulsus bisferiens, 38–40
Pulsus paradoxus, 58–62
PVCs. See Premature ventricular contractions

Q
QM_1 interval, 206
QRS, 77
QS_2 and Hegglin syndrome, 143
Quincke sign, 62

R

Radial-femoral lag, 56, 57
Rales, 28, 118
Rapid-filling sound. *See* Heart sound, fourth
    (S₃)
RBBB. *See* Right bundle branch block
Red lunula, 18–19
Regurgitation
  aortic
    with arthritis, 299
    and bicuspid valves, 299
    bisferiens pulse, 38
    blood pressure in, 43
    causes of, 299–300
    differential diagnosis of, 304
    in discrete subvalvular AS, 228
    and fenestrations, 299
    hypertension in, 299
    leg pulses in, 56
    and Marfan syndrome, 300
    and midsystolic sound, 258
    and MR in, 240
    murmurs in. *See* Murmurs, diastolic, aortic
    and opening snap, 174
    and osteogenesis imperfecta, 300
    and prosthetic valves, 300
    and S₂
      loudness, 151
      split, 162
    and S₃, 189
    and S₄, 200
    sudden
      severe
        cause of, 303–304
        and middiastolic S₁, 189
    with supracristal PS, 266
    in supravalvular AS, 227
    syphilitic, 300
    ticktack rhythm in, 152
    with VSD, 266
  mitral
    brisk pulse, 34
    and diastolic murmurs, 190
    in HSS or HOCM, 223. 226–227
    left parasternal movement in, 106–107
    and M₁, 141
    murmurs in. *See* Murmurs, systolic,
      regurgitant
    and myxomatous valves, 240
    and S₃, 187–188
    and S₄, 200
    and S₂OS interval, 174
    and split S₂ wide, 155
    systole, 35

  pulmonary
    and annular distortion, 308
    in ASD, 306
    and Austin Flint murmur, 293
    vs. Graham Steell murmur, 305–307
    primary, 306–308
    in tetralogy of Fallot, 306
  tricuspid
    in corrected transposition, 267
    and exophthalmos, 23
    jugular veins in, 68
    and jugular waves, 85, 87, 88
    lateral retraction in, 104
    and S₃, 191
    X′ descent abnormalities in, 83
Reiter's syndrome and AR, 299
Renal artery stenosis, 313–314
Rendu-Osler-Weber disease, murmurs in, 276
Respiration, evaluation of, 27–28
Reversed split. *See* Heart sounds, second (S₂)
Rheumatic fever, and Carey Coombs, 296
Rheumatic heart disease
  and AR, 300
  history in, 3
  Jaccoud's arthritis with, 26
Rheumatic MR, *vs.* papillary muscle MR, 243
Rheumatoid arthritis, and AR, 300
Right bundle branch block
  S₁ and S₂ split in, 130
  wide, 154
Right ventricle
  ejection, *vs.* LV ejection, 77
  enlargement
    ASD in, with pulmonary hypertension,
      105
    in constrictive pericarditis, 104, 105
    failure of, and split S₂, 163
    normal chest movement, 104
Right ventricular enlargement, 102–105
  identification of
    in left lateral decubitus position, 104
    by palpation, 102–103
Right ventricular failure
  history in, 2
  venous tone in, 74
Right ventricular hypertrophy
  apex beat in, 101
  PS or PH, left parasternal impulse in,
    104–105
Right ventricular impulse, tetralogy of Fallot,
    102–103
Rubella syndrome, 21
Ruptured chordae. *See also* Murmurs, systolic,
    mitral

and S_4, 200
Ruptured septum *vs.* MR, 267
RV. *See* Right ventricle
RVH. *See* Right ventricular hypertrophy

S

Sarcoid cardiomyopathy and S_3, 189
Septal rupture *vs.* MR, 267
Shield chest, 28
Shock
  blood pressure in, 61
Sinus of Valsalva rupture
  and AR murmur, 302, 303
  and continuous murmurs, 269, 277–278
  into right heart, 156
Situs inversus, 102
Situs solitus, 102, 221
Skin, examination of, 16–19
Sounds, "masking" of, 120
Sphygmomanometer, 44
Splenic artery murmurs, 314
Splenic infarction rub, 314
Splitting of S_2. *See* Heart sounds, second
    (S_2)
Square root sign, 89, 90
Squatting
  for AR, 302
  and HSS or HOCM, 226
  and mitral stenosis murmur, 289
St. Jude valve, 292, 316. *See also* Prosthetic
    valves
Starling effect, 34, 35, 112, 320
Stenosis
  aortic
    anacrotic pulse in, 33
    arterial palpation in, 34
    "A" wave in, 112–113
    blood pressure in, 42–43
    calcific, 219
    discrete subvalvular, 227
    ejection sound in, 127, 131–132
    HSS or HOCM in, 222–227. *See also*
      Cardiomyopathy
    Kortokoff sounds in, 44
    murmurs, 209–210. *See also* Murmurs,
      ejection
    pressure tracing, 210
    pulse contours, 33
    and reversed split, 162–163, 165–166
    S_2, soft in, 152
    severity, 33

S_4 in, 204
  supravalvular
    and AR, 300
    facies, 19
    murmurs in, 227
    pathophysiology, 227
    radial-femoral lag in, 58
    rate of rise, 34
    summary of findings, 227
  mitral
    and annular calcium, 240
    apex beat in, 98, 102
    congenital, 291
    and constrictive pericardium, 291
    and displaced left ventricular impulse,
      102
    and endocarditis, 291
    and handgrip, 202
    imitations of, 291
    and Lutembacher syndrome, 215
    murmur. *See* Murmurs, diastolic
    and opening snap. *See* Opening snap
    and parachute valve, 291
    pathophysiology, 291
    and P_2 loudness, 151
    and S_4, 196
    silent, 291
    S_1 loudness in, 141
    and S_2OS interval, 173–175
    unusual causes of, 291
  pulmonary
    apex beat in, 101
    fixed split in, 157
    gradient estimation in, 229–230
    in infundibular, 152
    murmurs in. *See* Murmurs, systolic,
      ejection
    and P_2, soft, 152
    and presystolic click and murmur, 204
    RVH, left parasternal impulse in,
      104–105
    and S_3, 191
    and S_4, 204
    A_2P_2 interval in, 156–157
  relative, 215
  tricuspid, jugular pulse in, 83
Sternal angle, 69–72
Stethoscope, 119–122
  air leaks and eartips, 121, 122
  bell chestpiece, 119–120
  chestpiece placement, 45
  and S_3, 187
  smooth diaphragm, 120–121
  tubing, 121

Still's murmur, 217
STIs. *See* Systolic time intervals
Stokes-Adams attack, 18
Straight back syndrome, 216–217
Subclavian murmur, 269
Subclavian steal, 43
Summation gallop, 186, 206
Superior vena cava, obstruction, abdominal
    compression, 74, 75
Supraclavicular murmur, 233
Supravalvular AS. *See* Stenosis, aortic,
    supravalvular
Syncope, etiology, 10–11
Syphilis, and AR, 300
Systolic honk or whoop, 253
Systolic time intervals, 317–322
    and anemia, 322
    conduction defects and arrhythmias of, 321
    and constriction and tamponade, 321
    and coronary disease, 321
    correction for rate and sex, 318
    and drugs and hormones, 322
    ejection *vs.* LVET, 317
    and hypertension, 321
    myocardial damage and, 321
    PEP, 317
    shunt effects on, 322
    and valvular disease, 321

T

Tachycardia
    and physiologic S_3, 185–186
    ventricular, and jugular waves, 92
Takayasu arteritis (aortic arch syndrome)
    and anti-Hegglin syndrome, 143
    and AR, 300
Tambour S_2, 150
Tamponade
    blood pressure in, 60
    and jugular waves, 86, 88–90
    and pericardial knock, 192–193
    symptoms, 5
    wide split S_2 in, 156
Tetralogy of Fallot
    and audible P_2, 135
    ejection sound in, 135
    vs. muscle-bound right ventricle, 231
    with PDA, 276
    A_2P_2 in, 156
    vs. PS with intact septum, 230–231
    pulmonary regurgitation in, 306

right ventricular impulse, 102–103
severity and murmur loudness, 231
S_2 in, 149
and unilateral continuous murmur, 276
valvular *vs.* infundibular PS, 135
Thrills, 124
Thyrotoxicosis, QS_2, 143
Ticktack rhythm, 152
Tidal wave, 31–32
Tilting disc valves, 316
To-and-fro murmurs, 267
Tone-volume, 74
Total anomalous connection. *See* Anomalous
    pulmonary vein connection
TR. *See* Regurgitation, tricuspid
Train wheel rhythm, 202
Transposition
    corrected
        and MR *vs.* TR, 241
        and VSD plus mR, 267
    physiology of, 149
    soft P_2 in, 152
    and split S_2 on right, 149
Traumatic TR, 261
Tremulous iris, 23
Tricuspid opening snap. *See* Opening snap
Tricuspid regurgitation. *See* Regurgitation,
    tricuspid
Tricuspid stenosis
    jugular pulse in, 83
Tricuspid valve prolapse, 256
Trisomy, 270
Trisomy 21, 22
    facies, 20
Truncus. *See* Persistent truncus arteriosus
Tuberous sclerosis, 19
Tuft erythema, 18
Tumor. *See* Atrial myxoma
Tumor plop. *See* Atrial myxoma
Turbulence, 208–209
Turner syndrome, 22, 25

U

Ulcerative colitis and AR, 300
Ullrich-Noonan syndrome, 25
Uremia, and AR, 300

V

Valsalva
    and absent overshoot, 64

and cardiac function, 62–64
  and dicrotic wave, 40
  on HSS or HOCM murmur, 225–226
  and MS murmur, 289
  normal hemodynamics, 62–63
  on paradoxical split, 168
  PR *vs.* AR, 306
  PS *vs.* AS murmur, 232
  and reversed splits, 168
  sinus rupture. *See* Sinus of Valsalva rupture
  square wave response, 63
  TR *vs.* MR, 260
Valves
  aortic
    prolapse with VSD, 266
    rupture of, and musical murmur, 302
  mitral
    and annular calcium, 240
      and aortic sclerosis, 220
    cleft, 240
    myxomatous, 240
    prolapse of, 251–259
      amyl nitrite effect on, 254
      and ASD, 257
      auscultation of, 252
      and CHF development, 258
      and click, 251–259
        causes of, 255–257
        vs. friction rub, 258
      definition, 251
      maneuvers and drug effects on,
        253–255
      murmurs in. *See* Murmurs, systolic,
        regurgitant
      and nonejection click, 251–259
      opening snap in, 171
      and papillary muscle dysfunction, 256
      parachute analogy in, 253
      PVC effect on, 254
      slowing rate effect on, 254
      standing effect on, 253
      ST-T changes in, 251
      synonyms and floppy valve, 246
      Valsalva effect on, 253
    regurgitation. *See* Murmurs, systolic
    sphincter, 241
    stenosis. *See* Murmurs, diastolic; Stenosis,
      mitral
  pulmonary
    bicuspid and click, 258
    PR. *See* Regurgitation, pulmonary
Vascular murmurs, 232–236

and amyl nitrite, 313
  vs. bruit, 233
  in bypasses, 234–235
  in coarctation, 233–234
  continuous, causes of, 232
  epigastric, 314
  in hyperthyroidism, 234
  mammary souffle, 269
  renal and splenic artery stenosis, 313–314
  subclavian artery, 269
Velocardiofacial syndrome, 21
Venous hum. *See also* Murmurs, continuous
  in epigastrium, 314
  in groin, 268
Venous pressure
  chest angle, 69
  internal, 69–70
  measurement, 70–72
  normal, 69–70
Ventricular aneurysm and S_3, 189
Ventricular gallop. *See* Heart sounds, third (S_3)
Ventricular hypertrophy
  vs. enlargement, 94
  precordium examination for, 109–114
Ventricular septal defect
  asymptomatic, 266
  brisk pulse, 34
  and click, 263–264
  diastolic flow murmur, 265
  and Down syndrome, 20
  Eisenmenger syndrome, S_2
    single in, 165
  and jugular waves, 86
  and left ventricular to right atrium shunt,
    261–262
  maladie de Roger type, 266
  murmurs. *See* Murmurs, systolic, regurgitant
  muscular, 262
  A_2/P_2 loudness ratio, 165
  and presystolic murmur, 267
  vs. PS, 230–231
  right ventricular impulse, 102–103
  and S_3, 188–189
  and S_4, 200
  sites of, 261
  S_2 split, and shunt size, 157
Ventricular septum, as cause of RV
    displacement, 107
Ventricular tachycardia, and jugular waves, 92
Venturi effect, 223
Viscosity, effect on murmur, 208–209
VSD. *See* Ventricular septal defect

W

Whoop, systolic, 253
Williams syndrome, facies, 19
Wolff-Parkinson-White preexcitation, and split
    S$_2$, 165

X

X and X′ descent. *See* Jugular waves and
    contours

Xanthelasma, 24
X-ray, for cardiac size, 107–109
    by cardiac volume, 107–109
    by height and weight, 107, 108t

Y

Y descent. *See* Jugular waves and contours